Cardiomyopathies: Classification, Evaluation and Treatment

Cardiomyopathies: Classification, Evaluation and Treatment

Cardiomyopathies: Classification, Evaluation and Treatment

Edited by Elliot Miller

hayle
medical

New York

Hayle Medical,
750 Third Avenue, 9th Floor,
New York, NY 10017, USA

Visit us on the World Wide Web at:
www.haylemedical.com

ISBN: 978-1-63241-562-2

Cataloging-in-Publication Data

Cardiomyopathies : classification, evaluation and treatment / edited by Elliot Miller.
    p. cm.
Includes bibliographical references and index.
ISBN 978-1-63241-562-2
1. Myocardium--Diseases. 2. Myocardium--Diseases--Treatment.
3. Cardiology. I. Miller, Elliot.
RC685.M9 C37 2019
616.124--dc23

Table of Contents

Preface

Cardiomyopathy refers to a set of diseases which affect the heart muscle. Common symptoms include swelling of the lower extremities, shortness of breath, fainting, irregular heartbeat and increased tiredness. Individuals with cardiomyopathy are at a higher risk of sudden cardiac death. Some types of cardiomyopathy are dilated cardiomyopathy, hypertrophic cardiomyopathy, arrhythmogenic right ventricular dysplasia, restrictive cardiomyopathy, takotsubo cardiomyopathy, etc. A cardiomyopathy is determined through a physical examination, blood test, ECG, echocardiogram, genetic testing, etc. The treatment of cardiomyopathy depends on the type of the cardiomyopathy and its symptoms, which are treatable through medications, lifestyle changes and surgery. Pacemakers, defibrillators and ventricular assist devices are some of the tools used for the management of abnormal heart rates, fatal heart rhythms and heart failure. These are therefore useful for the treatment of cardiomyopathies. This book is a compilation of chapters that discuss the most vital concepts and principles in the classification, evaluation and treatment of cardiomyopathies. The various advancements in this domain are glanced at and their implications as well as ramifications are looked at in detail. This book aims to equip students and cardiologists with the advanced topics and upcoming concepts in this area.

The information shared in this book is based on empirical researches made by veterans in this field of study. The elaborative information provided in this book will help the readers further their scope of knowledge leading to advancements in this field.

Finally, I would like to thank my fellow researchers who gave constructive feedback and my family members who supported me at every step of my research.

Editor

Idiopathic Dilated Cardiomyopathy: Molecular Basis and Distilling Complexity to Advance

Santiago Roura, Carolina Gálvez-Montón,
Josep Lupón and Antoni Bayes-Genis

Abstract

Cardiomyopathies are heterogeneous diseases of the myocardium associated with abnormal findings of chamber size, wall thickness, and/or functional contractility. In particular, dilated cardiomyopathy (DCM) is mainly characterized by ventricular chamber enlargement with systolic dysfunction and normal left ventricular (LV) wall thickness. Although DCM is thought to be induced mainly by genetic or environmental factors, in the majority of cases, the cause is unknown. With an estimated prevalence of 1:2500 and an incidence of 1:18,000 per year in adults, DCM is the most frequent indication for heart transplantation, which represents an enormous cost burden on healthcare systems. These figures warrant greater accuracy in patient diagnosis and prognosis and further insight into the underlying basis of DCM. Here, we discuss past and recent findings on the molecular mechanisms involved in DCM. Dilated cardiomyopathy has been linked to the overactivation of extracellular signal-regulated kinase (ERK1/2), which in turn is related to activation of low-density lipoprotein receptor–related protein-1 (LRP-1). Moreover, a redistribution of LRP-1 into cholesterol-enriched plasma membrane domains (lipid rafts) and alterations in cardiac DNA methylation have been reported in failing hearts. In conclusion, more comprehensive analyses of myocardial lipid rafts and epigenetic mechanisms may advance our understanding of DCM causes and progression. In turn, this understanding may promote the development of innovative treatments.

Keywords: dilated cardiomyopathy, heart failure, lipid rafts, LRP-1, molecular basis, cardiac muscle, vasculature

1. Introduction

Cardiomyopathies are heterogeneous diseases of the myocardium associated with abnormal findings of chamber size, wall thickness, and/or functional contractility [1]. Currently, cardiomyopathy is classified based on the dominant pathophysiology or by aetiological/pathogenetic factors. This system defines four distinct categories of cardiomyopathy: dilated, hypertrophic, restrictive, and arrhythmogenic (**Figure 1**) [2]. In particular, dilated cardiomyopathy (DCM) is mainly characterized by ventricular chamber enlargement or dilatation with systolic dysfunction and normal left ventricular (LV) wall thickness. In general, these abnormalities lead to progressive heart failure, a decline in LV contractile function, abnormalities in ventricular and supraventricular rhythm and conduction, thromboembolism, and finally, sudden or heart failure-related death [3]. Indeed, DCM is a common, largely irreversible cause of myocardial damage. It is thought to be induced by genetic or environmental factors that may manifest clinically over a wide range of ages (most commonly in the third or fourth decade, but also in young children). Dilated cardiomyopathy affects both sexes and all ethnic groups; it is typically identified when patients exhibit severe limiting symptoms and incapacity [4].

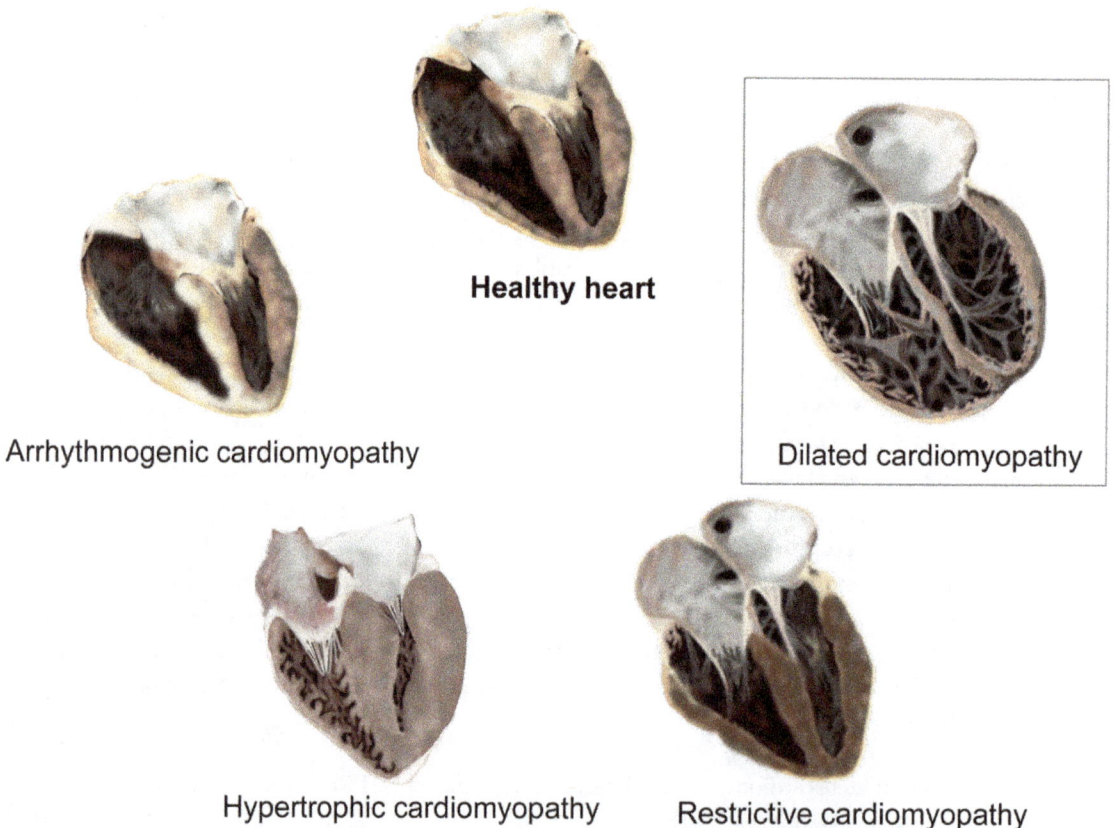

Healthy heart

Arrhythmogenic cardiomyopathy

Dilated cardiomyopathy

Hypertrophic cardiomyopathy   Restrictive cardiomyopathy

Figure 1. Heterogeneous diseases of the myocardium. The different types of cardiomyopathies fall into four principal categories, based on the muscle disorder involved. This chapter is confined to dilated cardiomyopathy.

This chapter summarizes the most important traits (aetiology, diagnosis, treatment, and pathophysiology) that characterize DCM. We focus on studies that provided novel insights into the underlying molecular basis of this extremely complex human disorder. In a sense, we will present new pieces of an intriguing puzzle, with the aim of bringing some order into the chaos of the molecular reality.

2. Dilated cardiomyopathy: characteristic features

Dilated cardiomyopathy has an estimated prevalence of 1:2500, an incidence of 1:15,000–18,000 per year in adults, and an estimated prevalence of 2:3 among children with unknown diseases [4, 5]. The clinical course of DCM can be progressive; one study reported that about 35% of individuals died within 5 years after diagnosis [1]. The origin of death is divided evenly between sudden death and pump failure. To date, prolonged survival has been achieved with neurohormone blockers (angiotensin-converting enzyme inhibitors and β-adrenoceptor antagonists) and devices (cardiac resynchronization and implanted defibrillators). Nevertheless, the only definitive treatment is heart transplantation, which is hampered in many instances by the limited number of heart donors and by graft rejection over time. Therefore, DCM is the most frequent indication for heart transplantation, which results in an enormous cost burden for healthcare systems throughout the world. Diagnosis is typically based on patient history and the presence of LV dilatation and impaired ejection fraction, with or without regurgitation; these signs are detected with echocardiography, cardiac magnetic resonance imaging, or both.

At the histological level, the main pathological derangements observed in explanted diseased hearts are patchy interstitial fibrosis surrounding myocardial filaments, marked lipid deposition, cardiac muscle atrophy, and lipid accumulation [6–8]. Moreover, further investigations of both patient samples and animal disease models have shown that DCM hearts exhibit marked vascular alterations [9, 10]. In most cases, the causal mechanism of disease is poorly understood. This reality has induced some authors to argue that heart disease in DCM arises from an obscure origin, and this viewpoint has given rise to the term 'idiopathic' DCM. Recently, relevant advances have been made in our understanding of the causes of this disease. The main causes include familial and genetic disorders, infectious and toxicity-related processes, autoimmunity, and inflammation [4].

Frequently, DCM has been defined as the result of an extremely complex genetic architecture that involves disruptions in a variety of myocardial proteins, which are provoked by rare variants in some genes; moreover, many of these genes are also involved in other cardiomyopathies, such as muscular dystrophy or syndromic diseases [11]. In brief, numerous DCM-associated genes have been identified. This information has provided a better understanding of disease pathogenesis, and it has promoted advances in mutation analytical techniques to facilitate the recognition of subjects and progeny that carry these mutations [12]. Alterations in more than 50 loci and genes have been identified, which mostly encode either cardiac myocyte-specific proteins or structural, nuclear membrane, and calcium metabolism proteins.

However, it is estimated that genetic disorders account for only 20–35% of DCM cases [12, 13]. Some researchers have predicted that genetic associations may have been missed due to the limited nature of previous studies; accordingly, they point to a need for more comprehensive studies in much larger cohorts of families that are rigorously phenotyped [11]. In addition, some cases of DCM are believed to be related to autoimmune and inflammatory processes [14–16]; metabolic, nutritional, and endocrine deficiencies; or heart muscle damage following exposure to viruses, exogenous drugs, or toxins (e.g., chronic alcohol consumption) [2]. Peripartum cardiomyopathy also represents a subset of LV systolic dysfunction. In the latter cases, initial symptoms of heart failure occur during the late stages of pregnancy [17]. Although there may be a variety of causes for DCM, the clinical presentation of this disease seems to be uniform, both in humans and in animal models that have been used to dissect DCM development, progression, and treatment [10].

Standard treatment of DCM involves neurohormonal inhibition of the renin-angiotensin-aldosterone system (i.e., angiotensin-converting enzyme inhibitors, angiotensin II receptor type 1 blockers, or mineralocorticoid receptor blockers) or blocking the sympathetic nervous system with β-blockers. In patients, it is crucial to focus on improving cardiac function and reducing mechanical stress. Although progress has been made in arrhythmia therapy and in sudden death prevention, many impediments for improving patient outcomes remain unresolved [4]. Innovative therapies, such as stem cell-based applications, are also being investigated [18].

3. Dilated cardiomyopathy affects both cardiac muscle and the vasculature

Dilated cardiomyopathy is associated with pronounced remodelling of one or both ventricles, which results in large changes in the shapes of ventricles and in the architecture of myocardial fibres. As mentioned previously, the main microscopic hallmarks of failing hearts are marked collagen deposition, patchy interstitial fibrosis, degenerated cardiac muscle cells, and sparse blood vessels. At the ultrastructural level, remodelling comprises mitochondrial abnormalities, T-tubular dilatation, and intracellular lipid droplet accumulation [10]. Because the mitochondrion is the main site of ATP production and cardiac myocytes are particularly sensitive to the supply of energy, deficits in mitochondrial function have been linked to DCM [19]. Additionally, altered levels of connexin-43 and modulation of its phosphorylation state can induce electromechanical uncoupling between neighbouring cardiac muscle cells [20].

A number of studies have indicated that programmed cell death or apoptosis contributes actively to human end-stage heart failure. Indeed, cell death occurs in myocardial ischemia-reperfusion [21], ischemia-reperfusion injury [22], and fatal myocarditis [23]. However, the role of apoptosis in the DCM myocardium remains controversial, due to some limitations in the techniques that have been used to measure apoptosis [24–26]. A positive Terminal deoxy-nucleotidyl transferase dUTP nick end labeling (TUNEL) signal seems to require fragmentation of only 10% of all DNA; as a result, the level of apoptosis may be highly overestimated [24]. Furthermore, cells that are apoptotic, necrotic, undergoing DNA repair, or living can emit equivalent signals in the TUNEL assay [27], which renders the use of this method even more questionable. Consequently, although some authors have reported putative increases in apoptotic markers with different methodologies, including caspase-3 activity, DNA fragmentation (TUNEL), and electron microscopy [28], others have failed to detect changes in apoptosis. For instance, Bott-Flügel *et al.* did not detect any correlations between caspase-3 activity, the induction of DNA fragmentation, and haemodynamic or echocardiographic variables in patients with end-stage heart failure, including DCM. Moreover, they did not find significant differences in caspase-3 activation between DCM and control myocardium [26]. **Figure 2** shows that only slight amounts of caspase-3 mRNA and protein were detected in LV samples from patients (unpublished results). These findings suggest that cardiac muscle cells might trigger apoptotic self-destruction, without completing the process. Hence, DCM is characterized by marked abnormalities in the function and integrity of cardiac muscle.

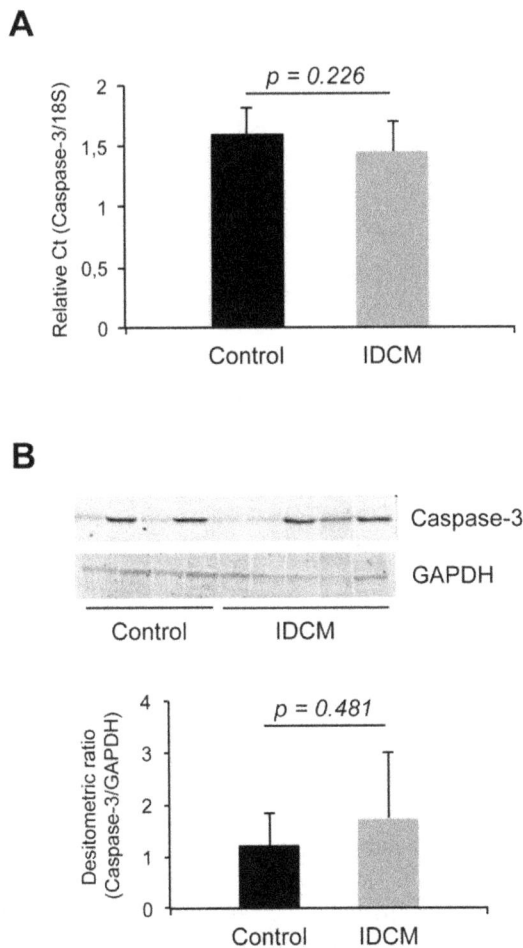

Figure 2. Comparative analysis of apoptosis in left ventricle samples collected from human explanted DCM hearts and control hearts from non-cardiac decedents. Representative caspase-3 gene (**A**) and protein (**B**) expression levels by quantitative RT-PCR and Western blotting, respectively.

Cardiac endothelial dysfunction was also associated with disease progression and a poor prognosis in patients with DCM. In the late 1940s, preliminary observations showed a correlation between heart weight and the total cross-sectional size of the main coronary vessels [29]. Since then, a number of studies have recognized that cardiac vasculature is a key regulator of the integrity and function of the myocardium. In an attempt to take this a step further, Brutsaert *et al.* studied the mechanical properties of the mammalian ventricular myocardium before and after damaging the endocardial surface [30]. Those authors speculated that the endocardium could affect myocardial performance by either forming an electrochemical barrier, releasing a chemical substance or messenger, or both. They subsequently demonstrated that nitric oxide synthase activity regulated the contractile responsiveness of ventricular myocytes [31]. Perhaps more significantly, additional studies in Langendorff-perfused and post-infarcted rat hearts confirmed that endothelial damage led to progressive myocardial dysfunction and that, conversely, protecting the associated vasculature preserved global myocardial homeostasis [32, 33].

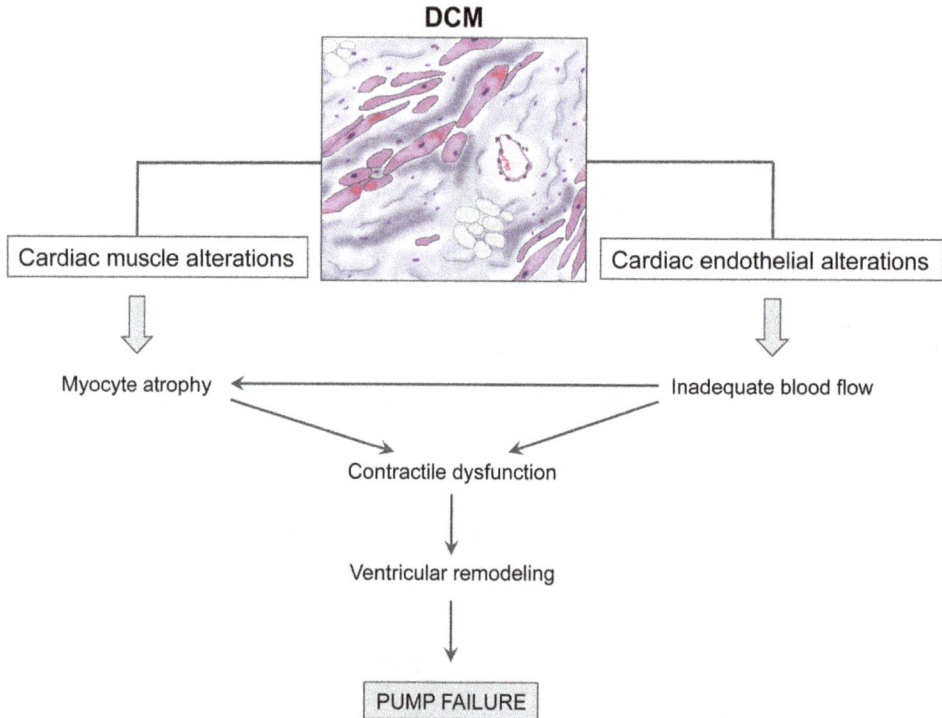

Figure 3. Foundation of DCM as a two-hit heart disease. The integrity and function of both cardiac muscle and vasculature are adversely compromised in DCM, which leads to LV remodelling and pump failure.

Advances in medical imaging techniques have become crucial for performing more comprehensive analyses of vascular derangements in DCM. Angiography revealed that a mismatch between artery size and LV mass in patients with DCM contributed to myocardial hypoperfusion [34–37]. Computed tomography measurements of DCM cardiac vasculature on a multislice scanner have also clearly shown side branch paucity and shortened, thinned epicardial arteries [9]. Therefore, the epicardial coronary arteries in patients with DCM are not adequately sized for the enlarged LV mass. Notably, a variety of studies described significantly reduced, sparse microvasculature in diseased myocardium samples [9, 38, 39]. In this context, numerous studies in patients with DCM have reported that the circulating levels of distinct bone marrow-derived cell populations are peripherally increased after vascular damage [40]. Although there is a correlation between the circulating levels of these progenitor cells and the progression and clinical outcomes of DCM, the clinical usefulness of this overrepresentation awaits further validation.

Collectively, these findings led to a re-examination of the pathophysiology of DCM. In 2009, Roura and Bayes-Genis [10] reviewed the extensive data from animal models and patients and concluded that DCM is a two-hit disease, where both cardiac muscle and endothelial alterations contribute equally to contractile deficiency and pump failure (**Figure 3**).

4. Molecular basis of dilated cardiomyopathy: past and new actors

Molecularly, in humans, DCM has been related to intramyocardial accumulation of α-2 macroglobulin (α-2M) [41] and increased activation of extracellular signal-regulated kinase (ERK1/2) [42]. In a mouse model of DCM, the disease was generated by a mutation in the lamin A/C gene [43, 44]. In these mice, chemically suppressing ERK1/2 activation prevented LV dilatation and greatly restored the cardiac ejection fraction.

The α-2M protein is a highly abundant plasma protease inhibitor, which has been shown to activate various tyrosine kinases and mitogen-activated protein kinases [45]. Moreover, α-2M was one of the first molecules to be described as a ligand of low-density lipoprotein (LDL) receptor-related protein 1 (LRP-1) [46]. A recent review described LRP-1 as a multifunctional receptor of the LDL-receptor family that mediates the clearance of a variety of structurally diverse extracellular molecules [47]. Moreover, LRP-1 plays key roles in various biological processes by interacting with multiple intracellular signalling pathways [48, 49]. As a result, LRP-1 tyrosine phosphorylation can be activated in response to diverse extracellular molecules, such as platelet-derived growth factor [50–52]. In particular, ERK1/2 activation is recognized as one of the main LRP-1 molecular relays [53–55]. In the following pages, we present and discuss novel data demonstrating that, together with the pivotal role of LRP-1 in the vascular wall and in the aetiology of atherosclerosis [56], LRP-1 is redistributed and overactivated within some specialized plasma membrane domains, termed lipid rafts, in DCM myocardium.

The decreased capillary density found in patients with DCM was shown to arise from impairments in myocardial endothelial cell survival and insufficient revascularization. These processes involve several intracellular signalling pathways, including those mediated by vascular endothelial (VE)-cadherin/β-catenin, angiopoietins, and vascular endothelial growth factors (VEGFs). In particular, VE-cadherin, β-catenin, angiopoietin-2, VEGF-A, VEGF-B, and VEGF receptor-1 (VEGFR-1) expression levels were downregulated in DCM [9, 57, 58]. Roura *et al.* [9] further demonstrated that reduced expression of β-catenin, an important angiogenic regulator [59], occurred exclusively in myocardial vascular cells in failing hearts.

Remarkably, different DNA methylation patterns have been detected in genes that regulate pathways related to heart disease and in genes with unknown functions in DCM. For example, variations in DNA methylation were observed in lymphocyte antigen 75, tyrosine kinase-type cell surface receptor HER3, homeobox B13, and adenosine receptor A2A [60]. These validated targets are most likely involved in modifying DCM rather than independently causing disease. Furthermore, other authors found differentially methylated gene promoters and a depletion of mitochondrial DNA that resulted in a thymidine kinase deficiency in DCM hearts [61, 62]. Indeed, investigating epigenetic mechanisms represents an attractive approach for finding novel mechanisms of disease.

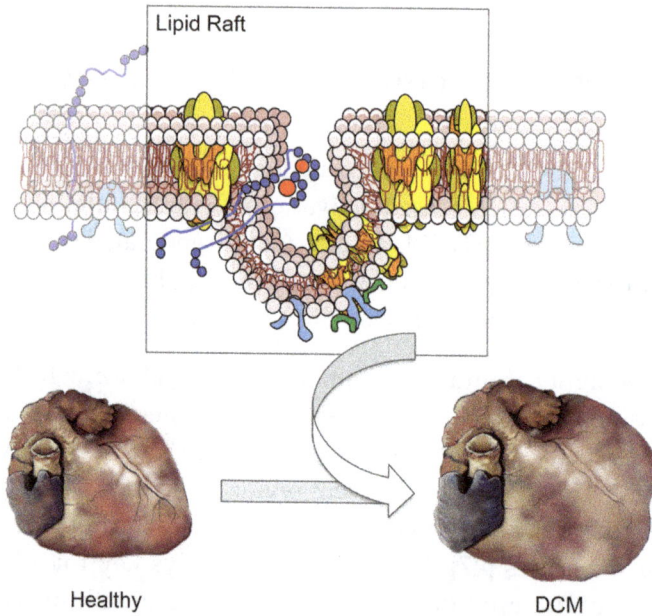

Figure 4. Potential impact of lipid raft–associated signalling on DCM. Schematic illustration of a lipid raft domain in a portion of the cell surface. Proteins potentially involved in disease progression are either packed into or excluded from these specialized plasma membrane areas.

For more than 40 years, the Singer and Nicolson model of the cell membrane, where proteins are viewed as icebergs floating in a sea of lipids, has provided a solid foundation for studying cell membrane properties [63]. This enduring model was subsequently reinterpreted with the discovery of localized, highly cholesterol- and glycosphingolipid-enriched plasma membrane areas, referred to as 'lipid rafts' [64]. Many proteins, particularly those involved in cell signalling and cytokine presentation, were found to be densely packed together in these specialized surface domains [65]. Accordingly, lipid rafts facilitate interactions between protein receptors and mediators by maintaining them tightly packed together in one location. Interestingly, LRP-1 was reported to be associated with lipid rafts [66, 67].

As previously mentioned, recent research has given us new molecular aspects of the disease. Particularly, in patients with DCM, LRP-1 was seen redistributed and further activated, through tyrosine phosphorylation, within lipid rafts enriched in caveolin-3 and flotillin-1 [68]. Of note, these observations suggested that movement of LRP-1 within these specialized membrane domains contribute to the overactivation of ERK1/2-mediated signalling described in DCM. However, further confirmatory exploration is warranted to determine whether this overactive signalling leads to the characteristic promotion of extracellular matrix metalloproteinase activity and subsequent LV remodelling (**Figure 4**) [69, 70].

To investigate this novel regulatory impact of lipid rafts on DCM, Roura *et al.* extracted lipid rafts from failing myocardium and detected elevated amounts of the mobilizing cytokine, stromal cell-derived factor (SDF)-1 [71]. In that same study, the authors showed that deficiencies in ILK and ERK1/2 signalling impeded SDF-1-mediated migration of circulating progenitor cells. As a result, impaired cell migration compromised endothelial maintenance and recovery, which contributed to the marked vascular derangements observed in diseased myocardium [72].

Taken together, these observations support the growing body of data that led to the recognition of myocardial lipid rafts and their associated proteins as modulators of cardiac performance and as novel therapeutic targets [73–75].

5. Conclusions

Heart failure has become an increasingly common disorder worldwide, and it is associated with substantial morbidity and mortality. Many causes of heart failure are easily identified in clinical practice, including abnormal heart valves, inherited cardiomyopathies, severe coronary artery disease, or hypertensive heart disease. However, the precise mechanisms that govern the progression of heart failure and ventricular remodelling in DCM remain obscure. Some authors have appropriately pointed out that, for both clinicians and researchers, attempting to discover the underlying genetic and environmental causes linked to complex human diseases, such as DCM, is like facing a drawer filled with thousands of puzzle pieces mixed together from an unknown number of jigsaw puzzles [76, 77]. The question remains, how can they begin to solve it?

There is a growing body of data that describes the multifaceted genetic diversity involved in DCM and the alterations in both cardiac muscle and vasculature that contribute to the disease. However, several crucial issues remain to be addressed. For example, it is not clear whether the marked vascular deficiencies observed in patients with DCM develop secondary to heart remodelling, or whether they directly contribute to myocardial alterations and to the temporal evolution of LV dilatation. Accordingly, researchers are providing novel mechanistic insights that might bring some order to this 'disordered' collection of data. For example, they have shown that lipid rafts participate in the mechanism underlying the spatial regulation of LRP-1-mediated ERK1/2 activity. Undoubtedly, further work is needed to increase our comprehension of the causes underlying this 'obscure' disease. To that end, the current state of knowledge summarized in the present review provides a starting point for addressing the remaining questions in the pathophysiology of this disease. Moreover, we highlight new avenues for discovering potentially effective treatments.

Funding sources

This work was supported by grants from the Ministerio de Educación y Ciencia (SAF2014-59892), Fundació La MARATÓ de TV3 (201502 and 201516), Fundació Daniel Bravo Andreu, Sociedad Española de Cardiología, Societat Catalana de Cardiologia, Generalitat de Catalunya (SGR 2014), and Acadèmia de Ciències Mèdiques i de la Salut de Catalunya i de Balears. This work was also funded by the Red de Terapia Celular - TerCel (RD12/0019/0029), Red de Investigación Cardiovascular - RIC (RD12/0042/0047), and Fondo de Investigación Sanitaria, Instituto de Salud Carlos III (FIS PI14/01682) projects as part of the Plan Nacional de I+D+I and cofounded by ISCIII-Sudirección General de Evaluación y el Fondo Europeo de Desarrollo Regional (FEDER).

Author details

Santiago Roura[1,2*], Carolina Gálvez-Montón[1], Josep Lupón[3,4] and Antoni Bayes-Genis[1,3,4]

*Address all correspondence to: sroura@igtp.cat

1 ICREC Research Program, Germans Trias i Pujol Health Science Research Institute, Badalona, Spain

2 Center of Regenerative Medicine in Barcelona, Barcelona,Spain

3 Cardiology Service, Germans Trias i Pujol University Hospital, Badalona, Spain

4 Department of Medicine, Autonomous University of Barcelona, Barcelona, Spain

References

[1] Towbin JA, Bowles NE: The failing heart. Nature. 2002;415:227-233.

[2] Maron BJ, Towbin JA, Thiene G, Antzelevitch C, Corrado D, Arnett D, Moss AJ, Seidman CE, Young JB; American Heart Association; Council on Clinical Cardiology, Heart Failure and Transplantation Committee; Quality of Care and Outcomes Research and Functional Genomics and Translational Biology Interdisciplinary Working Groups; Council on Epidemiology and Prevention. Contemporary definitions and classification

of the cardiomyopathies: an American Heart Association Scientific Statement from the Council on Clinical Cardiology, Heart Failure and Transplantation Committee; Quality of Care and Outcomes Research and Functional Genomics and Translational Biology Interdisciplinary Working Groups; and Council on Epidemiology and Prevention. Circulation. 2006;113:1807-1816.

[3] Towbin JA, Lorts A: Arrhythmias and dilated cardiomyopathy common pathogenetic pathways? J Am Coll Cardiol. 2011;57:2169-2171.

[4] Jefferies JL, Towbin JA: Dilated cardiomyopathy. Lancet. 2010;375:752-762.

[5] Towbin JA, Lowe AM, Colan SD, Sleeper LA, Orav EJ, Clunie S, Messere J, Cox GF, Lurie PR, Hsu D, Canter C, Wilkinson JD, Lipshultz SE: Incidence, causes, and outcomes of dilated cardiomyopathy in children. JAMA. 2006;296:1867-1876.

[6] Marijianowski MM, Teeling P, Mann J, Becker A: Dilated cardiomyopathy is associated with an increase in the type I/type III collagen ratio: a quantitative assessment. J Am Col Cardiol. 1995;25:1263–1272.

[7] Gunja-Smith Z, Gunja-Smith Z, Morales AR, Romanelli R, Woessner JF Jr: Remodeling of human myocardial collagen in idiopathic dilated cardiomyopathy. Role of metallo-proteinases and pyridinoline cross-links. Am J Pathol. 1996;148:1639-1648.

[8] Pauschinger M, Knopf D, Petschauer S, Doerner A, Poller W, Schwimmbeck PL, Kühl U, Schultheiss HP: Dilated cardiomyopathy is associated with significant changes in collagen type I/III ratio. Circulation. 1999;99:2750-2756.

[9] Roura S, Planas F, Prat-Vidal C, Leta R, Soler-Botija C, Carreras F, Llach A, Hove-Madsen L, Pons Lladó G, Farré J, Cinca J, Bayes-Genis A: Idiopathic dilated cardiomyopathy exhibits defective vascularization and vessel formation. Eur J Heart Fail. 2007;9:995-1002.

[10] Roura S, Bayes-Genis A: Vascular dysfunction in idiopathic dilated cardiomyopathy. Nat Rev Cardiol. 2009;6:590-598.

[11] Hershberger RE, Hedges DJ, Morales A: Dilated cardiomyopathy: the complexity of a diverse genetic architecture. Nat Rev Cardiol. 2013;10:531-547.

[12] Jacoby D, McKenna WJ: Genetics of inherited cardiomyopathy. Eur Heart J. 2012;33:296-304.

[13] Seidman JG, Seidman C: The genetic basis for cardiomyopathy: from mutation identification to mechanistic paradigms. Cell. 2001;104:557-567.

[14] Lappé JM, Pelfrey CM, Tang WH: Recent insights into the role of autoimmunity in idiopathic dilated cardiomyopathy. J Card Fail. 2008;14:521-530.

[15] Jahns R, Boivin V, Schwarzbach V, Ertl G, Lohse MJ: Pathological autoantibodies in cardiomyopathy. Autoimmunity. 2008;41:454-461.

[16]   Kaya Z, Katus HA: Role of autoimmunity in dilated cardiomyopathy. Basic Res Cardiol. 2010;105:7-8.

[17]   Bachelier-Walenta K, Hilfiker-Kleiner D, Sliwa K: Peripartum cardiomyopathy: update 2012. Curr Opin Crit Care. 2013;19:397-403.

[18]   Roura S, Gálvez-Montón C, Bayes-Genis A: Umbilical cord blood-derived mesenchymal stem cells: new therapeutic weapons for idiopathic dilated cardiomyopathy? Int J Cardiol. 2014;177:809-818.

[19]   Limongelli G, Masarone D, D'Alessandro R, Elliott PM: Mitochondrial diseases and the heart: an overview of molecular basis, diagnosis, treatment and clinical course. Future Cardiol. 2012;8:71-88.

[20]   Ai X, Pogwizd SM: Connexin 43 downregulation and dephosphorylation in nonischemic heart failure is associated with enhanced colocalized protein phosphatase type 2A. Circ Res. 2005;96:54-63.

[21]   Gottlieb RA, Engler RL: Apoptosis in myocardial ischemia-reperfusion. Ann N Y Acad Sci. 1999;874:412-426.

[22]   Saraste A, Pulkki K, Kallajoki M, Henriksen K, Parvinen M, Voipio-Pulkki LM: Apoptosis in human acute myocardial infarction. Circulation. 1997;95:320-323.

[23]   Kytö V, Saraste A, Saukko P, Henn V, Pulkki K, Vuorinen T, Voipio-Pulkki LM: Apoptotic cardiomyocyte death in fatal myocarditis. Am J Cardiol. 2004;94:746-750.

[24]   Schaper J, Lorenz-Meyer S, Suzuki K: The role of apoptosis in dilated cardiomyopathy. Herz. 1999;24:219-224.

[25]   Westphal E, Rohrbach S, Buerke M, Behr H, Darmer D, Silber RE, Werdan K, Loppnow H: Altered interleukin-1 receptor antagonist and interleukin-18 mRNA expression in myocardial tissues of patients with dilatated cardiomyopathy. Mol Med. 2008;14:55-63.

[26]   Bott-Flügel L, Weig HJ, Uhlein H, Nabauer M, Laugwitz KL, Seyfarth M: Quantitative analysis of apoptotic markers in human end-stage heart failure. Eur J Heart Fail. 2008;10:129-132.

[27]   Kanoh M, Takemura G, Misao J, Hayakawa Y, Aoyama T, Nishigaki K, Noda T, Fujiwara T, Fukuda K, Minatoguchi S, Fujiwara H: Significance of myocytes with positive DNA in situ nick end-labeling (TUNEL) in hearts with dilated cardiomyopathy: not apoptosis but DNA repair. Circulation. 1999;99:2757-2764.

[28]   Narula J, Haider N, Virmani R, DiSalvo TG, Kolodgie FD, Hajjar RJ, Schmidt U, Semigran MJ, Dec GW, Khaw BA: Apoptosis in myocytes in end-stage heart failure. N Engl J Med. 1996;335:1182-1189.

[29]   Harrison CV, Wood P: Hypertensive and ischaemic heart disease; a comparative clinical and pathological study. Br Heart J. 1949;11:205-229.

[30] Brutsaert DL, Meulemans AL, Sipido KR, Sys SU: Effects of damaging the endocardial surface on the mechanical performance of isolated cardiac muscle. Circ Res. 1988;62:358-366.

[31] Ungureanu-Longrois D, Balligand JL, Okada I, Simmons WW, Kobzik L, Lowenstein CJ, Kunkel SL, Michel T, Kelly RA, Smith TW: Contractile responsiveness of ventricular myocytes to isoproterenol is regulated by induction of nitric oxide synthase activity in cardiac microvascular endothelial cells in heterotypic primary culture. Circ Res. 1995;77:486-493.

[32] Qi XL, Nguyen TL, Andries L, Sys SU, Rouleau JL: Vascular endothelial dysfunction contributes to myocardial depression in ischemia-reperfusion in the rat. Can J Physiol Pharmacol. 1998;76:35-45.

[33] Qi XL, Stewart DJ, Gosselin H, Azad A, Picard P, Andries L, Sys SU, Brutsaert DL, Rouleau JL: Improvement of endocardial and vascular endothelial function on myocardial performance by captopril treatment in postinfarct rat hearts. Circulation. 1999;100:1338-1345.

[34] MacAlpin RN, Abbasi AS, Grollman JH Jr, Eber L: Human coronary artery size during life. A cinearteriographic study. Radiology. 1973;108:567-576.

[35] Dodge JT Jr, Brown BG, Bolson EL, Dodge HT: Lumen diameter of normal human coronary arteries. Influence of age, sex, anatomic variation, and left ventricular hypertrophy or dilation. Circulation. 1992;86:232-246.

[36] Mosseri M, Zolti E, Rozenman Y, Lotan C, Ershov T, Izak T, Admon D, Gotsman MS: The diameter of the epicardial coronary arteries in patients with dilated cardiomyopathy. Int J Cardiol. 1997;62:133-141.

[37] Mela T, Meyer TE, Pape LA, Chung ES, Aurigemma GP, Weiner BH: Coronary arterial dimension-to-left ventricular mass ratio in idiopathic dilated cardiomyopathy. Am J Cardiol. 1999;83:1277-1280, A9.

[38] Abraham D, Hofbauer R, Schäfer R, Blumer R, Paulus P, Miksovsky A, Traxler H, Kocher A, Aharinejad S: Selective downregulation of VEGF-A(165), VEGF-R(1), and decreased capillary density in patients with dilative but not ischemic cardiomyopathy. Circ Res. 2000;87:644-647.

[39] Schäfer R, Abraham D, Paulus P, Blumer R, Grimm M, Wojta J, Aharinejad S: Impaired VE-cadherin/beta-catenin expression mediates endothelial cell degeneration in dilated cardiomyopathy. Circulation. 2003;108:1585-1591.

[40] Roura S, Gálvez-Montón C, Fernández MA, Lupón J, Bayes-Genis A: Circulating endothelial progenitor cells: Potential biomarkers for idiopathic dilated cardiomyopathy. J Cardiovasc Transl Res. 2016;9:80-84.

[41] Sharma S, Adrogue JV, Golfman L, Uray I, Lemm J, Youker K, Noon GP, Frazier OH, Taegtmeyer H: Intramyocardial lipid accumulation in the failing human heart resembles the lipotoxic rat heart. FASEB J. 2004;18:1692-1700.

[42] Haq S, Choukroun G, Lim H, Tymitz KM, del Monte F, Gwathmey J, Grazette L, Michael A, Hajjar R, Force T, Molkentin JD: Differential activation of signal transduction pathways in human hearts with hypertrophy versus advanced heart failure. Circulation. 2001;103:670-677.

[43] Muchir A, Shan J, Bonne G, Lehnart SE, Worman HJ: Inhibition of extracellular signal-regulated kinase signaling to prevent cardiomyopathy caused by mutation in the gene encoding A-type lamins. Hum Mol Genet. 2009;18:241-247.

[44] Wu W, Muchir A, Shan J, Bonne G, Worman HJ: Mitogen-activated protein kinase inhibitors improve heart function and prevent fibrosis in cardiomyopathy caused by mutation in lamin A/C gene. Circulation. 2011;123:53-61.

[45] Herz J, Strickland DK: LRP: a multifunctional scavenger and signaling receptor. J. Clin Invest. 2001;108:779-784.

[46] Cáceres LC, Bonacci GR, Sánchez MC, Chiabrando GA: Activated $\alpha(2)$ macroglobulin induces matrix metalloproteinase 9 expression by low-density lipoprotein receptor-related protein 1 through MAPK-ERK1/2 and NF-kB activation in macrophage-derived cell lines. J Cell Biochem. 2010;111:607-617.

[47] Huang W, Dolmer K, Liao X, Gettins PG: NMR solution structure of the receptor binding domain of human alpha(2)-macroglobulin. J Biol Chem. 2000;275:1089-1094.

[48] Lillis AP, Van Duyn LB, Murphy-Ullrich JE, Strickland DK: LDL receptor-related protein 1: unique tissue-specific functions revealed by selective gene knockout studies. Physiol Rev. 2008;88:887-918.

[49] Franchini M, Montagnana M: Low-density lipoprotein receptor-related protein 1: new functions for an old molecule. Clin Chem Lab Med. 2011;49:967-970.

[50] Boucher P, Liu P, Gotthardt M, Hiesberger T, Anderson RG, Herz J: Platelet-derived growth factor mediates tyrosine phosphorylation of the cytoplasmic domain of the low density lipoprotein receptor-related protein in caveolae. J Biol Chem. 2002;277:15507-15513.

[51] Loukinova E, Ranganathan S, Kuznetsov S, Gorlatova N, Migliorini MM, Loukinov D, Ulery PG, Mikhailenko I, Lawrence DA, Strickland DK: Platelet-derived growth factor (PDGF)-induced tyrosine phosphorylation of the low density lipoprotein receptor-related protein (LRP). Evidence for integrated co-receptor function between LRP and the PDGF. J Biol Chem. 2002;18:15499-15506.

[52] van der Geer P: Phosphorylation of LRP-1: regulation of transport and signal transduction. Trends Cardiovasc Med. 2002;12:160-165.

[53] Langlois B, Perrot G, Schneider C, Henriet P, Emonard H, Martiny L, Dedieu S: LRP-1 promotes cancer cell invasion by supporting ERK and inhibiting JNK signaling pathways. PLoS One. 2010;5:e11584.

[54] Muratoglu SC, Mikhailenko I, Newton C, Migliorini M, Strickland DK: Low density lipoprotein receptor-related protein 1 (LRP1) forms a signaling complex with platelet-derived growth factor receptor-beta in endosomes and regulates activation of the MAPK pathway. J Biol Chem. 2010;285:14308-14317.

[55] Geetha N, Mihaly J, Stockenhuber A, Blasi F, Uhrin P, Binder BR, Freissmuth M, Breuss JM: Signal integration and coincidence detection in the mitogen-activated protein kinase/extracellular signal-regulated kinase (ERK) cascade: concomitant activation of receptor tyrosine kinases and of LRP-1 leads to sustained ERK phosphorylation via down-regulation of dual specificity phosphatases (DUSP1 and -6). J. Biol. Chem. 2011;286:25663-25674.

[56] Llorente-Cortés V, Badimon L: LDL receptor-related protein and the vascular wall: implications for atherothrombosis. Arterioscler Thromb Vasc Biol. 2005;25:497-504.

[57] Abraham D, Hofbauer R, Schäfer R, Blumer R, Paulus P, Miksovsky A, Traxler H, Kocher A, Aharinejad S: Selective downregulation of VEGF-A(165), VEGF-R(1), and decreased capillary density in patients with dilative but not ischemic cardiomyopathy. Circ Res. 2000;87:644-647.

[58] Schäfer R, Abraham D, Paulus P, Blumer R, Grimm M, Wojta J, Aharinejad S: Impaired VE-cadherin/beta-catenin expression mediates endothelial cell degeneration in dilated cardiomyopathy. Circulation. 2003;108:1585-1591.

[59] Reis M, Liebner S: Wnt signaling in the vasculature. Exp Cell Res. 2013;319:1317-1323.

[60] Haas J, Frese KS, Park YJ, Keller A, Vogel B, Lindroth AM, Weichenhan D, Franke J, Fischer S, Bauer A, Marquart S, Sedaghat-Hamedani F, Kayvanpour E, Köhler D, Wolf NM, Hassel S, Nietsch R, Wieland T, Ehlermann P, Schultz JH, Dösch A, Mereles D, Hardt S, Backs J, Hoheisel JD, Plass C, Katus HA, Meder B: Alterations in cardiac DNA methylation in human dilated cardiomyopathy. EMBO Mol Med. 2013;5:413-429.

[61] Koczor CA, Lee EK, Torres RA, Boyd A, Vega JD, Uppal K, Yuan F, Fields EJ, Samarel AM, Lewis W: Detection of differentially methylated gene promoters in failing and nonfailing human left ventricle myocardium using computation analysis. Physiol Genomics. 2013;45:597-605.

[62] Koczor CA, Torres RA, Fields EJ, Boyd A, He S, Patel N, Lee EK, Samarel AM, Lewis W: Thymidine kinase and mtDNA depletion in human cardiomyopathy: epigenetic and translational evidence for energy starvation. Physiol Genomics. 2013;45:590-596.

[63] Singer SJ, Nicolson GL: The fluid mosaic model of the structure of cell membranes. Science. 1972;175:720-731.

[64] Sonnino S, Prinetti A: Membrane domains and the "lipid raft" concept. Curr Med Chem. 2013;20:4-21.

[65] Chiantia S, London E: Sphingolipids and membrane domains: recent advances. Handb Exp Pharmacol. 2013;215:33-55.

[66] Simons K, Ikonen E: Functional rafts in cell membranes. Nature. 1997;387:569-572.

[67] Parton RG, Simons: The multiple faces of caveolae. Nat. Rev. Mol. Cell. Biol. 2007;8:185-194.

[68] Roura S, Cal R, Gálvez-Montón C, Revuelta-Lopez E, Nasarre L, Badimon L, Bayes-Genis A, Llorente-Cortés V: Inverse relationship between raft LRP1 localization and non-raft ERK1,2/MMP9 activation in idiopathic dilated cardiomyopathy: potential impact in ventricular remodeling. Int J Cardiol. 2014;176:805-814.

[69] Fedak PW, Moravec CS, McCarthy PM, Altamentova SM, Wong AP, Skrtic M, Verma S, Weisel RD, Li RK. Altered expression of disintegrin metalloproteinases and their inhibitor in human dilated cardiomyopathy. Circulation. 2006;113:238-245.

[70] Sivakumar P, Gupta S, Sarkar S, Sen S: Upregulation of lysyl oxidase and MMPs during cardiac remodeling in human dilated cardiomyopathy. Mol Cell Biochem. 2008;307:159-167.

[71] Roura S, Gálvez-Montón C, Pujal JM, Casani L, Fernández MA, Astier L, Gastelurrutia P, Domingo M, Prat-Vidal C, Soler-Botija C, Llucià-Valldeperas A, Llorente-Cortés V, Bayes-Genis A: New insights into lipid raft function regulating myocardial vascularization competency in human idiopathic dilated cardiomyopathy. Atherosclerosis. 2013;230:354-364.

[72] Roura S, Gálvez-Montón C, Bayes-Genis A. The challenges for cardiac vascular precursor cell therapy: lessons from a very elusive precursor. J Vasc Res. 2013;50:304-323.

[73] Insel PA, Patel HH: Membrane rafts and caveolae in cardiovascular signaling. Curr Opin Nephrol Hypertens. 2009;18:50-56.

[74] Tsutsumi YM, Kawaraguchi Y, Horikawa YT, Niesman IR, Kidd MW, Chin-Lee B, Head BP, Patel PM, Roth DM, Patel HH: Role of caveolin-3 and glucose transporter-4 in isoflurane-induced delayed cardiac protection. Anesthesiology. 2010;112:1136-1145.

[75] Gazzerro E, Bonetto A, Minetti C. Caveolinopathies: translational implications of caveolin-3 in skeletal and cardiac muscle disorders. Handb Clin Neurol. 2011;101:135-142.

[76] Hunter DJ: Gene-environment interactions in human diseases. Nat Rev Genet. 2005;6:287-298.

[77] Craig J: Complex diseases: Research and applications. Nature Education. 2008;1:1.

2

Advanced Treatments and Emerging Therapies for Dystrophin-Deficient Cardiomyopathies

Jordi Camps, Enrico Pozzo, Tristan Pulinckx,
Robin Duelen and Maurilio Sampaolesi

Abstract

Dystrophinopathies are characterized by skeletal and cardiac muscle complications because of a lack or shortened DYSTROPHIN protein. Ventilation assistance and corticosteroid treatment have positively affected life outcome but lead to an increased incidence of cardiomyopathy. Cardiomyopathy is now the leading cause of death in patients with dystrophinopathy. Thus, coherent guidelines for cardiac care have become essential and need to be communicated well. Progression of cardiac complications in patients with dystrophinopathy diverges from standard dilated cardiomyopathy development and monitoring and medical care for dystrophinopathy. This chapter summarizes current guidelines and recommendations for monitoring and clinical treatment of cardiac complications in patients with dystrophinopathy and provides a thorough survey of emerging therapies focusing on cardiac outcomes.

Keywords: dystrophin, Duchenne and Becker muscular dystrophy, dilated cardiomy-opathy, symptomatic treatment, exon skipping, gene and cell therapy

1. Introduction

Dystrophinopathies are a group of diseases comprising Duchenne muscular dystrophy (DMD), Becker muscular dystrophy (BMD) and X-linked dilated cardiomyopathy (XLDCM), characterized by a shortened or absent *DYSTROPHIN* gene. DMD is the most prominent, with an incidence around 1:5000 live male births [1]. BMD occurs about three times less than DMD [2], while XLDCM is extremely rare [3]. *DYSTROPHIN*—part of the dystrophin-glycoprotein complex (Appendix 1)—is located on the X chromosome, and therefore, only males are affected.

The main clinical feature of patients with dystrophinopathy is an early loss of ambulation depending on the availability of DYSTROPHIN. Patients with DMD completely lack DYS-TROPHIN—the pathological mechanisms are discussed in Appendix 2—and are presented with the most severe disease progression. This is indicated by a loss of ambulation around 10 years of age and consequent ventilation assistance, followed by death during the second or third decade [4]. Conversely, patients with BMD still express a truncated form of DYSTRO-PHIN. Although only partially functional, this still has an effect on disease progression and life expectancy, which are drastically prolonged [5]. Patients with XLDCM show the absence of DYSTROPHIN in the heart, while expression in skeletal muscles is conserved. Several hypotheses have been proposed for this peculiar genotype [3]. In patients with dystrophin-opathy, the routine use of corticosteroids and nocturnal ventilation support have dramatically improved the life expectancy and its quality. Unfortunately, this brings up other complications, as the incidence of cardiomyopathy is raising and is nearly ubiquitous in older patients with DMD. In this perspective, monitoring and treatment of cardiac complications becomes more and more important.

This chapter contains an overview of the current monitoring and treatment guidelines and state-of-the-art therapies for dystrophin-deficient cardiomyopathies. The clinical features of dystrophinopathies with an emphasis on cardiac disease progression will be discussed briefly, followed by a description of the diagnostic process and current management strategies. Conclusions from recent clinical trials on current symptomatic treatments will be summarized and emerging therapies will be discussed in detail, from promising preclinical research to ongoing clinical trials.

2. Clinical features

2.1. Duchenne and Becker muscular dystrophy

Neonate boys with DMD are rarely symptomatic, and the disease will not be recognized until the second or third year of life. The patient may show evidence of mild muscle weakness before the 12th month of life (i.e., poor head control after the 6th week, mild inability to sit unsup-ported at the 6th month). It is possible that he achieves the motor milestones of walking (12th month) and running (2nd year) during the toddler period, but he will eventually be brought to medical attention due to being less active than expected, as well as being prone to falling [6].

One of the earliest clinical signs of DMD is pseudohypertrophy of the gastrocnemii in the calves caused by hypertrophy of muscle fibers combined with fat infiltration and proliferation of collagen. The muscles have a firm and rubbery consistency, as well as being hypotonic compared with unaffected muscles. By the age of 3–5 years, the clinical picture of DMD gradually appears and "the patient straddles as he stands and waddles as he walks". In order to rise from the ground, the typical Gowers' sign (i.e., the child first extends the arms and legs assuming a four-point position and then works each hand alternately up the corresponding thigh) is present and it is fully expressed by the age of 5 or 6 years. While standing and walking, the patient places the feet wide apart to increase the base of support, and as a result of gluteus medius weakness, there is waddling when walking [7].

The typical posture of a patient with DMD is lumbar lordosis and scoliosis (due to weakness of abdominal muscles and paravertebral muscles) with hip flexion and abduction, knee flexion and plantar flexion, as well as winging of the scapulae. Other common presentations in toddlers include falling, troubles in running or using the stairs and developmental delays [7, 8]. As the muscular wasting progresses, the weakness will spread to the muscles of the legs and forearms and patients may end up being confined to a wheelchair by 7 years of age, while other patients may continue walking with increasing difficulty until 10 years of age. Death usually occurs around the second decade of life, caused by pulmonary infections, respiratory failure, aspiration, airway obstruction or heart failure [6].

In BMD, the weakness and hypertrophy appear in the same muscles as DMD, but the onset is later (5–45 years; mean age: 12 years) with most patients losing ambulation in the third or fourth decade. However, some patients may have a milder phenotype with the onset of muscular weakness in late adulthood [6].

In both DMD and BMD groups, the median age of diagnosis of cardiac involvement is 14 years, with all patients having cardiac problems after 18 years of age [8]. While in BMD, the cardiac involvement can be the presenting symptom at diagnosis [9], and in patients with DMD, the presentation at diagnosis is usually subclinical and asymptomatic. Patients often have unspecific symptoms including fatigue, weight loss, nausea, sleep disturbance, cough, palpitations, sweating, chest and abdominal discomfort, decreased urinary output, irritability and concentration difficulties [8].

The physical examination may present some problems in patients with advanced muscular dystrophy (MD) due to scoliosis, immobility or glucocorticoid-related obesity. Tachycardia will be present, unless treated with β-blockers. Hypotension may be present—as a result of DYSTROPHIN loss in both vascular smooth muscles and low oral fluid intake—causing altered cardiac pacemaker activity, altered myocardial contractility and altered vasomotor tone. Edema is not commonly present, even in the presence of advanced right and left cardiac failure [9].

At auscultation the cardiac apex may be displaced as a result of scoliosis, with S3 gallop and S4 gallop commonly heard as a result of acute congestive heart failure and left ventricular (LV) dysfunction, respectively [9]. Moderate mitral regurgitation (due to posterior wall fibrosis and LV thinning) and moderate tricuspid regurgitation may be present [10]. Neck venous engorgement may be seen as a result of abdominal compression caused by scoliosis [8].

As dystrophy progresses, the LV function worsens, leading to the clinical picture of dilated cardiomyopathy (DCM), which can be complicated by arrhythmias. DCM is an enlargement of one or both of the ventricles combined with systolic dysfunction, usually preceding signs and symptoms of congestive heart failure. The hallmarks of DCM are decreased LV function (decreased ejection fraction), LV dilation and mitral regurgitation. The latter manifests as palpitations, vertigo, dizziness, syncope or sudden cardiac death. Moreover, in DMD, the arrhythmia occurs even in the absence of myocardial fibrosis [11]. **Table 1** provides a summary with the most important clinical characteristics for DMD, BMD and XLDCM.

	DMD	BMD	XLDCM
Dystrophin	Absent	Partially functional	Absent (heart only)
Incidence	1 : 3500–6000 male births	1 : 18,000–19,000 male births	Very rare
Myopathy onset	3–5 years	12 years	Variable
Loss of ambulation	~12 years	~27 years	No loss
Life expectancy	Mid to late 20s	40s	Mid to late 10s
Cardiomyopathy onset	16–18 years	Variable, can precede skeletal muscle symptoms	Variable, from mild to severe cases

Table 1. Characteristics of Duchenne muscular dystrophy (DMD), Becker muscular dystrophy (BMD) and X-linked dilated cardiomyopathy (XLDCM).

2.2. X-linked dilated cardiomyopathy

XLDCM is a cardio-specific dystrophinopathy presenting with congestive heart failure (CHF) due to DCM in 10- to 20-year-old patients, without the dystrophinopathy-related involvement of skeletal muscles (**Table 1**). Patients show a brisk and progressive heart failure and ventricular arrhythmias, with untreated patients that may die of congestive heart failure not long after diagnosis [3].

3. Diagnosis and monitoring

Dystrophinopathy is generally underdiagnosed and definitive diagnosis can even take up to 2, 5 years from the onset of symptoms [12]. The first diagnostic test performed, when dystrophinopathy is expected, is a serum creatine kinase (CK) measurement. In most cases, CK levels are elevated, around 50–100 times in DMD, while in BMD levels are lower but still higher compared to healthy patients [13]. A second level diagnostic test is a mutation analysis, which reveals the specific genetic alteration and is useful to discriminate between DMD and BMD [14]. Differences between DMD and BMD are clarified by the reading frame concept (Appendix 3) [15]. For 5% of the cases, mutation analysis is not able to diagnose for dystrophinopathy [16]. In this circumstance, a muscle biopsy is taken and the reduction or the absence of DYSTROPHIN is analyzed by tissue staining (immunohistochemistry and immunofluorescence) or immunoblot (Western blot).

Recognizing cardiac complications in patients with dystrophinopathy is challenging, especially because of physical inactivity and respiratory complications [8]. Hence, cardiomyopathies are underdiagnosed in these patients [17]. Clinical guidelines were created in 2010, recommending an echocardiogram every 2 years from the moment of diagnosis of dystrophinopathy or from the age of 6 years. From 10 years of age, a yearly screening to asses LV function is suggested [14]. Recently, it has been documented that cardiac MRI is more sensitive and can distinguish cardiac complications in an earlier stage for patients with dystrophinopathy [18]. Therefore, it is recommended to perform a cardiac MRI instead of echocardiography, also because patients with dystrophinopathy can suffer from scoliosis, which makes diagnosis with echocardiography more complicated. However, cardiac MRI can also be challenging for pediatric patients because of the need for sedation, cost and lack of accessibility. Sinus tachycardia is also known to precede any cardiac complications in patients with DMD [19].

As mentioned before, early diagnosis of cardiomyopathy onset is essential in patients with dystrophinopathy. Hence, clinical trials are still undertaken to study whether electrocardiogram (ECG), echocardiography, cardiac MRI and sera biomarkers can improve early detection of myocardial involvement and clinical outcome (NCT02020954).

4. Clinical management

4.1. Pharmacological treatment

Early diagnosis of dystrophinopathies—before the onset of cardiac complications—gives the opportunity to treat patients in a presymptomatic stage (**Figure 1**). However, for dystrophinopathy there is no general agreement on the treatment of cardiomyopathy [20]. There are some guidelines published to guide the decision-making process; however, still a huge variability in treatments exists between centers and clinicians [11].

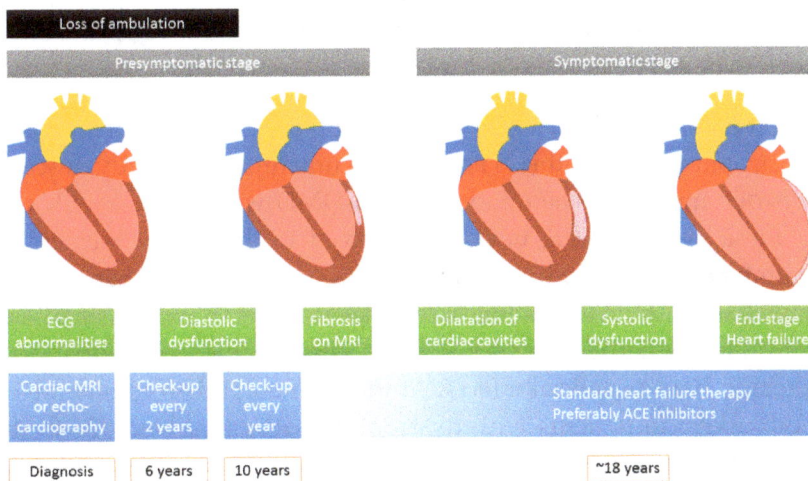

Figure 1. Progression of dystrophin-deficient cardiomyopathy and guidelines for monitoring and treatment. ACE, angiotensin-II-converting enzyme.

Corticosteroids improve muscle performance and delay loss of ambulation and also have beneficial effects on ventilation and scoliosis. However, this is accompanied by many side effects such as weight gain, delay of puberty, decrease of vertebral bone mass, increase of vertebral fragility, cataract formation and growth-failure [11]. Evidence exists that corticosteroids also have advantageous effects on the heart of patients with DMD, several clinical trials suggest a delayed onset of cardiomyopathy in patients with dystrophy [21]. However, these results have to be interpreted with caution; all studies were retrospective without the objective to treat for cardiomyopathic complications. In addition, corticosteroids treatment in X-linked muscular dystrophy (*mdx*) mice—an animal model for DMD with a stop codon in exon 23— led to cases of heart failure, myocardial fibrosis and sarcolemmal damage [22]. Prospective clinical trials are necessary to address the effect of corticosteroids on heart functionality. Preclinical results in dystrophic mice and hamsters are concerning, especially given the broad use of corticosteroids for treating dystrophinopathies, and reveal the gap in our understanding about effects of corticosteroids on the heart [11]. In addition, the most suitable duration of corticosteroid therapy still has to be determined.

The effect of angiotensin-converting enzyme inhibitors (ACEIs) is more clear-cut and proved to postpone cardiomyopathy onset in both preclinical animal models and patients. A three-year treatment did not show any effect among a group of DMD patients treated with perindopril and another placebo-treated group. However, after 2 additional years of perindopril treatment – in which both of these groups now received this drug - a significant reduction in LV ejection fraction was observed between the 5 year-treated and 2 year-treated group [23]. A 10-year follow-up study, observed a significantly higher survival rate in a group of DMD patients that received a presymptomatic treatment with perindopril for 3 years [24]. Current guidelines propose a start of ACEIs for DMD patients only after development of LV dysfunction [14]. However, because aforementioned results demonstrated a clear beneficial effect of presymptomatic treatment, it is now recommended to initiate treatment with ACEIs before the onset of LV dysfunction in patients with DMD [25] (**Figure 1**). In case of observed intolerance against ACEIs, angiotensin-II receptor blockers (ARBs) could be used instead, since they have been shown to be as effective as ACEIs [26].

The use of β-blockers as a combined therapy with ACEIs is common for heart failure treatment; however, for dystrophinopathies, this is not well documented. One study described improvements in LV systolic function, when patients with DMD were treated with carvedilol [27]. Unfortunately, these findings were never reproduced in dystrophic *mdx* mice [28]. Study outcomes for combined therapy were mixed and showed additional beneficial effects for β-blockers in some cases, and no additional advantageous effects in others [29]. Future clinical trials need to evaluate whether the use of β-blockers for dystrophinopathy as mono- or combination therapy have beneficial effects. At the moment, it is recommended to initiate a therapy with β-blockers in patients with dystrophinopathy that have LV dysfunction [25]. Future studies will need to assess whether therapies combining corticosteroids with β-blockers and ACEIs could be of added benefit.

Mineralocorticoid receptor antagonists are a standard heart failure therapy due to their anti-fibrotic effect in DMD and ability to attenuate cardiomyopathy [30]. In a recent randomized double-blind clinical trial, one group of DMD patients with normal LV function were treated with only ACEIs or ARBs and the other group additionally also received eplerenone (aldosterone inhibitor). Results showed a lower LV circumferential strain in both treated groups compared to control, but not between treated groups [31]. This study is the only study of mineralocorticoid-receptor antagonists on dystrophin-deficient cardiomyopathy, and although it was not able to demonstrate a significant improvement, it is essential to investigate further whether aldosterone inhibitors could be of any benefit for delaying cardiomyopathy onset.

4.2. Nonpharmacological treatment

Heart transplantation is the only remedy for end-stage heart failure. Some cases have been published in which patients with DMD received a successful transplantation with no significant adverse effects [25]. Heart transplantation occurs more frequently in patients with BMD because of the higher incidence of cardiomyopathy and is only recommended for patients who have end-stage heart failure [25]. A deficit in surrogate organs complicates heart transplantation; therefore, left ventricular assist devices (LVADs) are an interesting substitution, demonstrating effectiveness in DMD and BMD patients with advanced heart failure [25]. However, possible postoperative complications, such as arrhythmias, bleeding, respiratory failure, stroke and rehabilitation, need to be further addressed [25].

4.3. Treatments with indirect effects

Treatments that have no direct effect on the heart can also have considerable benefits on cardiac function. For example, pain reduction lowers blood levels of catecholamines, which on its turn generates no further stress on the heart.

Lung and heart function are known to affect each other. When lung function needs to be assisted by noninvasive positive pressure ventilation (NIPPV)—because of breathing difficulties—it also has favoring results on cardiac function. It leads to less strain on the heart and a correspondingly reduced heart rate. Reduced lung function is also a strong negative predictor of survival when the vital capacity hits one liter [32]. In addition, assisted ventilation increased the mean survival of DMD patients with more than 10 years; however, patients who need constant ventilation will not exceed 20 years of age [32].

Although corticosteroids treatment has positively affected the incidence of scoliosis, it still occurs that thoracolumbar surgery becomes necessary to correct the spinal curvature [33]. In this case, timing is important and certain risk factors are bound to patients with DMD that have LV dysfunction [32]. Even when surgery is undertaken, it is not certain if scoliosis will not develop. This could lead into feeding and swallowing problems [32]. When surgery is able to prevent scoliosis onset, not only does it improve positioning and pulmonary function, but it also ameliorates cardiac function [33]. It is important to note that—although spinal surgery is performed in many neurological centers—it is not uniformly supported [11]. If patients with dystrophinopathy undergo surgery, an appropriate use of anesthetics is essential and needs to be assessed and monitored carefully before, during and after surgical intervention [34]. **Table 2** gives an overview of all current clinical interventions available for the treatment of dystrophin-deficient cardiomyopathy.

Method	Level of evidence	Recommendations	References
Pharmacological			
Corticosteroids	Mid	Initiation based on functional state and pre-existing risk factors for adverse side-effects	[14]
		Be aware of controversial cardiac results in animal studies and clinical trials	[83]
ACEIs and ARBs	High	First-line therapy upon development of LV dysfunction	[18]
		Initiate therapy from 10 years of age or earlier	[14]
β-Blockers	Low	Follow guidelines for adults with chronic heart failure	[84]
		Variable, normally initiation after ACEIs start on the basis of ventricular dysfunction or elevated heart rate	[18]
Mineralocorticoid -receptor antagonists	Low	Timing not adequately addressed and variation in clinical practice	[18]
Nonpharmacological			
LVAD	High	Currently bridge to heart transplantation but potential for destination therapy High-risk factor: scoliosis, respiratory muscle weakness and difficulties in recovery and rehabilitation	[85]
Heart transplantation	High	Should be considered for patient with end-stage heart failure	[25]
Indirect effects			
NIPPV	High	Main need for pulmonary care is from the onset of ambulation loss. Decisions for respiratory care must be taken by a care team including a physician and skilled therapist.	[86]
Thoracolumbar surgery	Mid	For patients not receiving glucocorticoids: surgery warranted when spinal curvature > 20°. For patients receiving glucocorticoids: surgery warranted upon further spinal curve progression.	[33]

ACEIs, angiotensin-converting enzyme inhibitor; ARBs, angiotensin II receptor blockers; LVAD, left ventricular assist device; NIPPV, noninvasive positive pressure ventilation.

Table 2. Clinical treatments of dystrophin-deficient cardiomyopathy.

5. Emerging therapies

5.1. Utrophin upregulation

In 1972, UTROPHIN—a DYSTROPHIN homolog with a shortened rod domain but many similar binding proteins—was discovered [35]. These resemblances started the speculation that UTROPHIN could partially compensate for DYSTROPHIN loss. More clarity was brought by the creation of a *DYSTROPHIN/UTROPHIN* double knockout (*mdx/utrn⁻/⁻*) mouse model, that showed a worsened skeletal and cardiac muscle phenotype with a drastically lower life expectancy of only 2–3 months compared to *mdx* mice [36]. Several studies have been performed testing UTROPHIN upregulation in preclinical models, the most promising one coming from a small molecule screening. SMT C1100 treatment demonstrated an increase of UTROPHIN levels in *mdx* mice and improved muscle function [37]. A phase Ia and recently also a phase Ib clinical trial were completed, concluding that no serious adverse effects were accompanied by SMT C1100 treatment in healthy controls and pediatric DMD patients, respectively [38]. It is important to mention that UTROPHIN will never be able to replace symptoms of DYSTROPHIN deficiency because of its structural differences and lack of a NO binding site (Appendix 1), presuming an incomplete surrogate effect.

5.2. Nonsense suppression

About 10–15% of patients with DMD carry a premature stop codon that abrogates translation of *DYSTROPHIN* [39]. Aminoglycosides are mainly used as antibiotic agents but are also able to cause a ribosomal read-through—meaning it is able to ignore premature stop codons while still detecting normal stop codons—and in this way generating a shortened, although functional DYSTROPHIN protein. Although promising, clinical results have been poor with inconclusive or very low expressed DYSTROPHIN levels and major concerns about side effects caused by Gentamicin and Negamicin [40]. Henceforth, PCT124 or ataluren was discovered by another small-molecule drug screening, showing promising results in preclinical animal models without skipping normal stop codons [41]. In addition, ataluren was considered safe and showed upregulation of DYSTROPHIN in certain subgroups of patients with DMD, although nothing was mentioned about the heart [42–44]. These clinical trials confirmed the need for further understanding and a division of patients with DMD in subgroups. Currently, ataluren is involved in a randomized, double-blind and placebo-controlled phase III trial, with the primary outcome being an improvement in the 6-minute walking test (6MWT) after 48 weeks; however, cardiac function will not be monitored (NCT01826487). A search for more effective read-through compounds (RTCs) ended up with two more drugs: RTC13 and RTC14. The highest efficiency was reached by RTC13. This compound restored DYSTROPHIN levels the most in the skeletal muscle and the heart compared to gentamicin, PTC124 and RTC14. Moreover, CK levels were reduced and muscle function was improved in *mdx* mice [45].

5.3. Exon skipping

The idea of exon skipping originated from BMD, due to the fact that these patients express a shorter isoform of DYSTROPHIN and show a much milder phenotype [46]. Skipping the genetic alteration of *DYSTROPHIN* so that an out-of-frame shift is turned into an in-frame shift would result in the expression of a truncated DYSTROPHIN isoform such as in BMD (Appendix 2) [47]. Antisense oligonucleotides (AONs) are short, single-stranded DNA sequences that are complementary to a target pre-mRNA splice site and able to skip exons by sterically hindering splice enhancers [48]. This procedure should be able to treat 35% of patients with

DMD by targeting one exon and even 83% when two exons are simultaneously targeted [49]. The downside is that AONs can only target one exon, for this reason research currently focuses only on the most frequently involved exons [49].

There are currently two different types of AONs undergoing clinical trials: 2'O methyl phosphorothioate (2'OMePS)—also called drisapersen [50]—and phosphorodiamidate morpholino oligomers (PMO)—also known as eteplirsen [51]. Both were unable to improve DYSTROPHIN expression in the heart [52, 53]. Recently, a high degree of DYSTROPHIN rescue was achieved in the respiratory and cardiac muscles with tricyclo DNA oligomers in *mdx* mice [54]. However, these results were accomplished by multiple injections and high doses of administration (200 mg/kg per week).

Previous clinical trials picked up the inefficiency of systemic delivery of naked AONs [50, 51, 55]. For this reason, attention quickly converted toward the development of delivery methods for AONs. Systems like cell-penetrating peptides (CPPs) or encapsulation techniques such as liposomes or nanoparticles appeared. CPPs are small peptides that are conjugated to AONs. They facilitate the penetration through the plasma membrane and can be divided into three groups: arginine rich, Pip (PNA/PMO internalization peptide) or phage and chimeric peptides. Arginine-rich CPPs associated with a PMO showed the first robust cardiac DYSTROPHIN expression and an improved cardiac function [56, 57]. More recently, Pip6 conjugated with a PMO also showed cardiac Dystrophin expression and functional improvement at low doses [55] and prevented exercise-induced cardiomyopathy after long-term treatment [58]. Phage peptides were less successful with the exception of a 7-mer phage conjugated to 2'OMePS that resulted in an enhanced uptake and exon skipping in the cardiac muscle [59].

Instead of a molecular approach with AONs conjugated to CPPs, it is also possible to deliver small nuclear RNAs (snRNAs) or nucleases to the cardiac muscle. These effectors need to be incorporated into the genome; recombinant adenoviral-associated viruses (rAAVs) are the preferred choice because of their long persistence in myonuclei. However, the disadvantage is their relatively small cloning capacity (5 kb). In addition, to safely apply AAV therapy, all viral genes have to be removed except for the components necessary for replication [60].

Delivery of U7snRNA by rAAV6 has shown to restore cardiac DYSTROPHIN expression, even one year after injection higher DYSTROPHIN levels were still found [61]. The safety profile and optimal concentrations of rAAV8 U7snRNA delivery in the forelimb of a large cohort of GRMD dogs have been monitored carefully and concluded that this treatment is safe, since no adverse immunologic responses were observed [62]. Recently, an observational study was initiated, monitoring clinical and radiological changes of patients eligible for exon 53 skipping, while testing their immunization against viral serotypes (NCT01385917).

Exon skipping with nucleases such as "clustered regularly interspaced short palindromic repeats" (CRISPR) together with a Cas9 nuclease brought new insights and possibilities for gene-editing treatments. CRISPR/Cas9 is an immune protection system originating from bacteria that is able to edit the genome by introducing a double-strand break. Afterwards genomic damage is repaired by one of the two possible repair mechanisms: nonhomologous end-joining (NHEJ) or homology-directed repair (HDR). NHEJ was used as a technique for

DYSTROPHIN exon skipping in *mdx* mice, a CRISPR/Cas9 was designed targeting exon 23, leading into a removal of this exon by double-strand breaks where after these two ends are linked back together again by NHEJ [63]. Gene-editing components were delivered by rAAV9 through different administration routes and showed in all cases improved Dystrophin expression in the cardiac and skeletal muscle [63].

5.4. Gene therapy

Differently from exon skipping, it is also possible to incorporate *DYSTROPHIN* into the genome instead of designing techniques to modulate native *DYSTROPHIN*. The advantage of this therapy is that it is not patient specific, all patients can benefit from the same technique. However, due to the enormous size of *DYSTROPHIN*, it is impossible to compact it entirely into viral capsids. Because of the observation that short isoforms of only 45% of full-length DYSTROPHIN can lead to a very mild phenotype, mini- and microdystrophin were created, leaving behind redundant parts [64, 65].

Some different rAAV types have shown huge promise in delivering mini- or microdystrophin to the heart. Microdystrophin delivered by rAAV6 was able to incorporate itself in the skeletal, cardiac and respiratory muscles of *mdx* mice; however, heart function did not recover, while DYSTROPHIN was clearly expressed [66]. A subtype that has shown to be particularly efficient in transfecting the heart is rAAV9 [67]. Systemic injection of minidystrophin encapsulated in rAAV9 has shown widespread expression, also in the heart of the GRMD dogs [68].

While only one phase I clinical trial for minidystrophin has been executed [69] and another one for microdystrophin is ongoing (NCT02376816), it is clear that this field is still at its starting point. Many difficulties that need to addressed in the future are immunological responses and the necessity of high viral titers [70]. However, novel techniques like fetal transduction [71], chimeric vectors [72] and plasmapheresis [73] have already shown a drastic decrease in immunologic responses in preclinical animal models. In addition, viral gene therapy struggles with compaction size and eventually delivers smaller *DYSTROPHIN* constructs in comparison to skipped *DYSTROPHIN*. Nevertheless, full-length *DYSTROPHIN* was recently successfully incorporated into the skeletal muscle of a *mdx* mouse through the usage of three vectors carrying "intandem" sequential exonic parts of *DYSTROPHIN* [74].

5.5. Cell-based therapy

Cell therapy has some advantages compared to the aforementioned therapies. The idea of cell therapy is to produce healthy cells, which express full length DYSTROPHIN that are able to integrate into the tissue upon injection. In an optimal situation, these cells should also be able to repopulate the progenitor populations such as the satellite cell pool in the skeletal muscle. Many trials have been performed with adult stem cells like myoblasts, bone marrow-derived stem cells, CD133+ stem cells and mesoangioblasts (MABs). MABs are vessel-associated progenitors that are able to migrate across the vessel wall and have been shown to repopulate the skeletal muscle of GRMD dogs upon systemic injection, resulting into a variable improvement of muscle function [75]. Treatment of *mdx/utrn$^{-/-}$* mice with aorta-derived MABs led into a delay of DCM onset and promotion of angiogenesis [76]. Recently, a completed phase I clinical trial with MABs in patients with DMD showed no sign of DYSTROPHIN expression after treatment [77]. Multiple reasons could explain this observation, such as the late age of the patients and the lengthy procedure of isolation, which does not ensure that the cells are delivered in an optimal way. However, systemic treatment with MABs has shown to be safe and efforts are being made to start a phase II clinical trial.

Method	Phase	Model/patients	References
Utrophin upregulation			
Arginine butyrate	Preclinical	*Mdx* mice	[87]
SMT C1100	I	Healthy controls	[38]
Read-through therapy			
Aminoglycosides	I, completed	Patients with DMD and BMD	[40]
Ataluren (PTC124)	III, ongoing	Patients with DMD	NCT01826487
RTC13/14	Preclinical	*Mdx* mice	[45]
Exon skipping			
Drisapersen (2'OMePS)	III, recruiting	Patients with DMD	[51], NCT01803412
Eteplirsen (PMO)	III, recruiting	Patients with DMD	[50, 88], NCT02255552
Tricyclo-DNA	Preclinical	*Mdx* mice	[54]
Cell-penetrating peptide/AON	Preclinical	*Mdx* mice	[55–58]
Phage peptide/AON	Preclinical	*Mdx* mice	[59]
rAAV6/U7snRNA	Preclinical	GRMD	[61]
rAAV9/CRISPR/cas9	Preclinical	*Mdx* mice	[63]
Gene therapy			
rAAV6-microdystrophin	Preclinical	*Mdx* mice	[66]
rAAV9-minidystrophin	Preclinical	GRMD	[67, 89]
Cell-based therapy			
Mesoangioblast	Preclinical	*Mdx/utrn* mice	[76]
	I, completed	Patients with DMD	[77]
iPSC-derived cells	Preclinical	Sgcb-null mice	[78]

Mdx, X-linked muscular dystrophy; DMD, Duchenne muscular dystrophy; BMD, Becker muscular dystrophy; RTC, read-through compound; AON, antisense oligonucleotide; rAAV, recombinant adenoviral-associated viruses; CRISPR, clustered regularly interspaced short palindromic repeats; GRMD, golden retriever muscular dystrophy; utrn, Utrophin; iPSC, induced pluripotent stem cell; Sgcb, sarcoglycan beta.

Table 3. Preclinical treatments of MD-associated cardiomyopathy.

Recently, treatments with derivatives of induced pluripotent stem cells (iPSCs) are being explored. iPSCs are basically (patient-derived) somatic cells that are reprogrammed into pluripotent stem cells that possess similar features as embryonic stem cells. These cells have been differentiated into mesodermal-like progenitors and injected directly into the skeletal and cardiac muscles of *Sgcb-null* mice, a model for limb girdle muscular dystrophy with a worsened phenotype compared to *mdx* mice. Data showed that these unique iPSC-derived myogenic progenitors are able to integrate into heart and limb muscles and functionally ameliorate both cardiac and skeletal muscles of injected dystrophic mice [78].

Another advantage of cell therapy is the possibility of correcting patient-derived cells and reinjecting them, bypassing immunological responses. Novel strategies with CRISPR/Cas9 have been developed to repair DYSTROPHIN in iPSCs, showing functional recovery upon differentiation [79]. Eventually, differentiation of iPSCs towards cardiomyocytes can also be used to set up high-throughput screenings for detecting novel patient-tailored therapeutic molecules.

Nevertheless, there are still many aspects in cell-based therapy that need to be addressed. As of yet, there is no consensus about timing of injection, which is hypothesized to be crucial. As for integration, many cell therapies suffer from extremely low integration efficiencies. Future studies should focus on tracing the injected cells, to follow their trajectory and fate during treatment [80]. **Table 3** provides an overview of all the discussed preclinical therapies.

6. Conclusion

Since the utilization of ventilation support and corticosteroids treatment, cardiac complications in dystrophinopathies have become more prominent, being responsible for 40% of mortality in patients with DMD [11]. Cardiomyopathy development in patients with dystrophinopathy is highly variable and can be asymptomatic for a long period of time. The earlier onset of skeletal muscle symptoms and the sequential diagnosis can be used as an advantage for cardiac treatment. At the moment, it is recommended to perform a cardiac MRI at the age of 6 or right at the time of diagnosis, followed by two-year check-ups till the age of 10 where after annual check-ups are required. Momentarily, no consensus exists about initiation of treatment. It is advised to start symptomatic treatment as soon as possible because of the beneficial effects on cardiomyopathic progression. ACEIs are the preferred choice for treatment, because of their clear and advantageous effects on cardiomyopathy in patients with dystrophinopathy. Effects of corticosteroids treatment on the heart remain distrustful and cardiac deterioration should be monitored with care, while β-blockers are shown to be effective as stand-alone therapy, but additive effects together with ACEIs are not observed. In addition, transparent results about mineralocorticoid-receptor antagonist treatment on patients with dystrophinopathy are still missing. In the case of end-stage heart failure, heart transplantation or LVADs should be considered. While treatments with indirect effects on the heart like pain reduction, NIPPV and thoracolumbar surgery could also be of added benefit for cardiac health.

Many emerging therapies exist that are being investigated in preclinical models and clinical trials. These studies aim to enhance UTROPHIN expression, read through a stop codon mutation, skip the exon—that is holding the genetic alteration in DMD to express a shorter form of DYSTROPHIN corresponding to BMD—or bring in shortened *DYSTROPHIN* variants by viral or cell-based therapy. Several of these therapies already made it into clinical trials with some undergoing phase III trials. However, as skeletal muscle complications are the most prominent, effects on the heart have not been taken up into the expected outcomes of these trials. This also because in most preclinical treatments beneficial effects on the heart were absent. Novel approaches were necessary to deliver constructs to the cardiac muscle and some preclinical studies have shown DYSTROPHIN expression in the heart together with functional improvements in small and large animal models. Emerging literature is also showing that IPSC-derived myogenic progenitors from patients with dystrophy provide an attractive model to get new insights on gene-editing treatments. This novel technology offers possibilities for autologous therapy and eventually targeting both cardiac and skeletal dystrophic muscles with a single myogenic progenitor population. It is assumed that all these preclinical therapies will make it into clinical studies and hopefully subsequently into dystrophinopathy therapies. However, many issues still exist and need to be addressed such as immunogenic reactions toward the administered cells or viruses, the need for high-dosing regimens and bodywide delivery.

Appendix

Appendix 1: The dystrophin-glycoprotein complex

DYSTROPHIN functions as a linkage rod between the actin cytoskeleton and the cell membrane, where it is connected to β-DYSTROGLYCAN, which in turn associates with the extracellular matrix via LAMININ. The SARCOGLYCAN complex is in close proximity to β-DYSTROGLYCAN and is important in signaling, which occurs through SYNTROPHIN and DYSTROBREVIN. Together these proteins are part of the dystrophin-glycoprotein complex (DGC). DYSTROPHIN also accommodates a neuronal nitric oxide synthase (nNOS)-binding site.

Appendix 2: The molecular mechanisms of dystrophin deficiency

The 24 spectrin-like repeats within DYSTROPHIN neutralizes contraction-induced stress. The absence of DYSTROPHIN leads into a loss of muscle structural integrity, which generates membrane microruptures, leading to elevated CK levels in the serum and a high intracellular Ca^{2+} concentration that subsequently activates calcium-dependent proteases [81]. Because of the lack of experimental proof, researchers have started questioning this theory. It became evident that activation of stretch-induced Ca^{2+} channels corresponds with elevated intracellular Ca^{2+} levels, although the responsible channel has still to be found [82]. Repeated contraction-induced damage leads to a continuous muscle breakdown and regeneration, with an increased build-up of fatty and fibrotic tissue, followed by an eventual loss of muscle contractility.

Appendix 3: The reading-frame concept

A reading frame consists out of codons—three nucleotide-based sequences—which translate into a specific amino acid. A shift of the reading frame basically means that the reading frame is altered, for example by a deletion of nucleotides. If the genetic code is extended or shortened by a multitude of "3 nucleotides", the reading frame is sustained. Therefore, this is called an "in-frame shift" resulting in a partially functional protein, which corresponds to BMD. When genetic alteration occurs by a multiplication of "1–2 nucleotides", the reading-frame shifts, leading to post-translational disintegration of DYSTROPHIN; hence, this is called an "out-of-frame shift" and corresponds to DMD.

Acknowledgements

We would like to apologize to all authors whose work has not been reported here due to space limitations. This work has been supported with the contribution of "Opening The Future" Campaign [EJJ-OPTFUT-02010] CARIPLO 2015_0634, FWO (#G088715N, #G060612N, #G0A8813N), GOA (EJJ-C2161-GOA/11/012), IUAP-VII/07 (EJJ-C4851-17/07-P) and OT#09-053 (EJJ-C0420-OT/09/053) grants. We thank Christina Vochten and Vicky Raets for professional administrative assistance. We would also like to thank Rondoufonds voor Duchenne Onderzoek for kind donations.

Author details

Jordi Camps[1], Enrico Pozzo[1,2], Tristan Pulinckx[1], Robin Duelen[1] and Maurilio Sampaolesi[1,2*]

*Address all correspondence to: maurilio.sampaolesi@kuleuven.be

1 Translational Cardiomyology Lab, Stem Cell Biology and Embryology Unit, Department of Development and Regeneration, KU Leuven, Leuven, Belgium

2 Division of Human Anatomy, Department of Public Health, Experimental and Forensic Medicine, University of Pavia, Pavia, Italy

References

[1] Mendell JR, Shilling C, Leslie ND, Flanigan KM, al-Dahhak R, Gastier-Foster J, et al. Evidence-based path to newborn screening for duchenne muscular dystrophy. Ann. Neurol. 2012;71:304–13. DOI:10.1002/ana.23528

[2] Bushby KMD, Thambyayah M, Gardner-Medwin D. Prevalence and incidence of Becker muscular dystrophy. Lancet. 1991;337:1022–4. DOI:10.1016/0140-6736(91)92 671-N

[3] Nakamura A. X-linked dilated cardiomyopathy: a cardiospecific phenotype of dystro-phinopathy. Pharmaceuticals. 2015;8:303–20. DOI:10.3390/ph8020303

[4] Eagle M, Baudouin SV, Chandler C, Giddings DR, Bullock R, Bushby K. Survival in Duchenne muscular dystrophy: Improvements in life expectancy since 1967 and the impact of home nocturnal ventilation. Neuromuscul. Disord. 2002;12:926–9. DOI: 10.1016/S0960-8966(02)00140-2

[5] Bradley WG, Jones MZ, Mussini JM, Fawcett PR. Becker-type muscular dystrophy. Muscle Nerve. 1978;1:111–32. DOI:10.1002/mus.880010204

[6] Sarnat HB. Muscular dystrophies. In: Kliegman R, Stanton B, St. Geme J, editors. Nelson Textb. Pediatr. 19th ed. p. 2119–29. DOI:10.1016/B978-1-4377-0755-7.00601-1

[7] Ropper A, Sanuels MA. The muscular dystrophies. In: Ropper, AH, Samuels, MA, editors. Adams Victor's Princ. Neurol. 9th ed. p. 687–95. DOI:10.1055/s-0032-1329199

[8] Romfh A, McNally EM. Cardiac assessment in duchenne and becker muscular dystro-phies. Curr. Heart Fail. Rep. 2010;7:212–8. DOI:10.1007/s11897-010-0028-2

[9] Spurney CF. Cardiomyopathy of duchenne muscular dystrophy: Current understand-ing and future directions. Muscle Nerve. 2011;44:8–19. DOI:10.1002/mus.22097

[10] Connuck DM, Sleeper LA, Colan SD, Cox GF, Towbin JA, Lowe AM, et al. Character-istics and outcomes of cardiomyopathy in children with Duchenne or Becker muscular dystrophy: a comparative study from the Pediatric Cardiomyopathy Registry. Am. Heart J. 2008;155:998–1005. DOI:10.1016/j.ahj.2008.01.018

[11] Finsterer J, Cripe L. Treatment of dystrophin cardiomyopathies. Nat. Rev. Cardiol. 2014;11:168–79. DOI:10.1038/nrcardio.2013.213

[12] Ciafaloni E, Fox DJ, Pandya S, Westfield CP, Puzhankara S, Romitti PA, et al. Delayed diagnosis in Duchenne muscular dystrophy: data from the muscular dystrophy surveillance, tracking, and research network (MD STARnet). J. Pediatr. 2009;155:380–5. DOI:10.1016/j.jpeds.2009.02.007

[13] Zatz M, Rapaport D, Vainzof M, Passos-Bueno MR, Bortolini ER, Pavanello R de CM, et al. Serum creatine-kinase (CK) and pyruvate-kinase (PK) activities in Duchenne (DMD) as compared with Becker (BMD) muscular dystrophy. J. Neurol. Sci. 1991;102:190–6. DOI:10.1016/0022-510X(91)90068-I

[14] Bushby K, Finkel R, Birnkrant DJ, Case LE, Clemens PR, Cripe L, et al. Diagnosis and management of Duchenne muscular dystrophy, part 1: diagnosis, and pharmacological and psychosocial management. Lancet Neurol. 2010;9:77–93. DOI:10.1016/S1474-4 422(09)70271-6

[15] Monaco AP, Bertelson CJ, Liechti-Gallati S, Moser H, Kunkel LM. An explanation for the phenotypic differences between patients bearing partial deletions of the DMD locus. Genomics. 1988;2:90–5. DOI:10.1016/0888-7543(88)90113-9

[16] Dent KM, Dunn DM, Von Niederhausern AC, Aoyagi AT, Kerr L, Bromberg MB, et al. Improved molecular diagnosis of dystrophinopathies in an unselected clinical cohort. Am. J. Med. Genet. 2005;134:295–8. DOI:10.1002/ajmg.a.30617

[17] Spurney C, Shimizu R, Morgenroth LP, Kolski H, Gordish-Dressman H, Clemens PR. Cooperative international neuromuscular research group duchenne natural history study demonstrates insufficient diagnosis and treatment of cardiomyopathy in duchenne muscular dystrophy. Muscle Nerve. 2014;50:250–6. DOI:10.1002/mus.24163

[18] McNally EM, Kaltman JR, Benson DW, Canter CE, Cripe LH, Duan D, et al. Contemporary cardiac issues in Duchenne muscular dystrophy. Working Group of the National Heart, Lung, and Blood Institute in collaboration with parent project muscular dystrophy. Circulation. 2015;131:1590–8. DOI:10.1161/CIRCULATIONAHA.114.0151 51

[19] Thomas TO, Morgan TM, Burnette WB, Markham LW. Correlation of heart rate and cardiac dysfunction in Duchenne muscular dystrophy. Pediatr. Cardiol. 2012;33:1175–9. DOI:10.1007/s00246-012-0281-0

[20] Politano L, Nigro G. Treatment of dystrophinopathic cardiomyopathy: review of the literature and personal results. Acta. Myol. 2012;31:24–30. DOI:10.1016/S0960-896 6(00)00174-7

[21] Barber BJ, Andrews JG, Lu Z, West NA, Meaney FJ, Price ET, et al. Oral corticosteroids and onset of cardiomyopathy in Duchenne muscular dystrophy. J. Pediatr. 2013;163:1080–4.e1. DOI:10.1016/j.jpeds.2013.05.060

[22] Bauer R, Straub V, Blain A, Bushby K, MacGowan GA. Contrasting effects of steroids and angiotensin-converting-enzyme inhibitors in a mouse model of dystrophin-deficient cardiomyopathy. Eur. J. Heart. Fail. 2009;11:463–71. DOI:10.1093/eurjhf/hfp028

[23] Duboc D, Meune C, Lerebours G, Devaux JY, Vaksmann G, Bécane HM. Effect of perindopril on the onset and progression of left ventricular dysfunction in Duchenne muscular dystrophy. J. Am. Coll. Cardiol. 2005;45:855–7. DOI:10.1016/j.jacc.2004.09.078

[24] Duboc D, Meune C, Pierre B, Wahbi K, Eymard B, Toutain A, et al. Perindopril preventive treatment on mortality in Duchenne muscular dystrophy: 10 years' follow up. Am. Heart J. 2007;154:596–602. DOI:10.1016/j.ahj.2007.05.014.

[25] Kamdar F, Garry DJ. Dystrophin-deficient cardiomyopathy. J. Am. Coll. Cardiol. 2016;67:2533–46. DOI:10.1016/j.jacc.2016.02.081

[26] Allen HD, Flanigan KM, Thrush PT, Dvorchik I, Yin H, Canter C, et al. A randomized, double-blind trial of lisinopril and losartan for the treatment of cardiomyopathy in Duchenne muscular dystrophy. PLoS. Curr. 2013;5. DOI:10.1371/currents.md. 2cc69a1dae4be7dfe2bcb420024ea865

[27] Kwon HW, Kwon BS, Kim GB, Chae JH, Park JD, Bae EJ, et al. The effect of enalapril and carvedilol on left ventricular dysfunction in middle childhood and adolescent

patients with muscular dystrophy. Korean Circ. J. 2012;42:184–91. DOI:10.4070/kcj. 2012.42.3.184

[28] Blain A, Greally E, Laval SH, Blamire AM, MacGowan GA, Straub VW. Absence of cardiac benefit with early combination ACE inhibitor and beta blocker treatment in mdx mice. J. Cardiovasc. Transl. Res. 2015;8:198–207. DOI:10.1007/s12265-015-9623-7

[29] Viollet L, Thrush PT, Flanigan KM, Mendell JR, Allen HD. Effects of angiotensin-converting enzyme inhibitors and/or beta blockers on the cardiomyopathy in Duchenne muscular dystrophy. Am. J. Cardiol. 2012;110:98–102. DOI:10.1016/j.amjcard.2012. 02.064

[30] Rafael-Fortney JA, Chimanji NS, Schill KE, Martin CD, Murray JD, Ganguly R, et al. Early treatment with lisinopril and spironolactone preserves cardiac and skeletal muscle in Duchenne muscular dystrophy mice. Circulation. 2011;124:582–8. DOI: 10.1161/CIRCULATIONAHA.111.031716

[31] Raman S V, Hor KN, Mazur W, Halnon NJ, Kissel JT, He X, et al. Eplerenone for early cardiomyopathy in Duchenne muscular dystrophy: a randomised, double-blind, placebo-controlled trial. Lancet. Neurol. 2015;14:153–61. DOI:10.1016/S1474-4422(14) 70318-7

[32] Wollinsky KH, Kutter B, Geiger PM. Long-term ventilation of patients with Duchenne muscular dystrophy: Experiences at the Neuromuscular Centre Ulm. Acta Myol. 2012;31:170–8.

[33] Bushby K, Finkel R, Birnkrant DJ, Case LE, Clemens PR, Cripe L, et al. Diagnosis and management of Duchenne muscular dystrophy, part 2: implementation of multidisciplinary care. Lancet. Neurol. 2010;9:177–89. DOI:10.1016/S1474-4422(09)70272-8

[34] Cripe LH, Tobias JD. Cardiac considerations in the operative management of the patient with Duchenne or Becker muscular dystrophy. Paediatr. Anaesth. 2013;23:777–84. DOI: 10.1111/pan.12229

[35] Tinsley JM, Blake DJ, Roche A, Fairbrother U, Riss J, Byth BC, et al. Primary structure of dystrophin-related protein. Nature. 1992;360:591–3. DOI:10.1038/360591a0

[36] Deconinck AE, Rafael JA, Skinner JA, Brown SC, Potter AC, Metzinger L, et al. Utrophin-dystrophin-deficient mice as a model for Duchenne muscular dystrophy. Cell. 1997;90:717–27. DOI:10.1016/S0092-8674(00)80532-2

[37] Tinsley JM, Fairclough RJ, Storer R, Wilkes FJ, Potter AC, Squire SE, et al. Daily treatment with SMTC1100, a novel small molecule utrophin upregulator, dramatically reduces the dystrophic symptoms in the mdx mouse. PLoS One. 2011;6:e19189. DOI: 10.1371/journal.pone.0019189

[38] Ricotti V, Spinty S, Roper H, Hughes I, Tejura B, Robinson N, et al. Safety, tolerability, and pharmacokinetics of SMT C1100, a 2-arylbenzoxazole utrophin modulator, following single- and multiple-dose administration to pediatric patients with Duch

enne muscular dystrophy. PLoS One. 2016;11:e0152840. DOI:10.1371/journal.pone. 0152840

[39] Finkel RS. Read-through strategies for suppression of nonsense mutations in Duchenne/Becker muscular dystrophy: aminoglycosides and ataluren (PTC124). J. Child Neurol. 2-010;25:1158–64. DOI:10.1177/0883073810371129

[40] Malik V, Rodino-Klapac LR, Viollet L, Wall C, King W, Al-Dahhak R, et al. Gentamicin-induced readthrough of stop codons in Duchenne muscular dystrophy. Ann. Neurol. 2010;67:771–80. DOI:10.1002/ana.22024

[41] Welch EM, Barton ER, Zhuo J, Tomizawa Y, Friesen WJ, Trifillis P, et al. PTC124 targets genetic disorders caused by nonsense mutations. Nature. 2007;447:87–91. DOI: 10.1038/nature05756

[42] Hirawat S, Welch EM, Elfring GL, Northcutt VJ, Paushkin S, Hwang S, et al. Safety, tolerability, and pharmacokinetics of PTC124, a nonaminoglycoside nonsense mutation suppressor, following single- and multiple-dose administration to healthy male and female adult volunteers. J. Clin. Pharmacol. 2007;47:430–44. DOI:10.1177/00912700 06297140

[43] Finkel RS, Flanigan KM, Wong B, Bönnemann C, Sampson J, Sweeney HL, et al. Phase 2a study of ataluren-mediated dystrophin production in patients with nonsense mutation Duchenne muscular dystrophy. Sawada H, editor. PLoS One. 2013;8:e81302. DOI:10.1371/journal.pone.0081302

[44] Bushby K, Finkel R, Wong B, Barohn R, Campbell C, Comi GP, et al. Ataluren treatment of patients with nonsense mutation dystrophinopathy. Muscle Nerve. 2014;50:477–87. DOI:10.1002/mus.24332

[45] Kayali R, Ku JM, Khitrov G, Jung ME, Prikhodko O, Bertoni C. Read-through compound 13 restores dystrophin expression and improves muscle function in the mdx mouse model for Duchenne muscular dystrophy. Hum. Mol. Genet. 2012;21:4007–20. DOI:10.1093/hmg/dds223

[46] Hoffman EP, Fischbeck KH, Brown RH, Johnson M, Medori R, Loike JD, et al. Characterization of dystrophin in muscle-biopsy specimens from patients with Duchenne's or Becker's muscular dystrophy. N. Engl. J. Med. 1988;318:1363–8. DOI:10.1056/ NEJM198805263182104

[47] Wilton SD, Lloyd F, Carville K, Fletcher S, Honeyman K, Agrawal S, et al. Specific removal of the nonsense mutation from the mdx dystrophin mRNA using antisense oligonucleotides. Neuromuscul. Disord. 1999;9:330–8. DOI:10.1016/S0960-8966(99)0 0010-3

[48] Cartegni L, Chew SL, Krainer AR. Listening to silence and understanding nonsense: exonic mutations that affect splicing. Nat. Rev. Genet. 2002;3:285–98. DOI:10.1038/ nrg775

[49] Aartsma-Rus A, Fokkema I, Verschuuren J, Ginjaar I, van Deutekom J, van Ommen GJ, et al. Theoretic applicability of antisense-mediated exon skipping for Duchenne muscular dystrophy mutations. Hum. Mutat. 2009;30:293–9. DOI:10.1002/humu.20918

[50] Mendell JR, Goemans N, Lowes LP, Alfano LN, Berry K, Shao J, et al. Longitudinal effect of eteplirsen versus historical control on ambulation in Duchenne muscular dystrophy. Ann. Neurol. 2016;79:257–71. DOI:10.1002/ana.24555

[51] Voit T, Topaloglu H, Straub V, Muntoni F, Deconinck N, Campion G, et al. Safety and efficacy of drisapersen for the treatment of Duchenne muscular dystrophy (DEMAND II): an exploratory, randomised, placebo-controlled phase 2 study. Lancet. Neurol. 2014;13:987–96. DOI:10.1016/S1474-4422(14)70195-4

[52] Malerba A, Thorogood FC, Dickson G, Graham IR. Dosing regimen has a significant impact on the efficiency of morpholino oligomer-induced exon skipping in mdx mice. Hum. Gene Ther. 2009;20:955–65. DOI:10.1089/hum.2008.157

[53] Malerba A, Boldrin L, Dickson G. Long-term systemic administration of unconjugated morpholino oligomers for therapeutic expression of dystrophin by exon skipping in skeletal muscle: implications for cardiac muscle integrity. Nucleic Acid Ther. 2011;21:293–8. DOI:10.1089/nat.2011.0306

[54] Goyenvalle A, Griffith G, Babbs A, El Andaloussi S, Ezzat K, Avril A, et al. Functional correction in mouse models of muscular dystrophy using exon-skipping tricyclo-DNA oligomers. Nat. Med. 2015;21:270–5. DOI:10.1038/nm.3765

[55] Betts C, Saleh AF, Arzumanov AA, Hammond SM, Godfrey C, Coursindel T, et al. Pip6-PMO, A new generation of peptide-oligonucleotide conjugates with improved cardiac exon skipping activity for DMD treatment. Mol. Ther. Nucleic Acids. 2012;1:e38. DOI: 10.1038/mtna.2012.30

[56] Wu B, Moulton HM, Iversen PL, Jiang J, Li J, Li J, et al. Effective rescue of dystrophin improves cardiac function in dystrophin-deficient mice by a modified morpholino oligomer. Proc. Natl. Acad. Sci. 2008;105:14814–9. DOI:10.1073/pnas.0805676105

[57] Yin H, Moulton HM, Seow Y, Boyd C, Boutilier J, Iverson P, et al. Cell-penetrating peptide-conjugated antisense oligonucleotides restore systemic muscle and cardiac dystrophin expression and function. Hum. Mol. Genet. 2008;17:3909–18. DOI:10.1093/hmg/ddn293

[58] Betts CA, Saleh AF, Carr CA, Hammond SM, Coenen-Stass AML, Godfrey C, et al. Prevention of exercised induced cardiomyopathy following Pip-PMO treatment in dystrophic mdx mice. Sci. Rep. 2015;5:8986. DOI:10.1038/srep08986

[59] Jirka SMG, Heemskerk H, Tanganyika-de Winter CL, Muilwijk D, Pang KH, de Visser PC, et al. Peptide Conjugation of 2'-O-methyl phosphorothioate antisense oligonucleotides enhances cardiac uptake and exon skipping in mdx mice. Nucleic Acid Ther. 2014;24:25–36. DOI:10.1089/nat.2013.0448

[60] Scott JM, Li S, Harper SQ, Welikson R, Bourque D, DelloRusso C, et al. Viral vectors for gene transfer of micro-, mini-, or full-length dystrophin. Neuromuscul. Disord. 2002;12:S23–9. DOI:10.1016/S0960-8966(02)00078-0

[61] Bish LT, Sleeper MM, Forbes SC, Wang B, Reynolds C, Singletary GE, et al. Long-term restoration of cardiac dystrophin expression in golden retriever muscular dystrophy following rAAV6-mediated exon skipping. Mol. Ther. 2012;20:580–9. DOI:10.1038/mt.2011.264

[62] Le Guiner C, Montus M, Servais L, Cherel Y, Francois V, Thibaud J-L, et al. Forelimb treatment in a large cohort of dystrophic dogs supports delivery of a recombinant AAV for exon skipping in Duchenne patients. Mol. Ther. 2014;22:1923–35. DOI:10.1038/mt.2014.151

[63] Long C, Amoasii L, Mireault AA, McAnally JR, Li H, Sanchez-Ortiz E, et al. Postnatal genome editing partially restores dystrophin expression in a mouse model of muscular dystrophy. Science. 2015;351:400–3. DOI:10.1126/science.aad5725

[64] England SB, Nicholson L V, Johnson MA, Forrest SM, Love DR, Zubrzycka-Gaarn EE, et al. Very mild muscular dystrophy associated with the deletion of 46% of dystrophin. Nature. 1990;343:180–2. DOI:10.1038/343180a0

[65] Koenig M, Beggs AH, Moyer M, Scherpf S, Heindrich K, Bettecken T, et al. The molecular basis for Duchenne versus Becker muscular dystrophy: correlation of severity with type of deletion. Am. J. Hum. Genet. 1989;45:498–506.

[66] Gregorevic P, Allen JM, Minami E, Blankinship MJ, Haraguchi M, Meuse L, et al. rAAV6-microdystrophin preserves muscle function and extends lifespan in severely dystrophic mice. Nat. Med. 2006;12:787–9. DOI:10.1038/nm1439

[67] Bostick B, Shin JH, Yue Y, Duan D. AAV-microdystrophin therapy improves cardiac performance in aged female mdx mice. Mol. Ther. 2011;19:1826–32. DOI:10.1038/mt.2011.154

[68] Kornegay JN, Li J, Bogan JR, Bogan DJ, Chen C, Zheng H, et al. Widespread muscle expression of an AAV9 human mini-dystrophin vector after intravenous injection in neonatal dystrophin-deficient dogs. Mol. Ther. 2010;18:1501–8. DOI:10.1038/mt.2010.94

[69] Bowles DE, McPhee SWJ, Li C, Gray SJ, Samulski JJ, Camp AS, et al. Phase 1 gene therapy for Duchenne muscular dystrophy using a translational optimized AAV vector. Mol. Ther. 2012;20:443–55. DOI:10.1038/mt.2011.237

[70] Mendell JR, Rodino-Klapac L, Sahenk Z, Malik V, Kaspar BK, Walker CM, et al. Gene therapy for muscular dystrophy: lessons learned and path forward. Neurosci. Lett. 2012;527:90–9. DOI:10.1016/j.neulet.2012.04.078

[71] Hayashita-Kinoh H, Yugeta N, Okada H, Nitahara-Kasahara Y, Chiyo T, Okada T, et al. Intra-amniotic rAAV-mediated microdystrophin gene transfer improves canine X-

linked muscular dystrophy and may induce immune tolerance. Mol. Ther. 2015;23:627–37. DOI:10.1038/mt.2015.5

[72] Foster H, Sharp PS, Athanasopoulos T, Trollet C, Graham IR, Foster K, et al. Codon and mRNA sequence optimization of microdystrophin transgenes improves expression and physiological outcome in dystrophic mdx mice following AAV2/8 gene transfer. Mol. Ther. 2008;16:1825–32. DOI:10.1038/mt.2008.186

[73] Chicoine L, Montgomery C, Bremer W, Shontz K, Griffin D, Heller K, et al. Plasmaphe-resis eliminates the negative impact of AAV antibodies on microdystrophin gene expression following vascular delivery. Mol. Ther. 2014;22:338–47. DOI:10.1038/mt.2013.244

[74] Koo T, Popplewell L, Athanasopoulos T, Dickson G. Triple trans-splicing adeno-associated virus vectors capable of transferring the coding sequence for full-length dystrophin protein into dystrophic mice. Hum. Gene Ther. 2014;25:98–108. DOI:10.1089/hum.2013.164

[75] Sampaolesi M, Blot S, D'Antona G, Granger N, Tonlorenzi R, Innocenzi A, et al. Mesoangioblast stem cells ameliorate muscle function in dystrophic dogs. Nature. 2006;444:574–9. DOI:10.1038/nature05282

[76] Chun JL, O'Brien R, Song MH, Wondrasch BF, Berry SE. Injection of vessel-derived stem cells prevents dilated cardiomyopathy and promotes angiogenesis and endogenous cardiac stem cell proliferation in mdx/utrn$^{-/-}$ but not aged mdx mouse models for duchenne muscular dystrophy. Stem. Cells. Transl. Med. 2013;2:68–80. DOI:10.5966/sctm.2012-0107

[77] Cossu G, Previtali SC, Napolitano S, Cicalese MP, Tedesco FS, Nicastro F, et al. Intra-arterial transplantation of HLA-matched donor mesoangioblasts in Duchenne muscu-lar dystrophy. EMBO Mol. Med. 2015;7:1513–28. DOI:10.15252/emmm.201505636

[78] Quattrocelli M, Swinnen M, Giacomazzi G, Camps J, Barthélemy I, Ceccarelli G, et al. Mesodermal iPSC-derived progenitor cells functionally regenerate cardiac and skeletal muscle. J. Clin. Invest. 2015;125:4463–82. DOI:10.1172/JCI82735

[79] Young CS, Hicks MR, Ermolova N V, Nakano H, Jan M, Younesi S, et al. A single CRISPR-Cas9 deletion strategy that targets the majority of DMD patients restores dystrophin function in hiPSC-derived muscle cells. Cell. Stem. Cell. 2016;18:533–40. DOI:10.1016/j.stem.2016.01.021

[80] Holvoet B, Quattrocelli M, Belderbos S, Pollaris L, Wolfs E, Gheysens O, et al. Sodium iodide symporter PET and BLI noninvasively reveal mesoangioblast survival in dystrophic mice. Stem. Cell. Rep. 2015;5:1183–95. DOI:10.1016/j.stemcr.2015.10.018

[81] Petrof BJ. Molecular pathophysiology of myofiber injury in deficiencies of the dystro-phin-glycoprotein complex. Am. J. Phys. Med. Rehabil. 2002;81:S162–74. DOI:10.1097/01.PHM.0000029775.54830.80

[82] van Westering TLE, Betts CA, Wood MJA. Current understanding of molecular pathology and treatment of cardiomyopathy in duchenne muscular dystrophy. Molecules. 2015;20:8823–55. DOI:10.3390/molecules20058823

[83] Hoffman EP, Reeves E, Damsker J, Nagaraju K, McCall JM, Connor EM, et al. Novel approaches to corticosteroid treatment in Duchenne muscular dystrophy. Phys. Med. Rehabil. Clin. N. Am. 2012;23:821–8. DOI:10.1016/j.pmr.2012.08.003

[84] Hunt SA. ACC/AHA 2005 Guideline update for the diagnosis and management of chronic heart failure in the adult: a report of the American College of Cardiology/ American Heart Association Task Force on Practice Guidelines (Writing Committee to Update the 2001 Guideli. Circulation. 2005;112:e154–235. DOI:10.1161/CIRCULATIO-NAHA.105.167586

[85] Geller G, Harrison KL, Rushton CH. Ethical challenges in the care of children and families affected by life-limiting neuromuscular diseases. J. Dev. Behav. Pediatr. 2012;33:548–61. DOI:10.1097/DBP.0b013e318267c62d

[86] Finder JD, Birnkrant D, Carl J, Farber HJ, Gozal D, Iannaccone ST, et al. Respiratory care of the patient with Duchenne muscular dystrophy. Am. J. Respir. Crit. Care. Med. 2004;170:456–65. DOI:10.1164/rccm.200307-885ST

[87] Vianello S, Yu H, Voisin V, Haddad H, He X, Foutz AS, et al. Arginine butyrate: A therapeutic candidate for Duchenne muscular dystrophy. FASEB J. 2013;27:2256–69. DOI:10.1096/fj.12-215723

[88] Mendell JR, Rodino-Klapac LR, Sahenk Z, Roush K, Bird L, Lowes LP, et al. Eteplirsen for the treatment of Duchenne muscular dystrophy. Ann. Neurol. 2013;74:637–47. DOI: 10.1002/ana.23982

[89] Bostick B, Yue Y, Lai Y, Long C, Li D, Duan D. Adeno-associated virus serotype-9 microdystrophin gene therapy ameliorates electrocardiographic abnormalities in mdx mice. Hum. Gene. Ther. 2008;19:851–6. DOI:10.1089/hum.2008.058.

3

Cardiomyopathies in Animals

Kazumasu Sasaki, Tatsushi Mutoh, Kinji Shirota and

Ryuta Kawashima

Abstract

A wide variety of animal models in cardiomyopathy have been established for the discovery of pathophysiological mechanisms, diagnosis, and treatment of human myocardial disease. Experimentally, several species including rodents, rabbit, canine, pig, and sheep have been involved in the fundamental research in medical field. However, knowledge about naturally occurring myocardial disease in animals is limited in the veterinary medicine. Among small and large animals that develop myocardial disease, to the best of authors' knowledge, naturally occurring cardiomyopathy in canine and feline is commonly encountered in veterinary clinical setting. Their pathophysiology is not fully described; specific pathophysiology is documented in both species, which resembles those of humans. These conditions are hypertrophic cardiomyopathy (HCM) in feline and dilated cardiomyopathy (DCM) in canine. Each has distinct etiology and pathophysiology. In order to translate new findings from naturally occurring cardiomyopathies in small and large animals into medical applications, knowledge gained through animals with cardiomyopathies becomes a necessary approach. The purpose of this chapter is to introduce the overview of findings on small and large animals with naturally occurring cardiomyopathies already investigated.

Keywords: animal model, canine dilated cardiomyopathy, feline hypertrophic cardiomyopathy, naturally occurring cardiomyopathies

1. Introduction

Several animal models in cardiomyopathy have been established for the discovery of pathophysiological mechanisms, diagnosis, and treatment of human myocardial disease. Experimentally, rodents, rabbit, canine, pig, sheep, and other species have been involved in the fundamental research in medical field [1–7]. Although anatomic and biochemical differences between species are critical, each experimentally induced animal model plays an important role for translation to clinical practice in human. In addition to experimentally induced animal models, naturally occurring cardiomyopathies in small and large animals offer an excellent opportunity to evaluate novel therapies for those of human. However, knowledge about naturally occurring myocardial disease in animals is limited in the veterinary medicine. Among animals that develop myocardial disease, to the best of authors' knowledge, cardiomyopathy in canine and feline is commonly encountered in veterinary clinical setting [8–12]. Their pathophysiology is not always clearly described yet; however, specific features are documented in both canine and feline. Briefly, naturally occurring myocardial disease is one of the most common heart diseases in canine and feline. A number of remarkable similarities have been reported between these animals and humans [13, 14]. Several causes concerning genetic, metabolic, inflammatory, nutritional, infectious, and drug-induced myocardial disease have been reported as canine and feline idiopathic or secondary myocardial disease [15, 16]. Generally speaking, treatment strategy of these naturally occurring diseases in veterinary clinical setting is based on those of humans. Therefore, this chapter provides pathophysiological aspects of these diseases.

Dilated cardiomyopathy (DCM) was first reported in 1970, as congestive heart failure (CHF). It is characterized by chamber dilation and myocardial systolic and diastolic dysfunction. DCM appears to be common in canine, which has been suspected to be inherited defects and mainly affects the certain large- to giant-sized pure-bred such as English Cocker Spaniels, Doberman Pinschers, Irish Wolfhounds, Newfoundlands, Boxers, German Short-haired Pointers, Portuguese Water Dog, Airedale Terriers, St. Bernards, Standard Poodles, Scottish Deerhounds, Afghan Hounds, and other breeds [8, 15–17]. Myocardial dysfunction results from ischemia, tachycardia, and trauma in canine myocardial disease. An underlying disease associated with neoplasia, renal disease, immune-mediated hemolytic anemia, acute pancreatitis, disseminated intravascular coagulopathy (DIC), myocardial infarction, mitral insufficiency, and other disease results in ischemic myocardial disease. Atrioventricular nodal-reciprocating tachycardias can lead to the tachycardia-induced cardiomyopathy in several breeds. However, hypertrophic cardiomyopathy (HCM) occurs less often in canine [15–17].

On the other hand, HCM is being the most commonly diagnosed cardiomyopathy in feline [10, 18, 19]. It is prevalent in certain populations. The disease is known to be inherited in some breeds, most notably The Domestic Shorthair, Turkish Van, Maine Coon, Persian, Ragdoll, Sphynx, Scottish Fold Cats, Chartreux, British Shorthair, Norwegian Forest Cat, Persian, and other breeds [14–16, 18]. The pathogenic mechanisms responsible for the development of HCM remain unclear; however, causal genetic mutations in genes encoding the sarcomere protein myosin-binding protein C (MYBPC3) have been identified in specific breeds such as Maine Coons and Ragdolls [14, 19–21].

Limited information exists on naturally occurring cardiomyopathies in large animals such as swine, cattle, and other species. Generally, these large animals are classified as farm animals and treated under group control. Compared with small animal veterinary practice, which mainly treats canine and feline, large animals are not potentially therapeutic objectives. From this circumstance, few opportunities exist for veterinarian to treat the disease. Even though numerous anatomic and biochemical differences exist, naturally occurring disease in large animal species can provide significant advantages for understanding those human conditions.

2. Canine DCM

2.1. Etiology and pathogenesis

The canine DCM can be divided into two categories: idiopathic and secondary (**Table 1**). The exact underlying molecular and biochemical mechanisms for canine DCM are generally not established in all cases. However, the etiology concerning genetic, nutritional, infectious, metabolic, inflammatory, drug- or toxin-induced myocardial hypokinesis have been proposed in canine DCM [17]. In idiopathic cases, genetic basis is thought to exist especially in certain breeds with high prevalence or familial occurrence of disease [15–17]. Large and giant breeds such as Great Danes, Scottish Deerhounds, Boxers, St. Bernards, Newfoundlands, Dalmatians, Doberman Pinschers, Irish Wolfhounds, and other breeds have been documented [8, 15, 16]. Newfoundlands, Irish Wolfhounds, Boxers, and Doberman Pinschers appear to have an autosomal dominant mode of transmission pattern of inheritance [8, 22, 23]. An autosomal recessive transmission has been documented in the inherited form of DCM in juvenile Portuguese Water Dogs [24, 25]. The disease is rapidly progressive and fatal in puppies. In some German Short-haired Pointer littermates, DCM appears to be an X-linked disorder caused by mutations in the Duchenne muscular dystrophy (DMD) gene [8, 26]. This gene codes for dystrophin, which is thought to strengthen muscle fiber membranes.

Myocardial function can impair result from a variety of causes including infections, inflammation, nutritional deficiencies, metabolic abnormalities, certain drugs, and other factors. These factors can lead to canine secondary myocardial disease. The antineoplastic drug doxorubicin and ethyl alcohol can cause severe myocardial damage and death. Plant toxins (e.g., *Taxus*, foxglove, black locust, buttercup, gossypol), cocaine, cobalt, catecholamines, and anesthetic drug can also affect the myocardial function [8, 15–17]. Carnitine and taurine deficiencies have been described in canine DCM [8]. L-Carnitine deficiency is not a primary cause of canine DCM; however, in Boxers, Doberman Pinschers, American Cocker Spaniels, Irish Wolfhounds, Newfoundlands, and Great Danes, low myocardial L-carnitine concentration has been reported [15]. L-Carnitine is an essential component of the long-chain fatty acids, which is an important energy-producing substrate of the myocardium. Taurine is known to regulate calcium influx across membranes in heart muscle. However, most cases with canine DCM are not taurine deficient; a reversible canine DCM associated with low plasma taurine concentration was reported in Cocker Spaniels [27]. Low plasma taurine level has also been described in Golden Retrievers, Labrador Retrievers, St. Bernards, Dalmatians, and other breeds with DCM.

Etiology/pathogenesis	Breed	References
Idiopathic DCM		
Genetic disorder		
Dystrophin	German Short-haired Pointers	Schatzberg et al. [47]
Desmin	Doberman Pinschers	Stabej et al. [48]
Titin-cup	Irish Wolfhounds	Philipp et al. [49]
α-actinin	Doberman Pinschers	O'Sullivan et al. [50]
Striatin	Boxers	Cattanach et al. [51]
Secondary DCM		
Nutritional disorder		
L-Carnitine	Doberman Pinschers, Boxers	Keene et al. [52]
	American Cocker Spaniels	Kittleson et al. [53]
Metabolic disorder		
Thyroid hormone	Great Dane	Phillips and Harkin [54]
	Alaskan Malamute	Flood and Hoover [55]
	Doberman Pinschers	Beier et al. [56]
Immunological disorder		
Anti-mitochondrial antibodies	English Cocker Spaniel	Day [57]
Canine adenovirus type 1	Crossed breed	Maxson et al. [58]

Table 1. Possible factors of naturally occurring canine DCM.

2.2. Pathophysiology

Dilation of all cardiac chambers is typical in canine DCM [8, 15, 16, 28]. Decreased ventricular contractility is the major functional defect. Compensatory mechanisms become activated as progressive cardiac chamber dilation and remodeling develop as cardiac output worsens. Development of higher end-diastolic pressure, venous congestion, and congestive heart failure occurs in response to increased diastolic stiffness. Valve insufficiency also occurs because of cardiac enlargement and papillary muscle dysfunction. Arterial fibrillation (AF) is typical in canine DCM [15].

2.3. Histologic description

Gross anatomically, canine idiopathic DCM reveals marked dilation of all four cardiac chambers and/or predominantly dilation of the left chambers [8, 29–31]. Generally, myocardial hypertrophy is evident in the lesion. Distinct two histological forms of canine DCM have been reported: the fatty infiltration-degenerative type observed in specific breeds such as Boxers and Doberman Pinschers, and the attenuated wavy fiber type reported in medium-, large-, and giant-sized breed (**Table 2**). Histological forms such as vacuolar degeneration of myofibers, atrophic myofibers, lipid deposits, and fatty infiltration replacing myofibers are evident for the fatty infiltration-degenerative type. On the other hand, the attenuated wavy fiber type seems to be a major histological form of canine DCM. The myofibers are stretched and thinner than normal with wavy appearance. The morphological alterations including myofiber atrophy, impairing wavy appearance to the fibers, and diffuse infiltration of subendocardial fibrosis were reported [8]. These lesions were most abundant in the lateral wall of the left ventricle (LV) [32, 33].

References	Breed
Fatty infiltration-degenerative type	
Calvert et al. [59]	Doberman Pinschers
Harpster et al. [34]	Boxers
Hazlet et al. [60]	Doberman Pinschers
Tidholm and Jünsson [61]	Newfoundland
Calvert et al. [62]	Doberman Pinschers
Dambach et al. [25]	Portuguese Water Dogs
Everett et al. [63]	Doberman Pinschers
Vollmar et al. [64]	Doberman Pinschers
Lobo et al. [65]	Estrela Mountain Dogs
Attenuated wavy fiber type	
Tilley and Liu [66]	Great Dane, Doberman Pinschers, Irish Wolfhound
Sandusky et al. [67]	Afghan Hound, Doberman Pinschers, Great Dane
Tidholm et al. [33]	Large- and medium-size breeds
Dambach et al. [25]	Portuguese Water Dogs
Tidholm et al. [32]	Newfoundlands
Alroy et al. [68]	Portuguese Water Dogs
Vollmar et al. [69]	Doberman Pinschers
Sleeper et al. [24]	Portuguese Water Dogs

Table 2. Two distinct histological forms of canine idiopathic DCM.

2.4. Survival and prognosis

Prognosis in canine DCM varies from weeks to several years. Sudden death may occur before the development of disease. Survival rate of Doberman Pinschers with fatty infiltration-degenerative type of DCM is shorter than attenuated wavy fiber type of those with DCM [8].

3. Cardiomyopathy in Boxers

Inherited cardiomyopathy in Boxers has similar features to arrhythmogenic right ventricular cardiomyopathy (ARVC) [15, 23]. Three forms were originally described by Harpster in 1983 including the cases with asymptomatic arrhythmias, ventricular tachyarrhythmias, cardiac arrhythmias, and congestive heart failure [34]. The disease appears to have an autosomal dominant inherited pattern. The Boxers with cardiac arrhythmias and congestive heart failure is considered to be a form of canine DCM, which is characterized by left and right ventricular myocardial systolic dysfunction [15, 23]. Histologic form of the disease includes myofibers atrophy, fibrosis, and fatty infiltration in the right ventricular wall. Deletion in the desmosomal striatin gene is associated with the disease developed in Boxer with ARVC [23]. The prognosis is varied in the forms of disease but survival is less than 6 months in case of CHF. Sudden death is common in asymptomatic cases.

4. Feline HCM

4.1. Etiology and pathogenesis

Recent report suggested that feline cardiomyopathy may be classified as HCM, hypertrophic obstructive cardiomyopathy (HOCM), restrictive cardiomyopathy (RCM), dilated cardiomyopathy, arrhythmogenic right ventricular cardiomyopathy, and unclassified cardiomyopathy (UCM) based on echocardiography and other factors [12]. However, diagnosis is quite challenging because of complexity of the disease. Feline idiopathic HCM is the most commonly diagnosed heterogeneous disease, which is transmitted in autosomal dominant trait in some specific breeds [15]. The disease is more frequent in male than in female. Genetic mutations in gene encoding in sarcomere protein myosin-binding protein C (MYBPC3) is associated with the development of disease in Manine Coon Cats (A31P mutation) and Ragdoll Cats (R820W mutation) [18]. Other breeds including Domestic Short Hair, Norwegian Forest Cats, Sphinx, Bengals, Chartreux, British Shorthairs, European, Scottish Folds, Cornish Rex, and Persian breeds are also high in disease prevalence but causative mutations associated with disease have yet to be documented [11, 15, 16]. In addition to specific gene mutation, feline myocardial hypertrophy results from possible causes such as an excessive production of catecholamines, myocardial ischemia, fibrosis, primary collagen abnormality, and abnormalities in myocardial calcium-handling process [15].

4.2. Pathophysiology

The disease is characterized by papillary muscle and LV hypertrophy, systolic anterior motion (SAM) of the mitral valve, diastolic dysfunction, end-systolic cavity obliteration, and enlargement of the left atrium [14, 35]. Abnormal sarcomere function results from myocyte hypertrophy and increased collagen synthesis. Asymmetric or symmetric LV free-wall concentric hypertrophy with interventricular septum is the characteristic form of the disease [36]. Some have limited abnormality in the basal septum and/or papillary muscles. These different patterns of hypertrophy may be caused by different phenotypic expression between different breeds.

Myocardial hypertrophy and reduced ventricular distensibility result in increased diastolic pressure and LV filling accompanying increased left arterial (LA) and pulmonary venous pressure. Secondary right-sided congenital heart failure (CHF) may occur in response to prolonged pulmonary vasoconstriction and increased pulmonary arterial pressure. LV outflow obstruction accompanying ejection murmur results from LV papillary muscle hypertrophy. Several factors contribute to myocardial ischemia, which leads to fibrosis, arrhythmias, and other complications. CHF, arterial thromboembolism (ATE), and sudden cardiac death are common clinical manifestation in end-stage feline HCM [15].

4.3. Histologic description

Gross anatomy is characterized by moderate to severe papillary muscle and LV concentric hypertrophy (**Figure 1**). Histologic findings based on hematoxylin and eosin (HE) staining and other specific markers revealed several abnormalities including multifocal myocardial interstitial fibrosis, myofiber disarray, diffuse myocyte hypertrophy with or without scattered individual cell necrosis, and arteriosclerosis in papillary muscles in the LV wall, interventricular septum, and intramural coronary artery [10, 37]. Recent evidence showed remodeling of the myofibrils and interfibrillar mitochondria, sarcolemmal remodeling with depletion of the subsarcolemmal mitochondria, changes of Z-disc morphology, myofibrillar degeneration, and endomysial fibrosis based on electron microscopic examination [10].

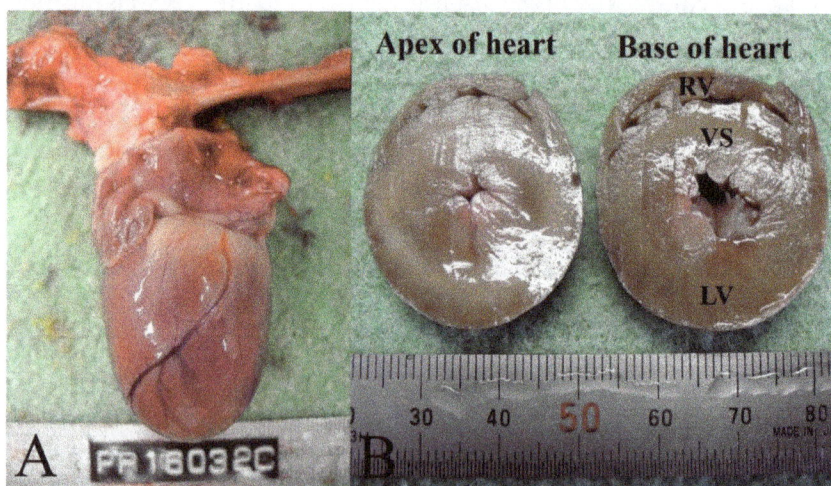

Figure 1. Gross morphologic features of heart from feline with HCM. (A) Overview of the heart from feline HCM. (B) Hypertrophy of ventricular septum (VS) in relation to left ventricular (LV) free wall. RV = right ventricle. Images courtesy of Prof. Kinji Shirota.

4.4. Survival and prognosis

Some prognostic factors such as heart rate and LA size are associated with survival time [12]. The prognosis is worse in case with ATE and/or CHF. Restrictive cardiomyopathy may be a consequence of the end stage of myocardial failure and infarction caused by HCM. Several factors cause a secondary RCM including tumor and infectious disease that were documented [15]. The prognosis is poor for feline with RCM accompanied by heart failure.

5. Other species

5.1. Swine

Experimentally induced porcine model of cardiomyopathy is widely used for medical applications [2, 38]. On the other hand, we have limited knowledge about naturally occurring swine cardiomyopathies. To date, naturally occurring porcine HCM and DCM have been described [39–41]. In addition to experimentally induced animal models, characteristics of naturally occurring affected pigs would be useful for translational research.

Several findings from swine HCM resemble those of humans with HCM. Higher incidence of specific breeds such as Landrace, Yorkshire, and Duroc were reported [39]. Pathological findings including increased number of mitochondria contained in the LV, increased amount of collagen matrix and abnormality in intramural coronary arteries, alternation of endogenous antioxidant enzymes, and decreased Ca^{2+}-ATPase activity in the LV are identical to those found in humans [39]. Histological abnormalities in swine HCM including abnormal intramural coronary arteries, subendocardial fibrosis in the ventricular septum, myocardial fibrosis, abnormalities in matrix connective tissue in myocardium, increased perimysial coil, and weave fibers of matrix connective tissue space between myocytes were documented [41, 42].

Recently, the case of spontaneous DCM was recognized in Yorkshire-Landrace crossbred [40]. The postmortem investigation after sudden death of this case revealed marked dilated ventricles and thinned ventricular walls and interventricular septum. Characteristics of gross anatomy and histological findings including multifocal myofiber attenuation and loss of myofiber cross striations supported the diagnosis of swine DCM. Cardiac lesions observed in the reported case were consistent with DCM as recognized in other species.

5.2. Cattle

Few reports on cardiomyopathies in cattle were descried [43, 44]. Hereditary cardiomyopathy in cattle has been described in some breeds including Japanese Black Calves, Holstein-Friesian-Cattle, Simmental/Red and White Holstein crossbreds, and Polled Hereford Calves [44, 45]. Recently, evidence suggested that specific breeds appear to have an autosomal dominant mode of transmission pattern of inheritance [45]. However, limited information exists about pathophysiological features compared with those of canine and feline. Affected cattle had multifocal myocardial degeneration and necrosis under histological investigation [46].

6. Conclusion

Naturally occurring inherited canine DCM and feline HCM are well-recognized myocardial disease in veterinary clinical setting. Although anatomic and biochemical differences between species are critical, reported findings resemble those of human disease condition. Little is known about naturally occurring cardiomyopathies in large animals but evidence suggested that they also develop spontaneous myocardial disease, which resembles those of other species including human. Given the similarities of cardiomyopathies in both human and other species, the knowledge of naturally occurring myocardial disease in small and large animals may help expand the understanding of disease pathophysiology.

Acknowledgements

The authors gratefully acknowledge the financial support: Sendai Animal Care and Research Center Foundation of Japan.

Author details

Kazumasu Sasaki[1,2*], Tatsushi Mutoh[3,4], Kinji Shirota[5] and Ryuta Kawashima[6]

*Address all correspondence to: kazumasu.sasaki.d8@tohoku.ac.jp

1 Department of Functional Brain Imaging and Preclinical Evaluation, Institute of Development, Aging and Cancer, Tohoku University, Sendai, Japan

2 Sendai Animal Care and Research Center, Sendai, Japan

3 Department of Nuclear Medicine and Radiology, Institute of Development, Aging and Cancer, Tohoku University, Sendai, Japan

4 Department of Surgical Neurology, Research Institute for Brain and Blood Vessels-AKITA, Akita, Japan

5 Department of Veterinary Pathology, School of Veterinary Medicine, Azabu University, Kanagawa, Japan

6 Department of Functional Brain Imaging, Institute of Development, Aging and Cancer, Tohoku University, Sendai, Japan

References

[1] Sirasaka T, Miyagawa S, Fukushima S, et al. Skeletal myoblast cell sheet implantation ameliorates both systolic and diastolic cardiac performance in canine dilated cardiomyopathy model. *Transplantation*. 2016;100:295–302.

[2]   Lacroix D, Gluais P, Marquié C, et al. Repolarization abnormalities and their arrhythmogenic consequences in porcine tachycardia-induced cardiomyopathy. *Cardiovasc Res.* 2002;54:42–50.

[3]   Mittal A, Sharma R, Prasad R, et al. Role of cardiac TBX20 in dilated cardiomyopathy. *Mol Cell Biochem.* 2016;414:129–36.

[4]   Wilder T, Ryba DM, Wieczorek DF, et al. N-acetylcysteine *reverses* diastolic dysfunction and hypertrophy in familial hypertrophic cardiomyopathy. *Am J Physiol Heart Circ Physiol.* 2015;309:1720–1730.

[5]   Frey N, Franz WM, Gloeckner K, et al. Transgenic rat hearts expressing a human cardiac troponin T deletion reveal diastolic dysfunction and ventricular arrhythmias. *Cardiovascular Res.* 2000;47:254–264.

[6]   Sanbe A, James J, Tuzcu V, et al. Transgenic rabbit model for human troponin I-based hypertrophic cardiomyopathy. *Circulation.* 2005;111:2330–2338.

[7]   Geens JH, Trenson S, Rega FR, et al. Ovine models for chronic heart failure. *Int J Artif Organs.* 2009;32:496–506.

[8]   Tidholm A, Jünsson L. Histologic characterization of canine dilated cardiomyopathy *Vet Pathol.* 2005;42:1–8.

[9]   Martin MW, Stafford Johnson MJ, Strehlau G, et al. Canine *dilated* cardiomyopathy: a retrospective study of prognostic findings in 367 clinical cases. *J Small Anim Pract.* 2010;51:428–436.

[10] Christiansen LB, Prats C, Hyttel P, Koch J. Ultrastructural myocardial changes in seven cats with spontaneous hypertrophic cardiomyopathy. *J Vet Cardiol.* 2015;17: 220–232.

[11] Maron BJ, Fox PR. Hypertrophic cardiomyopathy in man and cats. *J Vet Cardiol.* 2015;17:6–9.

[12] Ferasin L. Feline myocardial disease 2: *diagnosis,* prognosis and clinical management. *J Feline Med Surg.* 2009;11:183–194.

[13] Simpson S, Edwards J, Ferguson-Mignan TF, et al. Genetics of human and canine dilated cardiomyopathy. *Int J Genomics.* 2015;2015:204823.

[14] Kitteleson MD, Meurs KM, Harris SP. The genetic basis of hypertrophic cardiomyopathy in cats and humans. *J Vet Cardiol.* 2015;17:53–73.

[15] Nelson RW, Couto CG., editors. Small animal internal medicine. St. Louis, MO: Elsevier Mosby; 2014.

[16] Tilley LP, Smith, Jr FWK, Oyama MA, Sleeper MM. Manual of canine and feline cardiology. St. Louis, MO: Saunders Elsevier; 2008.

[17] Tidholm A, Häggstrüm J, Borgarelli M, et al. Canine idiopathic dilated cardiomyopathy. Part I: aetiology, clinical characteristics, epidemiology and pathology. *Vet J*. 2001;162:92–107.

[18] Longeri M, Ferrari P, Knafelz P, et al. Myosin-binding protein C DNA variants in domestic cats (A31P, A74T, R820W) and their association with hypertrophic cardiomyopathy. *J Vet Intern Med*. 2013;27:275–285.

[19] Häggstrüm J, Luis Fuentes V, Wess G. Screening for hypertrophic cardiomyopathy in cats. *J Vet Cardiol*. 2015;17:134–149.

[20] Meurs KM, Norgard MM, Ederer MM, et al. A substitution mutation in the myosin binding protein C gene in ragdoll hypertrophic cardiomyopathy. *Genomics*. 2007;90:261–264.

[21] Meurs KM, Sanchez X, David RM, et al. A cardiac myosin binding protein C mutation in the Maine Coon cat with familial hypertrophic cardiomyopathy. *Hum Mol Genet*. 2005;14:3587–3593.

[22] Meurs KM, Fox PR, Norgard M, et al. A prospective genetic evaluation of familial dilated cardiomyopathy in the Doberman Pinscher. *J Vet Intern Med*. 2007;21:1016–1020.

[23] Meurs KM, Stern JA, Sisson DD, et al. Association of dilated cardiomyopathy with the striatin mutation genotype in boxer dogs. *J Vet Intern Med*. 2013;27:1437–1440.

[24] Sleeper MM, Henthorn PS, Vijayasarathy C, et al. Dilated cardiomyopathy in juvenile Portuguese Water Dogs. *J Vet Intern Med*. 2002;16:52–62.

[25] Dambach DM, Lannon A, Sleeper MM, et al. Familial dilated cardiomyopathy of young Portuguese water dogs. *J Vet Intern Med*. 1999;13:65–71.

[26] Towbin JA, Hejtmancik JF, Brink P, et al. X-linked dilated cardiomyopathy. Molecular genetic evidence of linkage to the Duchenne muscular dystrophy (dystrophin) gene at the Xp21 locus. *Circulation*. 1993;87:1854–1865.

[27] Gavaghan BJ, Kittleson MD. Dilated cardiomyopathy in an American cocker spaniel with taurine deficiency. *Aust Vet J*. 1997;75:862–868.

[28] Borgarelli M, Tarducci A, Tidholm A, et al. Canine idiopathic dilated cardiomyopathy. Part II: pathophysiology and therapy. *Vet J*. 2001;162:182–195.

[29] Liu SK, Roberts WC, Maron BJ. Comparison *of morphologic* findings in spontaneously occurring hypertrophic *cardiomyopathy in* humans, cats and dogs. *Am J Cardiol*. 1993;72:944–951.

[30] Legge CH, López A, Hanna P, *et al*. *Histologic*al characterization of dilated cardiomyopathy in the juvenile toy Manchester terrier. *Vet Pathol*. 2013;50:1043–1052.

[31] Janus I, Noszczyk-Nowak A, Nowak M, et al. A comparison of the histopathologic pattern of the left atrium in canine dilated cardiomyopathy and chronic mitral valve disease. *BMC Vet Res*. 2016;12:3.

[32] Tidholm A, Häggström J, Jünsson L. Detection of attenuated wavy fibers in the myocardium of Newfoundlands without clinical or echocardiographic evidence of heart disease. *Am J Vet Res*. 2000;61:238–241.

[33] Tidholm A, Häggström J, Jünsson L. Prevalence of attenuated wavy fibers in myocardium of dogs with dilated cardiomyopathy. *J Am Vet Med Assoc*. 1998;212:1732–1734.

[34] Harpster N. Boxer cardiomyopathy. *Vet Clin North Am Small Anim Pract*. 1991;21:989–1004.

[35] Granstrüm S, Godiksen MT, Christiansen M, et al. Prevalence of hypertrophic cardiomyopathy in a cohort of British Shorthair cats in Denmark. *J Vet Intern Med*. 2011;25:866–871.

[36] Gundler S, Tidholm A, Häggströmm J. Prevalence of myocardial hypertrophy in a population of asymptomatic Swedish Maine coon cats. *Acta Vet Scand*. 2008;50:22.

[37] Cesta MF, Baty CJ, Keene BW, et al. Pathology of end-stage remodeling in a family of cats with hypertrophic cardiomyopathy. *Vet Pathol*. 2005;42:458–467.

[38] Saito Y, Suzuki Y, Kondo N, et al. Direct epicardial assist device using artificial rubber muscle in a swine model of pediatric dilated cardiomyopathy. *Int J Artif Organs*. 2015;38:588–594.

[39] Lin JH, Huang SY, Lee WC, et al. Echocardiographic features of pigs with spontaneous hypertrophic cardiomyopathy. *Comp Med*. 2002;52:238–242.

[40] Collins DE, Eaton KA, Hoenerhoff MJ. Spontaneous dilated cardiomyopathy and right-sided heart failure as a differential diagnosis for hepatosis dietetica in a production pig. *Comp Med*. 2015;65:327–332.

[41] Shyu JJ, Cheng CH, Erlandson RA, et al. Ultrastructure of intramural coronary arteries in pigs with hypertrophic cardiomyopathy. *Cardiovasc Pathol*. 2000;11:104–111.

[42] Liu SK, Chiu YT, Shyu JJ, et al. Hypertrophic cardiomyopathy in pigs: quantitative pathologic features in 55 cases. *Cardiovasc Pathol*. 1994;3:261–268.

[43] Horiuchi N, Kumagai D, Matsumoto K, et al. Detection of the nonsense mutation of OPA3 gene in Holstein Friesian cattle with dilated cardiomyopathy in Japan. *J Vet Med Sci*. 2015;77:1281–1283.

[44] Van Vleet JF, Ferrans VJ. Myocardial diseases of animals. *Am J Pathol*. 1986;124:98–178.

[45] Owczarek-Lipska M, Plattet P, Zipperle L, et al. A nonsense mutation in the optic atrophy 3 gene (OPA3) causes dilated cardiomyopathy in Red Holstein cattle. *Genomics*. 2011;97:51–57.

[46] Furuoka H, Yagi S, Murakami A, et al. Hereditary dilated cardiomyopathy in Holstein-Friesian cattle in Japan: association with hereditary myopathy of the diaphragmatic muscles. *J Comp Pathol.* 2001;125:159–165.

[47] Schatzberg SJ, Olby NJ, Breen M, et al. Molecular analysis of a spontaneous dystrophin 'knockout' dog. *Neuromuscul Disord.* 1999;9:289–295.

[48] Stabej P, Imholz S, Versteeg SA, et al. Characterization of the canine desmin (DES) gene and evaluation as a candidate gene for dilated cardiomyopathy in the Doberman. *Gene.* 2004;340:241–249.

[49] Philipp U, Vollmar A, Distl O. Evaluation of the titin-cap gene (TCAP) as candidate for dilated cardiomyopathy in Irish wolfhounds. *Anim Biotechnol.* 2008;19:231–236.

[50] O'Sullivan ML, O'Grady MR, Pyle WG, Dawson JF. Evaluation of 10 genes encoding cardiac proteins in Doberman Pinschers with dilated cardiomyopathy. *Am J Vet Res.* 2011;72:932–939.

[51] Cattanach BM, Dukes-McEwan J, Wotton PR, et al. A pedigree-based genetic appraisal of Boxer ARVC and the role of the Striatin mutation. *Vet Rec.* 2015;176:492.

[52] Keene BW, Panciera DP, Atkins CE, et al. Myocardial L-carnitine deficiency in a family of dogs with dilated cardiomyopathy. *J Am Vet Med Assoc.* 1991;198:647–650.

[53] Kittleson MD, Keene B, Pion PD, et al. Results of the multicenter spaniel trial (MUST): taurine- and carnitine-responsive dilated cardiomyopathy in American cocker spaniels with decreased plasma taurine concentration. *J Vet Intern Med.* 1997;11:204–211.

[54] Phillips DE, Harkin KR. Hypothyroidism and myocardial failure in two Great Danes. *J Am Anim Hosp Assoc.* 2003;39:133–137.

[55] Flood JA, Hoover JP. Improvement in myocardial dysfunction in a hypothyroid dog. *Can Vet J.* 2009;50:828–34.

[56] Beier P, Reese S, Holler PJ, et al. The role of the hypothyroidism in the etiology and progression of dilated cardiomyopathy in Doberman Pinschers. *J Vet Intern Med.* 2015;29:141–149.

[57] Day MJ. Inheritance of serum autoantibody, reduced serum IgA and autoimmune disease in a canine breeding colony. *Vet Immunol Immunopathol.* 1996;53:207–219.

[58] Maxson TR, Meurs KM, Lehmkuhl LB, et al. Polymerase chain reaction analysis for viruses in paraffin-embedded myocardium from dogs with dilated cardiomyopathy or myocarditis. *Am J Vet Res.* 2001;62:130–135.

[59] Calvert CA, Chapman WL, Toal RL. Congestive cardiomyopathy in Doberman Pinscher dogs. *J Am Vet Med Assoc.* 1982;181:598–602.

[60] Hazlett MJ, Maxie MG, Allen DG, et al. A retrospective study of heart disease in Doberman Pinscher dogs. *Can Vet J.* 1983;24:205–210.

[61] Tidholm A, Jünsson L. Dilated cardiomyopathy in the Newfoundland: a study of 37 cases (1983–1994). *J Am Anim Hosp Assoc.* 1996;32:465–470.

[62] Calvert CA, Pickus CW, Jacobs GJ, et al. Signalment, survival and prognostic factors in Doberman Pinschers with end-stage cardiomyopathy. *J Vet Intern Med.* 1997;11:323–326.

[63] Everett RM, McGann J, Wimberly HC, et al. Dilated cardiomyopathy of Doberman Pinschers: retrospective histomorphologic evaluation of heart from 32 cases. *Vet Pathol.* 1999;36:221–227.

[64] Vollmar AC, Fox PR, Meurs KM, et al. Dilated cardiomyopathy in juvenile Doberman Pinscher dogs. *J Vet Cardiol.* 2005;5:23–27.

[65] Lobo L, Carvalheira J, Canada N, et al. Histologic characterization of dilated cardio-myopathy in Estrela mountain dogs. *Vet Pathol.* 2010;47:637–642.

[66] Tilley LP, Liu S-K. Cardiomyopathy in the dog. *Recent Adv Stud Cardiac Struct Metab.* 1975;10:641–653.

[67] Sandusky GE, Capen CC, Kerr KM. Histological and ultrastructural evaluation of cardiac lesions in idiopathic cardiomyopathy in dogs. *Can J Comp Med.* 1984;48:81–86.

[68] Alroy J, Rush JE, Freeman L, et al. Inherited infantile dilated cardiomyopathy in dogs: genetic, clinical, biochemical, and morphologic findings. *Am J of Med Genet.* 2000;95:57–66.

[69] Vollmar AC, Fox PR, Meurs KM, et al. Dilated cardiomyopathy in juvenile Doberman Pinscher dogs. *J Vet Cardiol.* 2005;5:23–27.

4

Arrhythmogenic Right Ventricular Cardiomyopathy/Dysplasia

Bandar Al-Ghamdi

Abstract

Arrhythmogenic right ventricular cardiomyopathy/dysplasia (ARVC/D) is a rare disease characterized by progressive fibrofatty replacement of the myocardium, primarily involving the right ventricle (RV). The structural changes in the ventricular myocardium form a substrate for ventricular arrhythmia ranging from premature ventricular complexes to ventricular tachycardia typically of RV origin and may result in RV failure and progress to congestive heart failure at a later stage. ARVC/D is a recognized cause of sudden cardiac death in young people, but it may occur at any age. With the discovery of underlying pathogenic mutations involved in the disease development and insight from long-term follow-up of ARVC/D patients, ARVC/D is an inherited cardiomyopathy. Mutations in at least eight genes have been involved in ARVC/D genesis in 30–50% of patients. Most of these genes are involved in the function of desmosomes, which are structures that attach heart muscle cells to one another. Desmosomes provide strength to the myocardium and play a role in signaling between neighboring cells. Mutations in the genes responsible for ARVC/D often impair the normal desmosomal function. There has been significant advancement in the diagnosis and management of ARVC/D in the past few decades. This chapter provides an overview of ARVC/D pathophysiology, clinical presentations, diagnosis, and management.

Keywords: cardiomyopathy, arrhythmia, right ventricle, sudden cardiac death, heart failure

1. Introduction

Arrhythmogenic right ventricular cardiomyopathy/dysplasia (ARVC/D) is a rare disease characterized by progressive fibrofatty replacement of the myocardium, primarily involving the right ventricle (RV) [1–4].

The typical age of presentation is between the second and the fourth decade of life. The structural changes in the ventricular myocardium form a substrate for ventricular arrhythmia ranging from premature ventricular complexes (PVCs) to ventricular tachycardia (VT), typically of RV origin and may result in RV failure, and progress to congestive heart failure at a later stage. ARVC/D is a recognized cause of sudden cardiac death (SCD) in young individuals, but it may occur at any age [4].

ARVC/D was first described by Frank et al. [1], and the first clinical profile of the disease was published in 1982 [2]. It was described as a disease in which "the right ventricular musculature is partially or totally absent and is replaced by fatty and fibrous tissue [2]." With the discovery of underlying pathogenic mutations involved in the disease development and insight from long-term follow-up of ARVC/D patients, the ARVC/D is currently considered to be an inherited cardiomyopathy [4–6]. However, the presence of sporadic cases of ARVC/D increased the possibility of nongenetic causes.

Mutations in at least eight genes have been involved in the ARVC/D genesis in 30–50% patients. Most of these genes are involved in the function of desmosomes, which are structures that attach heart muscle to one another. Desmosomes provide strength to the myocardium and also play a role in signaling between neighboring cells. Mutations in the genes responsible for ARVC/D often impair the normal desmosomal function. This results in cells of the myocardium detaching from one another and dying (apoptosis). They are then replaced with fibrous and fibrofatty tissue. The apoptosis occurs predominantly when the heart muscle is placed under stress (such as during vigorous exercise). Most of these gene code for desmosome proteins— plakoglobin (JUP), desmoplakin (DSP), plakophilin-2 (PKP2), the desmoglein-2 (DSG2), and desmocollin-2 (DSC2)—and other genes that code for nondesmosomal protein (e.g., RYR2 and TMEM43) have also been associated with ARVC/D [7]. Additionally, an autosomal recessive variant of ARVC/D has been described. The first disease-causing gene, encoding the desmosomal protein plakoglobin (JUP), was identified in patients with Naxos disease and is an autosomal recessive variant of ARVC/D. It was first reported from the Greek island of Naxos and is associated with palmoplantar keratoderma and wooly hair [8]. Another recessive mutation of DSP has been reported and associated with Carvajal syndrome, another cardiocutaneous disease [9].

In the past few decades, there has been a significant improvement in our understanding of this disease pathogenesis, natural course, diagnosis, and management.

This chapter provides an overview of ARVC/D pathophysiology, clinical presentations, diagnosis, and management.

2. Epidemiology

The estimated prevalence of ARVC/D in the general population ranges from 1 in 2000 to 1 in 5000 individuals; men are more frequently affected than women, with an approximate ratio of 3:1 [10, 11].

The median age at onset of the disease is about 30 years, whereas it rarely manifests before the age of 12 or after the age of 60 years [12, 13]. ARVC/D is a leading cause of sudden cardiac death (SCD) accounting for 11–22% of cases of SCD in the young athlete patient population 8 [13–15]. However, this varies based on the geographic area as it accounts for approximately 22% of SCD cases in athletes in northern Italy [5] and about 17% of SCD in young people in the United States [16]. The genes involved and different mode of inheritance may explain the ARVC/D ethnic variations [17]. The most prevalent mode of inheritance of ARVC/D is an autosomal dominant; however, autosomal recessive form has also been described such as Naxos disease. This disease was first described in Naxos Island, Greece, and it is associated with cutaneous manifestations such as palmoplantar keratosis [8]. Although there are no genetic studies in ARVC/D Chinese patients, some studies showed a lower familial incidence of premature SCD among these patients [18].

3. Molecular genetics

ARVC/D is a genetically determined cardiac disease because one or more first-degree relatives also display signs of the disease in 30–50% of cases [2, 19].

A large majority of mutations in ARVC/D patients have been found in genes encoding different components of the cardiac desmosome, i.e., plakophilin 2 (PKP2), desmocollin 2 (DSC2), desmoglein 2 (DSG2), desmoplakin (DSP), and plakoglobin (JUP), suggesting that ARVC/D is primarily a disease of disturbed desmosomal function. However, mutations in other genes (nondesmosomal genes) have also been reported in ARVC/D, including transmembrane protein 43 (TMEM43), desmin (DES), and titin (TTN), indicating genetic heterogeneity. Several ARVC/D cases were found to be caused by multiple mutations in the same gene (compound heterozygosity) or mutations in different genes (digenic inheritance), which could result in an earlier onset and increased disease severity [7] (**Figure 1**).

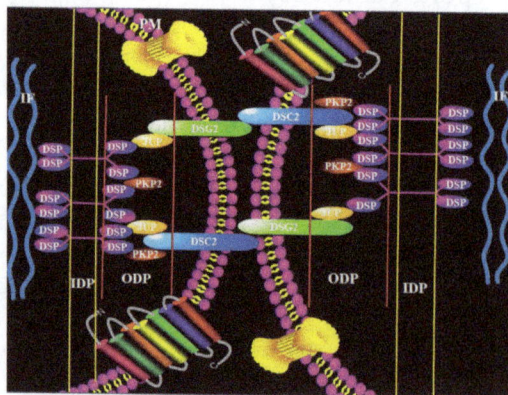

Figure 1. The structural schematic diagram of desmosome. IDP, inner dense plaque; ODP, outer dense plaque; PM, plasma membrane; DSG2, desmoglein-2; DSC2, desmocollin-2; JUP, plakoglobin; PKP2, plakophilin-2; DSP, desmoplakin; IF, intermediate filaments. Adapted with permission from Que et al. [186].

The ARVC/D is inherited predominantly as an autosomal dominant (the classical form), and as autosomal recessive (nonclassical form) such as Naxos disease and Carvajal syndrome [8, 9]. **Table 1** summarizes ARVC/D genes and corresponding phenotypes.

ARVC/D subtype	Location (chromosome/locus)	Inheritance	Gene/locus (encoded protein)
ARVC/D 1	14q24.3	AD	TGFβ3
ARVC/D 2	1q43	AD	RyR2
ARVC/D 3	14q12-q22	AD	–
ARVC/D 4	2q32.1-q32.3	AD	–
ARVC/D 5	3p25.1	AD	TMEM43
A\RVC/D 6	10p14-p12	–	–
ARVC/D 7	10q22.3	AD	DES
ARVC/D 8	6p24.3	AD	DSP
ARVC/D 9	12p11.21	AD	PKP2
ARVC/D 10	18q12.1	AD	DSG2
ARVC/D 11	18q12.1	AR/AD	DSC2
ARVC/D 12	17q21.2	AD	JUP
Naxos disease	17q21.2	AR	JUP
ARVC/D 13	10q21.3	AD	CTNNA3

Abbreviations: AD: autosomal-dominant; AR: autosomal-recessive; ARVC/D: arrhythmogenic right ventricular cardiomyopathy/dysplasia; CTNNA3: catenin Alpha; DSC2: desmocollin-2; DSG2: desmoglein-2; DES: desmin; DSP: desmoplakin; JUP: junction plakoglobin; PKP2: plakophilin-2; RyR2: Ryanodine receptor 2; TGF: transforming growth factor; TMEM43: transmembrane protein 43.

Table 1. Arrhythmogenic ventricular cardiomyopathy/dysplasia genetics from OMIM®and Online Mendelian Inheritance in Man®.

3.1. Desmosomal ARVC/D

3.1.1. Autosomal dominant disease

3.1.1.1. Plakophilin-2

Plakophilin-2 is a protein that in humans is encoded by the PKP2 gene [20]. Plakophilin 2 is expressed in cardiac muscle as well as skin, where it functions to link cadherins to intermediate filaments in the cytoskeleton. In cardiac muscle, plakophilin-2 is found in desmosome structures located within intercalated discs [21]. In 2004, Syrris et al. [22] was the first to show that mutations in PKP2 are a major cause of ARVC/D. The disease was incompletely penetrant in most mutation carriers as confirmed by subsequent studies [23–26]. It is estimated that up to 70% of all mutations associated with ARVC/D are within the PKP2 gene [27, 28]. This finding is consistent with this chapter author's experience of ARVC/D patients in Saudi Arabia [29]. Specific and sensitive markers of PKP2 and plakoglobin mutation carriers in ARVC/D have been identified to include T-wave inversions, right ventricular wall motion abnormalities, and ventricular extrasystoles [30]. Investigations looking at the clinical and genetic characterization of ARVC/D to understand the penetrance associated with PKP2 mutations, as well as other genes encoding desmosomal proteins, in disease progression and outcome, are of major interest [31–40]. PKP2 mutations were also found to coexist with sodium channelopathies in patients with Brugada syndrome [41, 42].

3.1.1.2. Desmoplakin

Desmoplakin is a protein in humans that is encoded by the DSP gene [43, 44]. Desmoplakin is a critical component of desmosome structures in cardiac muscle and epidermal cells, which function to maintain the structural integrity at adjacent cell contacts. In cardiac muscle, desmoplakin is localized to intercalated discs, which mechanically couple cardiac cells to function in a coordinated syncytial structure. Mutations in this gene are the cause of several cardiomyopathies, including dilated cardiomyopathy (DCM) [9, 45], and ARVC/D [46–50]. Mutations in DSP have also been associated with striate palmoplantar keratoderma [9, 48, 51]. Carvajal syndrome results from an autosomal recessive mutation in DSP gene [45] (see below).

3.1.1.3. Desmoglein-2

Desmoglein-2 is a protein that in humans is encoded by the DSG2 gene [52]. Desmoglein-2 is highly expressed in cardiomyocytes and epithelial cells. Desmoglein-2 is localized to desmosome structures at regions of cell-cell contact and functions to structurally adhere adjacent cells together. In cardiac muscle, these regions are specialized regions known as intercalated discs. Mutations in desmoglein-2 have been associated with ARVC/D [53] and familial dilated cardiomyopathy [54].

3.1.1.4. Desmocollin-2

Desmocollin-2 is a protein that in humans is encoded by the DSC2 gene [55]. Desmocollin-2 is a cadherin-type protein that functions to link adjacent cells together in desmosomes. Desmocollin-2 is widely expressed and is the only desmocollin isoform expressed in cardiac muscle, where it localizes to intercalated discs. Mutations in DSC2 have been causally linked to ARVC/D.

Syrri et al. [56] reported 4 DSC2 mutations in 77 probands who were negative for other mutations. Disease expression was variable, and most mutation carriers had LV involvement. Other studies show the same findings [33, 34, 57, 58].

3.1.1.5. Plakoglobin

The first dominant mutation in plakoglobin was described in a German family [59]. Affected individuals carried an insertion of an extra serine residue at position 39 in the N-terminus of plakoglobin (S39_K40insS) [59]. None of the individuals affected by the S39_K40insS mutation showed apparent cutaneous abnormalities, in contrast to abnormalities seen in patients with Naxos disease.

3.1.2. Autosomal recessive

3.1.2.1. Plakoglobin

Plakoglobin, also known as junction plakoglobin or gamma-catenin, is a protein that in humans is encoded by the JUP gene. Plakoglobin is a cytoplasmic component of desmosomes and adherens junctions structures located within intercalated discs of cardiac muscle that function to anchor sarcomeres and join adjacent cells in cardiac muscle. It is the first gene that was identified as a cause of ARVC/D by Protonotarios et al. [60] in 1986. The mutations in JUP specifically cause an autosomal recessive form of the disease referred to as Naxos disease. It was first described in patients originating from the Hellenic island of Naxos. Naxos disease is characterized phenotypically by cutaneous manifestations such as wooly hair plus palmar and plantar erythema that progresses to keratosis with physical activity involving the palms and soles of the feet [7, 36–38, 61–63]. Noninvasive cardiac screening identified T-wave inversion, abnormalities in RV wall motion, and frequent ventricular extrasystoles as sensitive and specific markers of a JUP mutation [30].

3.1.2.2 Desmoplakin

Carvajal syndrome is a variety of Naxos disease presenting at a younger age with more pronounced left ventricular involvement has been described in families from India and Ecuador [34, 35, 45, 64]. It results from an autosomal recessive mutation of a frameshift (7901delG) in DSP that results in a combination of above conditions, including dilated cardiomyopathy, keratoderma, and wooly hair [45]

3.2. Nondesmosomal ARVC/D

3.2.1. Cardiac ryanodine receptor (RyR2)

The RyR2 receptor is responsible for calcium release from the sarcoplasmic reticulum. Mutations in the cardiac ryanodine receptor RyR2 have been described in only one Italian ARVC/D family [65].

Mutations in the human RYR2 gene have been associated with three inherited cardiac diseases: arrhythmogenic right ventricular cardiomyopathy type 2 (ARVC/D2)[65, 66], catecholaminergic polymorphic ventricular tachycardia (CPVT) [67,68], and familial polymorphic ventricular tachycardia (FPVT) [69, 70].

3.2.2. Transforming growth factor beta-3 (TGFβ3)

The TGF-β superfamily of cytokines consists of proteins that regulate different physiological processes, such as embryonic development, chemotaxis, homeostasis, cell cycle control, and wound healing [71]. The gene has been mapped to chromosome 14. With the screening of the promoter and untranslated regions, a mutation of the TGFβ3 gene was found in all clinically affected members of a large family with ARVC/D [72]. TGFβs stimulate mesenchymal cells to proliferate and to produce extracellular matrix components [73]. It is, therefore, possible that enhanced TGFβ3 activity can lead to myocardial fibrosis.

3.2.3. Transmembrane protein 43 (TMEM43)

Transmembrane protein 43 (also called luma) is a protein that is encoded by the TMEM43 gene in humans [74]. TMEM43 may have an important role in maintaining a nuclear envelope structure by organizing protein complexes at the inner nuclear membrane.

A high-risk form of ARVC/D with a fully penetrant, and sex influenced inheritance has been identified in 15 unrelated families in a genetically isolated population in Newfoundland, Canada. The underlying mutation for this form of the disease was a missense mutation in the TMEM43 gene [75]. The TMEM43 gene contains the response element for PPAR gamma, which is an adipogenic transcription factor. The dysregulation of the adipogenic pathway regulated by PPAR gamma as a result of TMEM43 gene mutation may explain the fibrofatty replacement of myocardium in patients with ARVC/D [75]. Several other studies also show that mutations in TMEM43 are associated with ARCV/D [75–78].

3.2.4. Others

Only isolated reports showed causal mutations in other nondesmosomal genes, such as desmin (DES), titin (TTN), Lamin A/C (LMNA), phospholamban (PLN) and αT-catenin (CTNNA3), sometimes with a clinical phenotype similar but not identical to ARVC/D, as to be considered phenocopies or overlap syndromes [79].

4. Pathophysiology

The structural abnormalities in ARVC/D result from the fibrofatty infiltration of the RV myocardium, which leads to progressive RV dilatation and dysfunction (**Figure 2**). The gross

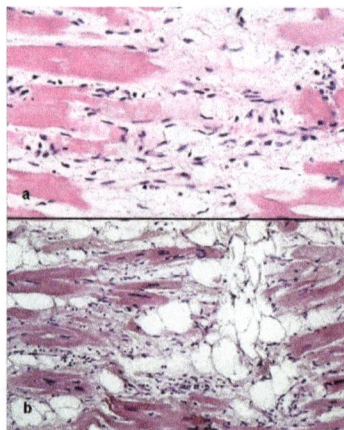

Figure 2. Typical histological features of ARVC/D. (a) Ongoing myocyte death and (b) early fibrosis and adipocytes infiltration. Adapted with permission from Thiene et al. [187].

pathognomonic features of ARVC/D consist of RV aneurysms, whether single or multiple, located in the so-called "triangle of dysplasia" which involve RV inflow, apex and outflow tract [4]. The left ventricle (LV) is less commonly involved, and the septum is relatively spared.

4.1. Early hypothesis

Basso et al. [4] suggested that the mechanism for myocardial loss and myocardial atrophy appeared to be the consequence of acquired injury (myocyte death) and repair (fibrofatty replacement), mediated by patchy myocarditis. The presence of apoptosis (programmed cell death) is confirmed in ARVC/D [80]. Inflammation, enhanced fibrosis, and loss of function are based on pathological reports of inflammatory infiltrates detected in the heart specimen collected from ARVC/D patients [81]. More recent studies showed that myocarditis might mimic ARVC/D, or it may be superimposed on existing disease in the affected heart muscle [82]. Another proposed mechanism was transdifferentiation of myocardium. This hypothesis assumes that myocardial cells can change from cardiac muscle to adipose tissue [83]. However, it was based on an observation in one patient only.

4.2. Current hypothesis

4.2.1. Abnormal cell-cell adhesion (desmosomal disease)

Our current understanding of ARCV/D indicates that it is a desmosomal disease. Desmosomes mediate cell-cell adhesion and provide cells with mechanical strength [84, 85]. They are present in tissues with mechanical stress like myocardium and epidermis. Desmosomes consist of three families of proteins: the armadillo proteins (junction plakoglobin and plakophilin), cadherins (desmocollins and desmogleins), and plakins (desmoplakin) [86]. Electron microscopy studies have demonstrated intercalated disc remodeling, which raised the hypothesis of an abnormal cell-cell adhesion in disease pathogenesis even before the discovery of desmosomal genes in ARVC/D [87, 88]. Reduced cell-cell adhesion was demonstrated using monolayers of neonatal rat ventricular myocytes in which PKP2 was silenced and subjected to a defined mechanical intervention [89]. However, when expressing mutant forms of either PKP2 or JUP, cells exhibited abnormal signaling in response to mechanical stress, but showed a preserved intercellular adhesion, which raised a question mark about the primary role of cell-cell adhesion in ARVC/D pathogenesis [90]. At the same time, the reduced junctional signal for JUP appears to have a significant role in the disease pathogenesis as demonstrated by Asimaki et al. [91] in myocardial samples from ARVC/D patients. This may indicate a possible role of intracellular signaling rather than adhesion, as suggested by other groups [92, 93].

4.2.2. Abnormal intercellular junction proteins and intracellular signaling

Suppression of the canonical Wnt/β-catenin signaling pathway is another proposed mechanism in the pathogenesis of ARVC/D. Plakoglobin (γ-catenin), a protein with functional similarities to catenin, can localize both to the plasma membrane and the nucleus [94]. Garcia-Gras et al. [92] demonstrated that disruption of desmoplakin frees plakoglobin from the plasma membrane allowing it to translocate to the nucleus and suppress canonical Wnt/-catenin signaling. Wnt/β-catenin signaling can inhibit adipogenesis by preventing mesodermal precursors from differentiating into adipocytes [95]. Suppression of Wnt/β-catenin signaling by plakoglobin nuclear localization could, therefore, promote the differentiation of adipose tissue in the cardiac myocardium in patients with ARVC/D [92] (**Figure 3**).

Recently, the Hippo/YAP signaling pathway has been associated with ARVC/D pathogenesis. The YAP interacts with β-catenin to drive Wnt-related gene expression in the nucleus. Chen et al. [96] demonstrated aberrant activation of the Hippo kinase cascade resulting in phosphorylation and cytoplasmic retention of YAP in ARVC/D myocardial samples, mouse models and pkp2 knockdown HL-1 myocytes.

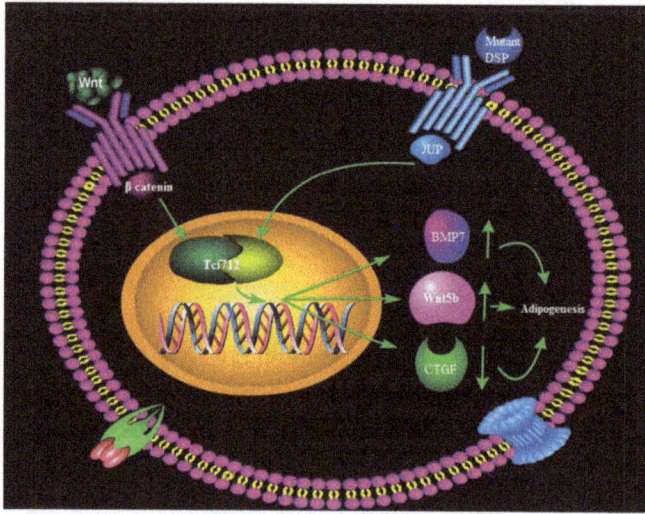

Figure 3. The suppression of the Wnt/β-catenin signal pathway. Mutant DSP frees JUP from the plasma membrane, allowing it to translocate to the nucleus. Nucleus location of JUP might be the initiator of the suppression of Wnt signaling. Plakoglobin competes against β-catenin for binding with Tcf712 (transcriptional factor 712), further leading to a series of consequences, increased expression of BMP7 and noncanonical Wnt5b and reduction of CTGF. Bone morphogenic protein 7 and Wnt5b are well-known promoters of adipogenesis as opposed to CTGF, which is inhibitor of adipogenesis. Ultimately, the pathological morphology of ARVC/D developed. Adapted with permission from Que et al. [186].

4.2.3. Gap junction and ion channel remodeling

At the cellular level, the functional triad of desmosomes, gap junctions and sodium channels is essential for normal function. The change in the composition of one component of this triad may affect the function and integrity of the others [97]. Impairment in mechanical coupling as expressed with diminished expression of connexin-43 at the intercellular junction was demonstrated in most of ARVC/D cases [98, 99].

Furthermore, in the ARVC/D experimental model, reduced cardiac sodium current was found [100–104]. These findings led researchers to hypothesize that life-threatening ventricular arrhythmias could occur in patients with ARVC/D even preceding the structural abnormalities due to electrical uncoupling and reduced sodium current, but this has yet to be proven.

Furthermore, animal studies using high-throughput drug screening identified as SB216763 showed an ability to restore the subcellular distribution of JUP, connexin-43 and Nav1.5 and of SAP97, a protein known to mediate the forward trafficking of Nav1.5 and Kir2.1. The SB216763 is already known as an activator of the canonical Wnt signaling pathway. This might be the beginning to move from experimental models to a target gene therapy [104].

5. Clinical presentation

In its initially described classical form of ARVC/D, the RV is primarily affected with possible LV involvement in a later stage. However, two additional patterns of disease have been identified by clinicogenetic characterization of families. These are the left dominant phenotype, with early and predominant LV manifestations, and the biventricular phenotype with equal involvement of both ventricles. Immunohistochemical studies at a molecular level indicated that ARVC/D is a global biventricular disease [95]. However, histologically and functionally overt manifestations of the disease usually start in the RV. There is no clear explanation for this finding, but the possible mechanism is that RV is less able to withstand pressure (over)load in the presence of impaired function of mechanical junctions due to their thin wall. The rare variant of the disease with cutaneous manifestations (palmoplantar keratoderma and wooly hair) has its features that will be discussed briefly later on.

5.1. Classic form of ARVC/D

ARVC/D patients typically present with monomorphic VT originating from the RV. However, rarely, sudden death at young age, or RV failure may be the first presentation. Patients' symptoms may include palpitations, shortness of breath, dizziness, and syncope or near syncope. Based on clinicopathologic and patients' follow-up studies, four different disease phases have been described for the classical form of ARVC/D, i.e., primarily affecting the RV (**Table 2**):

1. Concealed phase or early ARVC/D is characterized by the absence of obvious clinical changes, however, subtle RV structural changes may be found. Generally, these patients are asymptomatic but still at risk of SCD especially during heavy exercise.

2. The overt phase of the disease is characterized by the presence of patient's symptoms such as palpitations, syncope and ventricular arrhythmias ranging from isolated PVCs to sustained VT and ventricular fibrillation (VF).

3. The third phase is characterized by RV failure as manifest by RV dilatation and the reduced RV systolic function due to progressive loss of myocardium, with the preserved LV function.

4. Biventricular failure phase is characterized by LV involvement, which usually occurs at a late stage. This phase may mimic DCM and may require cardiac transplantation.

Phase	Characteristics
Concealed	No symptoms
	Subtle structural changes
Overt	Ventricular arrhythmias (PVCs/VT of LBBB morphology)
	RV structural abnormalities
RV failure	Symptoms and signs of RV failure
	Preserved LV function
Biventricular failure	Symptoms and signs of LV failure
	LV structural changes

Table 2. Clinicopathologic phases of ARVC/D.

5.2. Nonclassic form of ARVC/D

5.2.1. ARVC/D with cutaneous manifestations (cardiocutanous disease)

5.2.1.1. Naxos disease

Naxos disease is a recessively inherited stereotype association of arrhythmogenic cardiomy-opathy with a cutaneous phenotype, characterized by peculiar wooly hair and palmoplantar keratoderma [60]. It is a homozygous recessive JUP mutation. The cardiac manifestations of the disease are identical to ARVC/D in both clinical and histological studies [5, 105]. Since 1995, according to the classification of World Health Organization, Naxos disease has been considered as the recessive form of ARVC/D [106].

As mentioned earlier, the disease was first described by Protonotarios et al. [60] in families originating from the Greek island of Naxos. Later on the affected families were detected in other Greek Aegean islands, and other countries [106–108]. The typical clinical presentation of the disease includes appearance of wooly hair appears from birth, whereas palmoplantar keratoderma develops during the first year of life when infants start to use their hands and feet [109]. The cardiomyopathy clinically manifests by adolescence and shows 100% pene-trance [110]. Patients with Naxos disease is typically present with syncope and/or ventricular tachycardia of LBBB configuration. As with classic ARVC/D, sudden death may be the first manifestation of the disease. About one-third of patients become symptomatic before the 30th year of life, and a few clinical findings of an early heart disease can be detected during childhood in some cases [108]. They have ECG abnormalities, RV structural alterations, and LV involvement. In one series of 26 patients followed for 10 years, 62% had structural pro-gression of RV abnormalities and 27% developed heart failure due to LV involvement [110]. Naxos ARVC/D is a rather progressive heart disease with adverse prognosis, especially in young. The annual disease-related and sudden death mortality have been estimated at 3% and 2.3%, respectively [110]. The risk factors for sudden death based on a long-term study of an unselected population of patients with Naxos disease include the history of syncope, the appearance of symptoms and severely progressed disease to the right ventricle before the age of 35 years, and the involvement of the left ventricle [110].

5.2.1.2. Carvajal syndrome

Carvajal syndrome with the same cutaneous manifestations as Naxos disease but with predominantly LV involvement has been described in families from India and Ecuador [45, 111]. It is associated with a DSP gene mutation and is also a recessive disease. The cardiomyopathy is clinically manifested during childhood leading more frequently to a dilated cardiomyopathy and heart failure. In Carvajal syndrome, the heart disease is clinically manifested earlier during childhood [45, 111]. A significant proportion of patients developed heart failure at an early stage of the disease, and most of them died during adolescence. In a single case, gross cardiac pathologic examination showed aneurysms of the RV outflow tract, apex and posterior wall and involvement of the LV. In histologic examination, findings similar to ARVC/D pathology were found with areas of extensive myocardial loss and replacement fibrosis, particularly in subepicardial layers; however, there was no fatty infiltration [112].

5.2.2. Left-dominant arrhythmogenic cardiomyopathy (LDAC)

Patients with LDAC (also may refer to as left-sided ARVC/D or arrhythmogenic left ventricular cardiomyopathy) have fibrofatty changes, which predominantly involve the LV [113–117]. LDAC is characterized by ECG changes in the form of (infero)lateral T-wave inversion, arrhythmias of the LV origin. ARVC/D is distinguished from DCM by a propensity towards arrhythmia exceeding the degree of ventricular dysfunction [117]. Patients with LDAC may present with arrhythmias or chest pain, shortness of breath, syncope or presyncope at ages ranging from adolescence to over 80 years. In cardiac MRI, about one-third of patients show an LV ejection fraction less than 50% [117]. Furthermore, MRI with late gadolinium enhancement (LGE) of the LV demonstrated late enhancement extending through the outer one-third of the LV myocardium to the right side of the septum [117]. Some patients with LDAC have desmosomal gene mutations similar to ARVC/D (desmoplakin, plakophilin-2, and desmoglein-2) [64].

6. Diagnosis

The diagnosis of ARVC/D might be challenging in patients with early stages of the disease. The establishment of ARVC/D Task Force diagnostic criteria in 1994 and its modification in 2010 have improved the clinical diagnosis of the disease [118, 119]. The current Task Force criteria are the essential standard for classification of individuals suspected of ARVC/D. The Task Force criteria included six different categories: (1) global and regional dysfunction and structural alterations, (2) tissue characterization, (3) depolarization abnormalities, (4) repolarization abnormalities, (5) arrhythmias, and (6) family history, including pathogenic mutations. The diagnostic criteria within each category are further classified as major or minor according to their specificity for the disease. To fulfill ARVC/D diagnosis, it is required to have either two major or one major plus two minor or four minor criteria. The diagnosis of ARVC/D is regarded as definite with two major or one major and two minor criteria or four minor criteria from different categories; borderline with one major and one minor or three minor criteria from different categories; and possible with one major or two minor criteria from different categories. **Table 3** presents an overview of the 2010 modified Task Force criteria.

The Revised Task Force Criteria for ARVC/D	
I. Global or regional dysfunction and structural alterations[1]	
Major	**Minor**
By 2D echo:	**By 2D echo:**
• **Regional RV akinesia, dyskinesia, or aneurysm and 1 of the following (end diastole):**	• **Regional RV akinesia or dyskinesia and 1 of the following (end diastole):**
-PLAX RVOT ≥32 mm (corrected for body size [PLAX/BSA] ≥19 mm/m²)	-PLAX RVOT ≥29 to <32 mm (corrected for body size [PLAX/BSA] ≥16 to <19 mm/m²)
-PSAX RVOT ≥36 mm (corrected for body size [PSAX/BSA] ≥21 mm/m²)	-PSAX RVOT ≥32 to <36 mm (corrected for body size [PSAX/BSA] ≥18 to <21 mm/m²)
or	or
-fractional area change ≤33%	-fractional area change >33% to ≤40%
By MRI:	**By MRI:**
• **Regional RV akinesia or dyskinesia or dyssynchronous RV contraction and 1 of the following:**	• **Regional RV akinesia or dyskinesia or dyssynchronous RV contraction and 1 of the following:**
-Ratio of RV end-diastolic volume to BSA ≥110 mL/m² (male) or ≥100 mL/m² (female)	-Ratio of RV end-diastolic volume to BSA ≥100 to <110 mL/m² (male) or ≥90 to <100 mL/m² (female)
or	or
-RV ejection fraction ≤40%	-RV ejection fraction >40% to ≤45%
By RV angiography:	
Regional RV akinesia, dyskinesia, or aneurysm	
II. Tissue characterization of wall	
Major	**Minor**
• Residual myocytes<60% by morphometric analysis (or <50% if estimated), with fibrous replacement of the RV free wall myocardium in ≥1 sample, with or without fatty replacement	• Residual myocytes 60% to 75% by morphometric analysis (or 50% to 65% if estimated), with fibrous replacement of the RV free wall myocardium in ≥1 sample, with or without fatty replacement of tissue on endomyocardial biopsy

of tissue on endomyocardial biopsy

III. Repolarization abnormalities

Major	Minor
• Inverted T waves in right precordial leads (V_1, V_2, and V_3) or beyond in individuals >14 years of age (in the absence of complete right bundle-branch block QRS ≥120 ms)	• Inverted T waves in leads V_1 and V_2 in individuals >14 years of age (in the absence of complete right bundle-branch block) or in V_4, V_5, or V_6 • Inverted T waves in leads V_1, V_2, V_3, and V_4 in individuals >14 years of age in the presence of complete right bundle-branch block

IV. Depolarization/conduction abnormalities

Major	Minor
• Epsilon wave (reproducible low-amplitude signals between end of QRS complex to onset of the T wave) in the right precordial leads (V_1 to V_3)	• Late potentials by SAECG in ≥1 of 3 parameters in the absence of a QRS duration of ≥110 ms on the standard ECG • Filtered QRS duration (fQRS) ≥114 ms • Duration of terminal QRS <40 µV (low-amplitude signal duration) ≥38 ms • Root-mean-square voltage of terminal 40 ms ≤20 µV • Terminal activation duration of QRS ≥55 ms measured from the nadir of the S wave to the end of the QRS, including R′, in V_1, V_2, or V_3, in the absence of complete right bundle-branch block

V. Arrhythmias

Major	Minor
• **Nonsusta**ined or sustained ventricular tachycardia of left bundle-branch morphology with superior axis (negative or indeterminate QRS in leads II, III, and aVF and positive in lead aVL)	• Nonsustained or sustained ventricular tachycardia of RV outflow configuration, left bundle-branch block morphology with inferior axis (positive QRS in leads II, III, and aVF and negative in lead aVL) or of unknown axis • >500 ventricular extrasystoles per 24 hours (Holter)

VI. Family history

Major	Minor

- ARVC/D confirmed in a first-degree relative who meets current Task Force criteria

- ARVC/D confirmed pathologically at autopsy or surgery in a first-degree relative

- Identification of a pathogenic mutation[2] categorized as associated or probably associated with ARVC/D in the patient under evaluation

- History of ARVC/D in a first-degree relative in whom it is not possible or practical to determine whether the family member meets current Task Force criteria

- Premature sudden death (<35 years of age) due to suspected ARVC/D in a first-degree relative

- ARVC/D confirmed pathologically or by current Task Force Criteria in second-degree relative

- **Abbreviations:** PLAX indicates parasternal long-axis view; RVOT, RV outflow tract; BSA, body surface area; PSAX, parasternal short-axis view; aVF, augmented voltage unipolar left foot lead; and aVL, augmented voltage unipolar left arm lead.

- **Diagnostic terminology for original criteria:** This diagnosis is fulfilled by the presence of 2 major, or 1 major plus 2 minor criteria or 4 minor criteria from different groups. Diagnostic terminology for revised criteria: definite diagnosis: 2 major or 1 major and 2 minor criteria or 4 minor from different categories; borderline: 1 major and 1 minor or 3 minor criteria from different categories; possible: 1 major or 2 minor criteria from different categories.

---

[1] Hypokinesis is not included in this or subsequent definitions of RV regional wall motion abnormalities for the proposed modified criteria.

[2] A pathogenic mutation is a DNA alteration associated with ARVC/D that alters or is expected to alter the encoded protein, is unobserved or rare in a large non–ARVC/D control population, and either alters or is predicted to alter the structure or function of the protein or has demonstrated linkage to the disease phenotype in a conclusive pedigree. Modified from Marcus FI et al. Diagnosis of arrhythmogenic right ventricular cardiomyopathy/dysplasia: proposed modification of the task force criteria. Circulation. 2010;121(13):1533-41. DOI:10.1161/CIRCULATIONAHA.108.840827. Eur Heart J. 2010 Apr;31(7):806-14. DOI:10.1093/eurheartj/ehq025.)

Table 3. The 2010 revised Task Force criteria for the diagnosis of ARVC/D.

Evaluation of patients with suspected ARVC/D should include: a detailed medical history including a detailed family history, physical examination, 12-lead electrocardiogram (ECG), signal-averaged ECG (SAECG), 24-hours Holter monitoring, exercise testing, echocardiography (including RV functional evaluation and quantitative wall motion analysis), and when appropriate a more detailed analysis of the RV function by cardiac magnetic resonance imaging (MRI). Invasive tests with RV endomyocardial biopsy and RV angiogram are also useful for diagnostic purposes. Electrophysiology studies might be helpful in the evaluation of the VT site of origin and ablation of VT when indicated.

A brief description of diagnostic tests based on the Task Force criteria will be outlined below.

6.1. Global and regional dysfunction and structural alterations

Various imaging modalities have been used to evaluate RV (and LV) size and function, including echocardiography, cardiac MRI, computed tomography scan (CT scan) and/or RV angiography. According to the Task Force criteria, major criteria are defined as the presence of akinetic or dyskinetic areas in the RV combined with severe dilatation of the RV or RV ejection fraction 40% or lower [119]. In RV angiography the finding of only regional akinesia, dyskinesia or an aneurysm is considered to be sufficient for qualification as a major criterion. RV angiography has historically been considered the most sensitive method to visualize RV structural abnormalities, with a high specificity of 90% [120]. Compared to angiography, echocardiography is noninvasive, widely available, low in cost, and easy to perform and interpret, and has played a crucial role in imaging structural and functional abnormalities of the RV (**Figure 4**). It serves as the first-line imaging technique for evaluating patients suspected of ARVC/D and in family screening. There are numerous reports of the use of echocardiography to aid in the diagnosis of ARVC/D. These studies have found that the presence of right ventricular dysfunction by two-dimensional echocardiography has a high specificity and predictive value for ARVC/D [121–123]. The development of new echocardiographic techniques such as three-dimensional right ventricular (3D-RV), strain and tissue Doppler, and tissue deformation imaging, may improve the diagnostic, and prognostic performance of echocardiography in these patients, which help in minimizing the number of false-negative echocardiographic results and improve the sensitivity and specificity of this test [124]. Cardiac MRI has a significant role in the diagnosis of ARVC/D. It has the advantage of assessing the RV (and LV) function, size, global or regional wall motion abnormalities, and quantification of myocardial wall thinning and hypertrophy. The disadvantages of this technique are the lack of wide availability, and the need for interpretation by an expert specialized radiologist to prevent misdiagnosis. Incorrect interpretation of cardiac MRI is the most common cause of over diagnosis and physicians should be reluctant to diagnose ARVC/D when structural abnormalities are present only on MRI [125] (**Figure 5**). Quantitative analysis showed that RV end-diastolic diameter and outflow tract area were significantly higher and RV ejection fractions lower in ARVC/D patients when compared to controls. Although CMRI is a potentially useful test because it can distinguish fat from muscle, the sensitivity and specificity of CMRI detection of RV intramyocardial fat in the diagnosis of ARVC/D are variable, ranging from 22 to 100% [126–130]. Identifying fat can be challenging because of the thin RV wall; therefore, it is difficult to distinguish pathologic adipose infiltration from adjacent epicardial fat and it is not included in the Task Force diagnostic criteria.

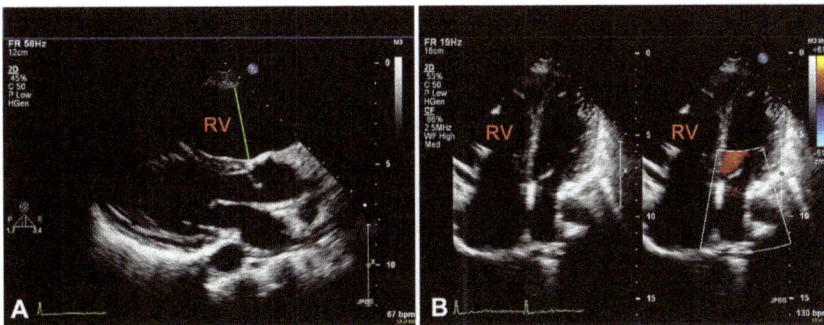

Figure 4. Parasternal long axis (A) and apical four-chamber (B) echocardiographic views showing RV dilatation.

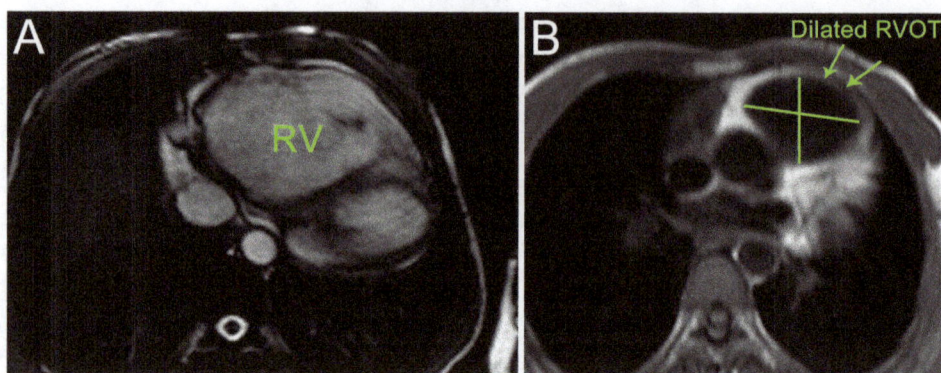

Figure 5. (A) Axial cine SSFP (steady-state free precession) MR imaging showing significant RV dilatation and (B) black-blood-prepared HASTE (Half-Fourier Acquired Single-shot Turbo spin Echo) axial slice MRI imaging at the level of RVOT showing RVOT dilatation.

6.2. Tissue characterization of wall (endomyocardial biopsy)

Endomyocardial biopsies (EMBs) are infrequently diagnostic, due to the focal nature of the lesions, and the fact that subendocardial layers of the myocardium are usually not affected in an early stage of the disease [131]. Furthermore, EMB sensitivity in ARVC/D is low if samples are taken from the septum, a region uncommonly involved by the disease [132]. Diagnostic values of EMB according to the new Task Force criteria are considered major if histomorphometric analysis of endomyocardial biopsies shows residual myocytes <60% by morphometric analysis (or <50% if estimated), with fibrous replacement of the RV free wall myocardium in ≥1 sample, with or without a fatty replacement of tissue (Task 2010). If the residual myocytes are 60–75% by morphometric analysis (or 50–65% if estimated), it is considered to be a minor criterion [129].

6.3. Electrocardiographic changes

The 12-lead ECG has a vital role in ARVC/D for diagnosis. The ECG changes and arrhythmias may precede the histological evidence of myocyte loss and RV changes in radiologic tests. Depolarization and repolarization ECG criteria have to be obtained during sinus rhythm and while off antiarrhythmic drugs.

6.3.1. Depolarization abnormalities

The hallmark of electrical changes in ARVC/D is the delayed RV activation. This delay may manifest with the presence of an epsilon wave, prolonged terminal activation duration (TAD) in the terminal part and after the QRS complex, and/or by recording late potentials on SAECG. Epsilon waves are defined as low amplitude potentials appearing after, and clearly separated from, the QRS complex in at least one of the precordial leads V1–V3 (**Figure 6**) [133]. Although epsilon waves are highly specific and considered to be one of the major diagnostic criteria, they are observed in only a small minority of patients [134, 135]. TAD has been defined as the longest value measured from the nadir of the S wave to the end of all depolarization deflections in V1–

V3, including the S wave upstroke and both late and fractionated signals and epsilon waves [136]. Prolonged TAD measured in V1–V3 greater than or equal to 55 ms, in the absence of complete RBBB, is considered to be a minor criterion. Prolonged TAD was recorded in 30 of 42 ARVC/D patients and only 1 of 27 patients with idiopathic VT [136]. The detection of late potentials on SAECG or late potentials detected during endocardial mapping in electrophysiologic studies (EPS) are frequently found in ARVC/D patients with documented VT; however, these late potentials can also be observed after myocardial infarction and with other structural heart diseases. Owing to this lack of specificity, SAECG abnormalities are considered a minor criterion. Common to all depolarization criteria is their correlation with disease severity. For instance, a positive correlation has been found between late potentials and the extent of RV fibrosis, reduced RV systolic function and significant morphological abnormalities on imaging [137–139].

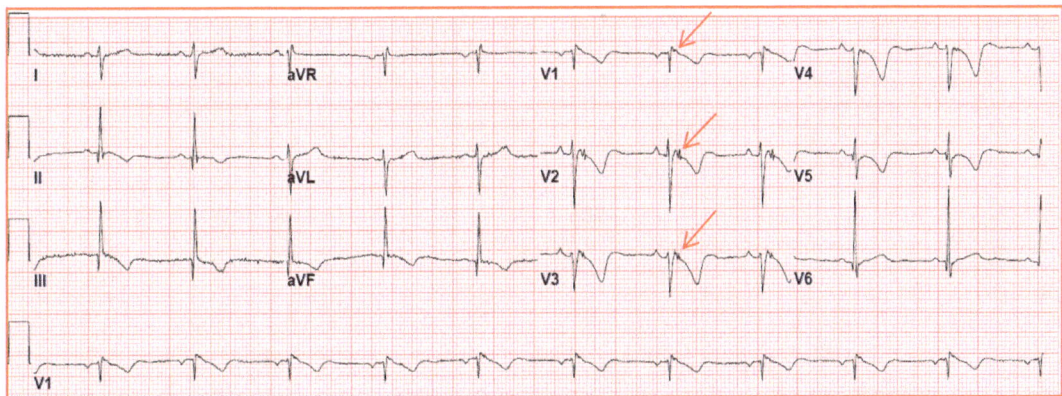

Figure 6. ECG of a patient with ARVC/D showing the presence of T-wave inversion in V1-V5 and an epsilon wave (electric potentials after the end of the QRS complex) (arrows).

6.3.2. Repolarization abnormalities

In the new Task Force criteria, negative T-waves in leads V1–V3 form a major ECG criterion in the absence of complete RBBB, but only if the patient is older than 14 years of age (**Figure 6**). T-wave inversion can be a normal feature of the ECG in children and early adolescence. Studies have reported variable prevalence of right precordial T-wave inversion, ranging from 19 to 94% [118–134, 140]. This variation may be due inclusion of family members in some studies and only index cases in others. In a study that considered only at ARVC/D index cases, 67% of them had this criterion but it was not found in patients with idiopathic RV-VT [136]. Other variants of T-wave inversion including T-wave inversion only in leads V1 and V2, T-wave inversion in V4–V6 among individuals older than 14 years of age in the absence of complete RBBB, and inverted T-waves in leads V1–V4 among individuals older than 14 years of age in the presence of RBBB, are considered to be minor repolarization criteria in the new Task Force criteria [119].

6.4. Arrhythmia

In ARVC/D, ventricular arrhythmias may range from PVCs to sustained VT or VF, leading to cardiac arrest [136, 141]. Typically, VT originating from RV has a LBBB-like morphology. Furthermore, VT with a superior axis (negative R waves in inferior leads) indicating RV inferior wall or apex origin (**Figure 7**) is considered a major criterion, while VT with inferior axis (positive R waves in inferior leads) indicating RV outflow tract (RVOT) origin is considered a minor criterion (**Figure 8**). VT with LBBB-like morphology and unknown axis is considered a minor criterion. Patients with the extensive disease often show multiple VT morphologies [136]. VT may degenerate into VF and lead to SCD especially in young and athletes individuals with ARVC/D. According to the new Task Force criteria, 500 or more PVCs in a 24-hour Holter recording are considered a minor criterion [119].

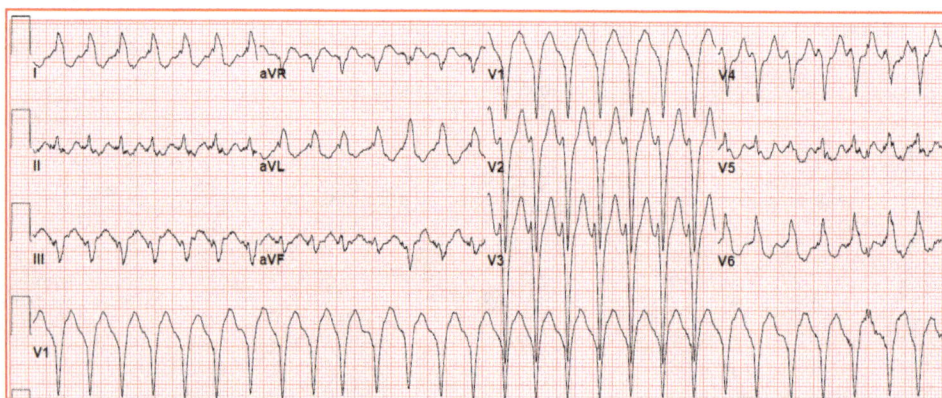

Figure 7. ECG showing ventricular tachycardia of RV inferior wall origin (LBBB and superior axis) in a patient with ARVC/D.

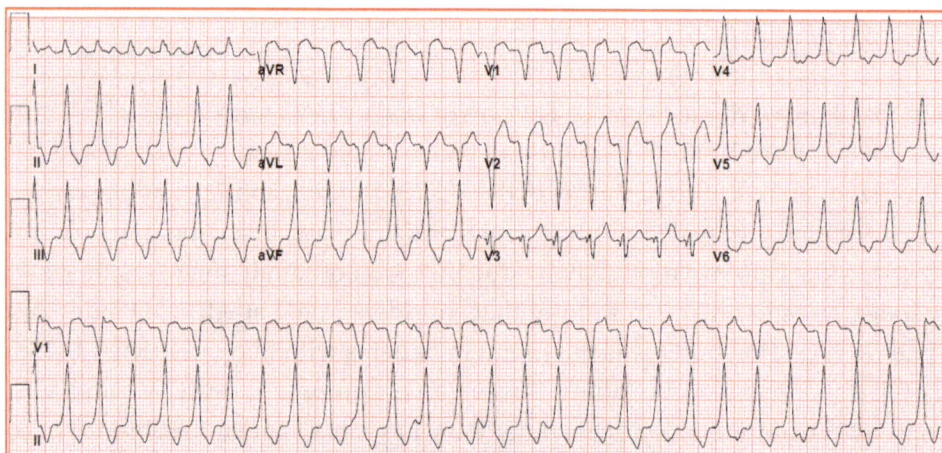

Figure 8. ECG showing ventricular tachycardia of RV outflow tract origin (LBBB and inferior axis) in a patient with ARVC/D.

6.5. Family history

ARVC/D is a familial disease. Having a first-degree family member with proven ARVC/D is considered an increased risk for other family members to be affected. ARVC/D confirmed in a first-degree relative who meets current Task Force criteria; ARVC/D confirmed pathologically at autopsy or surgery in a first-degree relative, or identification of a pathogenic mutation categorized as associated or probably associated with ARVC/D in the patient under evaluation is each considered as a major diagnostic criteria [119].

If a first-degree relative is diagnosed with ARVC/D but does not fulfill the diagnostic criteria, only a minor criterion is counted. Sudden death of a family member under the age of 35 years, presumably but not proven to be due to ARVC/D related arrhythmias, and ARVC/D confirmed pathologically or by current Task Force criteria in a second-degree relative is a minor criterion [119].

7. Differential diagnosis

It is crucial to differentiate ARVC/D from other diseases that primarily involve RV as the prognosis and management are very different. Differential diagnosis of ARVC/D includes:

1. **Right ventricular outflow tract VT (RVOT-VT):** RVOT-VT is a benign disorder that may cause exercise-induced left bundle branch block (LBBB) morphology VT with the inferior axis. In RVOT-VT there is no family history of ARVC/D or SCD, the ECG shows no depolarization or repolarization abnormalities and no RV structural changes can be detected. There is usually no reproducibly inducible VT by premature extrastimuli at programmed stimulation during electrophysiologic studies [142]. Idiopathic RVOT VT may be inducible by regular burst pacing and isoproterenol infusion [143]. The prognosis of RVOT-VT is usually good with very low risk of SCD. Furthermore, catheter ablation is usually curative in idiopathic RVOT-VT.

2. **Dilated cardiomyopathy:** Biventricular dilatation and congestive heart failure may mimic advanced ARVC/D with LV involvement. Characteristic ECG and cardiac MRI (CMRI) abnormalities in ARVC/D help to distinguish the two entities.

3. **Myocarditis:** Myocarditis due to viral infection or other causes may mimic ARVC/D. In general, endomyocardial biopsy is required to distinguish ARVC/D from myocarditis.

4. **Cardiac sarcoidosis:** Sarcoidosis is a disease of unknown etiology, characterized by the presence of noncaseating granulomas. It may affect mainly lungs, but other tissues such as heart, skin, eyes, reticuloendothelial system, kidneys, and central nervous system can be affected. About 5% of sarcoidosis patients may have cardiac involvement, which may manifest as conduction abnormalities, ventricular arrhythmias, valvular dysfunction or congestive heart failure. Although sarcoid patients typically have myocardial sarcoid granulomas and scarring in the LV and interventricular septum, the RV can also be affected. Patients can present with clinical features similar to those of ARVC/D including

arrhythmias, and SCD [144]. Visualization of granuloma in EMB can be a diagnostic value for cardiac sarcoidosis if granulomas are visualized [145]. Gadolinium-enhanced MRI may be beneficial by detecting located abnormalities in the septum, which is typical for sarcoidosis but seldom seen in ARVC/D. Positron emission tomography (PET) scans may show the active foci of sarcoidosis. Therapy with corticosteroids is recommended for patients diagnosed with cardiac sarcoidosis.

5. **Uhl anomaly:** This is a rare disorder characterized by the total lack of RV myocardium and results in a very thin-walled RV (parchment RV) [146]. In ARVC/D, the myocardium is not completely absent and is replaced by a variable degree of fibrosis.

8. Management

8.1. Risk stratification

The clinical objectives in ARVC/D management are prevention of SCD and death from heart failure; minimizing disease progression to RV, LV, or biventricular heart failure; improvement of quality of life by controlling palpitations, and minimizing appropriate or inappropriate implantable cardioverter defibrillator (ICD) discharges as much as possible; and improving functional capacity by optimization of heart failure management [147].

Therapeutic options consist of lifestyle changes, pharmacological treatment (beta-blockers, heart failure medications, antiarrhythmic medications), electrophysiological study (EPS) and catheter ablation, ICD implantation, and surgical intervention (e.g., RV isolation and heart transplantation).

8.2. Therapeutic options

8.2.1. Lifestyle changes

There is an established relationship between SCD and intense exertion in young individuals with ARVC/D. Competitive sports activity has been shown to increase the risk of SCD by fivefold in adolescent and young adults with ARVC/D [148]. Early identification of affected athletes by preparticipation screening and their disqualification from competitive sports activity may be "life-saving" [149]. Also, physical exercise has been implicated as a factor promoting development and progression of the ARVC/D phenotype [147]. In the animal study, it was demonstrated that in heterozygous plakoglobin-deficient mice, endurance training accelerated the development of RV dilatation, dysfunction, and ventricular ectopy, suggesting that chronically increased ventricular load might contribute to worsening of the ARVC/D phenotype [150].

Studies have shown that repetitive exercise and endurance sports increase age-related penetrance, the risk of VT/VF, and occurrence of heart failure in ARVC/D desmosomal-gene carriers [151, 152]. So, patients with a definite diagnosis of ARVC/D are encouraged not participate in endurance and/or competitive sports.

8.2.2. Pharmacological therapy

8.2.2.1. Beta-blockers

VTs and cardiac arrest in ARVC/D are frequently triggered by adrenergic stimulation and occur during or immediately after physical exercise [153–157]. Autonomic dysfunction with increased sympathetic stimulation of ventricular myocardium and subsequent reduction of β-adrenoceptor density were demonstrated with the use of radionuclide imaging and quantitative positron emission tomography [158, 159]. Beta-blockers are useful in the treatment of heart failure, preventing the effort-related VT, and possibly minimizing disease progression by lowering RV wall stress.

Beta-blocker therapy is recommended in ARVC/D patients with recurrent VT, as an adjunct to ICD therapy. It may also be a helpful addition to minimize inappropriate ICD shocks due to sinus tachycardia, supraventricular tachycardia, or atrial fibrillation/flutter with high-ventricular rate [147].

8.2.2.2. Heart failure therapy

For ARVC/D patients who developed right- and/or left-sided heart failure standard pharmacological treatment with angiotensin-converting-enzyme inhibitors, angiotensin II receptor blockers, β-blockers, and diuretics are recommended [147].

ARVC/D patients with severe RV dilatation are at risk of thromboembolism. A 0.5% annual incidence rate of thromboembolic complications is reported during a mean follow-up period of 99±64 months in a cohort of 126 ARVC/D patients [160]. Long-term oral anticoagulation is indicated for secondary prevention in patients with documented intra-cavitary thrombosis or venous/systemic thromboembolism [147].

8.2.2.3. Antiarrhythmic drugs

The aim of antiarrhythmic drug (AAD) therapy in patients with ARVC/D is to improve the quality of life by preventing symptomatic VT and ICD shocks. The data about AAD in ARVC/D are limited due to the lack of randomized control studies, the change in medication regimes over time and the common need for other modalities of treatment like VT ablation or ICD implantation [147, 161–163].

Although initial studies suggest that sotalol, administered at a dosage of 320–640 mg/day, is the most effective therapy with approximately 68% of patients achieving complete or partial arrhythmia suppression [164, 165], more recent available data suggest that amiodarone (loading dose of 400–600 mg daily for 3 weeks and then maintenance dose of 200–400 mg daily), alone or in combination with β-blockers, is the most effective drug for preventing symptomatic VTs and has relatively low proarrhythmic risk even in patients with ventricular dysfunction, although its ability to prevent SCD is unproven [166]. This variation in drugs effect may be partially a result of significant differences in design of the two studies, and the difference in sotalol doses, the difference in the amiodarone loading strategies and the method of medication selection [161]. There is relatively limited data about the combination of antiarrhythmic therapy. One recent report demonstrated the effective addition of flecainide to patients receiving sotalol with a resultant reduction in recurrent arrhythmias [167]. The addition of flecainide in this study was accomplished without significant adverse events. Several other studies have reported that the combination of amiodarone and beta-blockers may be effective in patients unable to achieve arrhythmia suppression with amiodarone alone [168, 169].

8.2.3. Catheter ablation

Fibrofatty replacement of RV myocardium creates scar regions that form a substrate for re-entry arrhythmias and VT.

Although VT catheter ablation is effective in the short term, the recurrence rate of VT after endocardial ablation procedures is about 50–75% in 3-year follow-up, which is likely secondary to the progressive nature of the disease [148, 170]. The discovery of the epicardial arrhythmogenic substrate in RVC/D patients makes epicardial VT ablation an attractive approach. The combination of endocardial and epicardial ablation approaches resulted in a higher success rate (77–83%) and lower recurrence of VTs over 18 and 36 month follow-up periods [171, 172]. However, this is at the expense of potential complications such as epicardial bleeding and coronary stenosis occurring in approximately 5% of cases [172]. Nevertheless, catheter ablation remains an important therapeutic modality for decreasing patient morbidity in conjunction with ICD implantation and antiarrhythmic medication especially in ARVC/D patients with incessant VT or frequent appropriate ICD interventions on VT despite maximal pharmacological therapy, including amiodarone [147, 161].

8.2.4. Implantable cardioverter defibrillator therapy

High-risk markers for mortality in ARVC/D include the history of syncope, sustained VT, severe RV dysfunction, and LV involvement [173–175]. ICD is the only treatment option that has been shown to reduce mortality. Over a 4-year follow-up period, the survival benefit of ICD implantation was about 25% in one study [176]. In a recent meta-analysis, the estimated annual mortality rate of patients with ARVC/D, who underwent ICD implantation, was 0.9%, significantly lower than those without ICDs [177]. A similar finding was noted in a large cohort of ARVC/D patients and family members where SCD during follow-up occurred more frequently among index-patients without an ICD (16% vs. 0.6%) [178]. The American College of Cardiology, American Heart Association and the European Society of Cardiology recommend ICD implantation for ARCV/D patients with high-risk features [179]. ICD Implantation is recommended in ARVC/D patients who have experienced hemodynamically unstable VT, sustained VT or VF (class I). Also, ICD implantation is recommended in ARVC/D patients with severe RV systolic dysfunction, LV systolic dysfunction or both (Class I). ICD implantation should be considered in ARVC/D patients who have experienced hemodynamically stable, sustained VT or who have "major" risk factors such as unexplained syncope, moderate ventricular dysfunction, or NSVT (Class IIa) [147] (**Figure 9**).

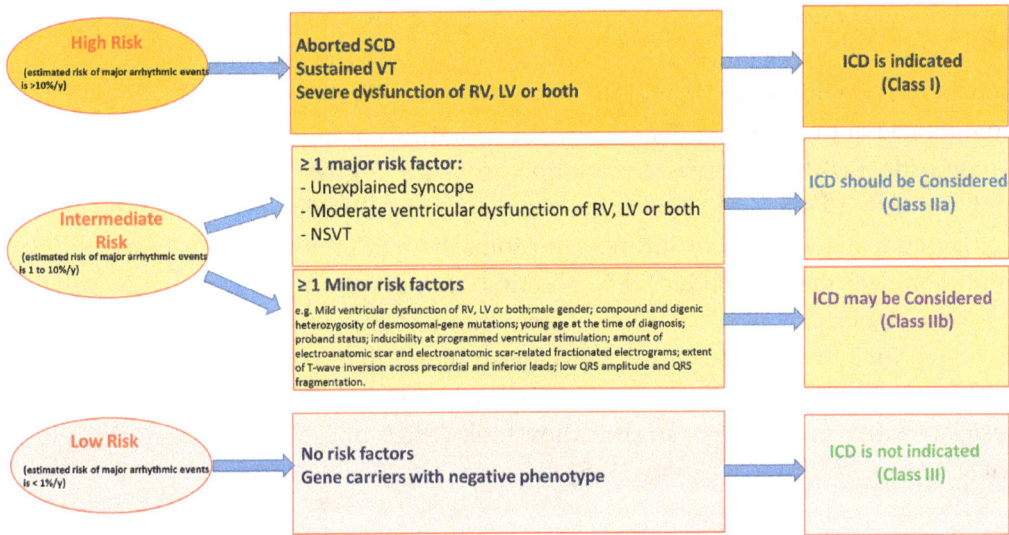

Figure 9. Indications for ICD in ARVC/D patients based on risk stratification. Modified with permission from Corrado et al. [147].

8.2.5. Surgical interventions

8.2.5.1. Heart transplantation

Heart transplantation is recommended as a final therapeutic option in ARVC/D patients with either severe, unresponsive congestive heart failure or recurrent episodes of VT/VF, which are refractory to catheter (and surgical) ablation and/or ICD therapy in experienced centers [147].

The most common indication for heart transplantation in ARVC/D patients is the progression of heart failure followed by intractable VTs [180]. Survival rates after 1-year post-heart transplant after were 94% and at an average follow-up of 6.2 ± 4.8 year it was 88%. In a recent study involving a large cohort of ARVC/D patients, the need for cardiac transplantation was 4% [178].

8.2.5.2. Other surgical therapies

There is currently no clinical role for surgical therapies such as beating heart cryoablation [181], RV disarticulation [182], RV cardiomyoplasty [183], and left cardiac sympathetic denervation [184] in the treatment of patients with ARVC/D.

9. Family screening

ARVC/D is a familial disease and screening the family of affected individuals is important. All first-degree family members of the affected individual should be screened for ARVC/D. Screening should begin during the teenage years unless otherwise indicated. Screening tests include ECG, signal-averaged ECG, Holter monitoring, echocardiogram, exercise stress test, and cardiac MRI. If a pathogenic mutation is identified in an ARVC/D patient, parents, siblings, and children of this patient can be tested for the mutation via the cascade method. In a recent study that looked at this matter it was found that one-third of family members fulfill conventional diagnostic Task Force criteria. Siblings are at the highest risk of disease even after correcting for age and sex, and an accurate prediction of ARVC/D diagnosis among relatives can be obtained using a model including symptoms, being a sibling, the presence of a pathogenic mutation, and female gender [185]. Meeting Task Force criteria independent of family history had a higher prognostic value for arrhythmic events than conventional Task Force criteria, which include family history. It was also noted that arrhythmic risk prediction is improved by applying modified Task Force criteria that exclude family history. This provides the physician with a reliable risk stratification tool, which does not require a difficult management scheme or additional testing [185].

10. Conclusions

ARVC/D is a rare cardiac disease characterized by fibrofatty replacement of myocardial tissue. It affects the RV primarily, but an extension to the LV in more advanced stages of the disease may occur. At the molecular level, both ventricles are affected, presumably in all stages of the disease. Its prevalence has been estimated to vary from 1:2000 to 1:5000. Patients typically present between the second and the fourth decade of life with VT episodes originating from the RV. It is also a major cause of SCD in the young patients and athletes.

The ARVC/D is an inherited cardiomyopathy and the causative genes encode proteins of mechanical cell junctions (e.g., plakoglobin, plakophilin-2, desmoglein-2, desmocollin-2, and desmoplakin) accounting for intercalated disk remodeling. The mode of inherence is mostly an autosomal dominant trait with variable penetrance. The rare recessively inherited variants are often associated with palmoplantar keratoderma and wooly hair. The diagnosis is made according to the modified Task Force criteria, based on functional and structural alterations of the RV, depolarization and repolarization abnormalities, fibrofatty replacement in the endomyocardial biopsy, VT with LBBB morphology, and family history. The use of the Task Force criteria helps to avoid under an overdiagnosis of the disease. Echocardiography and cardiac magnetic resonance imaging (MRI) are the main imaging tools to visualize structural and functional abnormalities. The ARVC/D should be differentiated from other cardiac diseases such as idiopathic RVOT-VT and myocarditis. ARVC/D therapy consists of lifestyle changes, antiarrhythmic drugs, and catheter ablation. Young age at diagnosis, family history of juvenile SCD, LV involvement, VT, syncope, and previous cardiac arrest are the major risk factors for adverse prognosis. Implantable cardioverter defibrillator (ICD) therapy has been demonstrated to affect positively patients' mortality, and it should be considered in all high-risk patients. Heart transplantation may be required in about 4% of the ARVC/D patients. Ongoing research is focused on the understanding of disease pathophysiology and providing a curative therapy that may be able to stop disease progression.

Acknowledgements

The author would like to express his appreciation to Ms. Sandra Keating and Mrs. Suzanne Tobias for editing the manuscript of this book chapter.

Author details

Bandar Al-Ghamdi

Address all correspondence to: balghamdi@kfshrc.edu.sa

Heart Centre, King Faisal Specialist Hospital and Research Centre, Alfaisal University, Riyadh, Saudi Arabia

References

[1] Frank R, Fontaine G, Vedel J, Mialet G, Sol C, Guiraudon G, Grosgogeat Y. Electrocardiologie de quatre cas de dysplasie ventriculaire droite arythmogène (Electrocardiology of 4 cases of right ventricular dysplasia inducing arrhythmia) [Article in French]. Arch Mal Coeur Vaiss. 1978 Sep;71(9):963–972.

[2] Marcus FI, Fontaine GH, Guiraudon G, Frank R, Laurenceau JL, Malergue C, Grosgeat Y. Right ventricular dysplasia: a report of 24 adult cases. Circulation. 1982 Feb; 65(2):384-398. DOI:10.1161/01.CIR.65.2.384.

[3] Corrado D, Basso C, Thiene G, McKenna WJ, Davies MJ, Fontaliran F, Nava A, Silvestri F, Blomstrom-Lundqvist C, Wlodarska EK, Fontaine G, Camerini F. Spectrum of clinicopathologic manifestations of arrhythmogenic right ventricular cardiomyopathy/dysplasia: a multicenter study. J Am Coll Cardiol. 1997 Nov 15;30(6):1512–1520. DOI:10.1016/S0735-1097(97)00332-X.

[4] Basso C, Thiene G, Corrado D, Angelini A, Nava A, Valente M. Arrhythmogenic right ventricular cardiomyopathy: dysplasia, dystrophy, or myocarditis? Circulation. 1996 Sep 1;94(5):983–991. DOI:10.1161/01.CIR.94.5.983.

[5] Thiene G, Nava A, Corrado D, Rossi L, Pennelli N. Right ventricular cardiomyopathy and sudden death in young people. N Engl J Med. 1988 Jan 21;318(3):129–133. DOI: 10.1056/NEJM198801213180301.

[6] Richardson P, McKenna W, Bristow M, Maisch B, Mautner B, O'Connell J, Olsen E, Thiene G, Goodwin J, Gyarfas I, Martin I, Nordet P. Report of the 1995 World Health Organization/International Society and Federation of Cardiology

Task Force on the Definition and Classification of cardiomyopathies. Circulation. 1996 Mar 1;93(5):841–842. DOI:10.1161/01.CIR.93.5.841.

[7] Lazzarini E, Jongbloed JD, Pilichou K, Thiene G, Basso C, Bikker H, Charbon B, Swertz M, van Tintelen JP, van der Zwaag PA. The ARVD/C genetic variants database: 2014 update.Hum Mutat. 2015 Apr;36(4):403–410. DOI:10.1002/humu.22765.

[8] McKoy G, Protonotarios N, Crosby A, Tsatsopoulou A, Anastasakis A, Coonar A, Norman M, Baboonian C, Jeffery S, McKenna WJ. Identification of a deletion in plakoglobin in arrhythmogenic right ventricular cardiomyopathy with palmoplantar keratoderma and woolly hair (Naxos disease). Lancet. 2000 Jun 17;355(9221):2119–2124. DOI:10.1016/S0140-6736(00)02379-5.

[9] Norgett EE, Hatsell SJ, Carvajal-Huerta L, Cabezas JC, Common J, Purkis PE, Whittock N, Leigh IM, Stevens HP, Kelsell DP. Recessive mutation in desmoplakin disrupts desmoplakin-intermediate filament interactions and causes dilated cardiomyopathy, woolly hair and keratoderma. Hum Mol Genet. 2000 Nov 1;9(18):2761–2766. DOI: 10.1093/hmg/9.18.2761.

[10] Gemayel C, Pelliccia A, Thompson PD. Arrhythmogenic right ventricular cardiomy-opathy. J Am Coll Cardiol. 2001;38(7):1773–1781. DOI:10.1016/S0735-1097(01)01654-0.

[11] Corrado D, Thiene G. Arrhythmogenic right ventricular cardiomyopathy/dysplasia: clinical impact of molecular genetic studies. Circulation. 2006;113(13):1634–1637. DOI: 10.1161/CIRCULATIONAHA.105.616490.

[12] Al-Ghamdi B, Shafquat A, Mallawi Y.Arrhythmogenic right ventricular cardiomyop-athy/dysplasia in Saudi Arabia: a single-center experience with long-term follow-up. Ann Saudi Med. 2014 Sep-Oct;34(5):415–426. DOI:10.5144/0256-4947.2014.415.

[13] Dalal D, Nasir K, Bomma C, Prakasa K, Tandri H, Piccini J, Roguin A, Tichnell C, James C, Russell SD, Judge DP, Abraham T, Spevak PJ, Bluemke DA, Calkins H. Arrhythmo-genic right ventricular dysplasia: a United States experience. Circulation. 2005;112:3823–3832. DOI:10.1161/CIRCULATIONAHA.105.542266.

[14] Corrado D, Fontaine G, Marcus FI, McKenna WJ, Nava A, Thiene G, Wichter T. Arrhythmogenic right ventricular dysplasia/cardiomyopathy: need for an international registry. Study Group on Arrhythmogenic Right Ventricular Dysplasia/Cardiomyop-athy of the Working Groups on Myocardial and Pericardial Disease and Arrhythmias of the European Society of Cardiology and of the Scientific Council on Cardiomyopa-thies of the World Heart Federation. Circulation. 2000 Mar 21;101(11):E101-6. DOI: 10.1161/01.CIR.101.11.e101.

[15] Corrado D, Basso C, Schiavon M, Thiene G. Screening for hypertrophic cardiomyop-athy in young athletes. N Engl J Med. 1998;339(6):364–369. DOI:10.1056/ NEJM199808063390602.

[16] Shen WK, Edwards WD, Hammill SC, Gersh BJ. Right ventricular dysplasia: a need for precise pathological definition for interpretation of sudden death (abstr). J Am Coll Cardiol. 1994; 23(Suppl):34A.

[17] Romero J, Mejia-Lopez E, Manrique C, Lucariello R. Arrhythmogenic right ventricular cardiomyopathy (ARVC/D): a systematic literature review. Clin Med Insights Cardiol. 2013 May 21;7:97–114. DOI:10.4137/CMC.S10940.

[18] Cheng TO. Ethnic differences in arrhythmogenic right ventricular dysplasia/cardio-myopathy. Int J Cardiol. 2002;83(3):293.Author reply 291. DOI:10.1016/S0167-5273(02)00068-2.

[19] Basso C, Corrado D, Marcus FI, Nava A, Thiene G. Arrhythmogenic right ventricular cardiomyopathy. Lancet. 2009;373:1289–300. DOI:10.1016/S0140-6736(09)60256-7.

[20] Mertens C, Kuhn C, Franke WW. Plakophilins 2a and 2b: constitutive proteins of dual location in the karyoplasm and the desmosomal plaque. J Cell Biol. 1996;135:1009–1025. DOI:10.1083/jcb.135.4.1009.

[21] Gerull B, Heuser A, Wichter T, Paul M, Basson CT, McDermott DA, Lerman BB, Markowitz SM, Ellinor PT, MacRae CA, Peters S, Grossmann KS, Drenckhahn J, Michely B, Sasse-Klaassen S, Birchmeier W, Dietz R, Breithardt G, Schulze-Bahr E, Thierfelder L. Mutations in the desmosomal protein plakophilin-2 are common in arrhythmogenic right ventricular cardiomyopathy. Nat Genet. 2004 Nov;36(11):1162–1164. Erratum in: Nat Genet. 2005 Jan;37(1):106. DOI:10.1038/ng1461.

[22] Syrris P, Ward D, Asimaki A, Sen-Chowdhry S, Ebrahim HY, Evans A, Hitomi N, Norman M, Pantazis A, Shaw AL, Elliott PM, McKenna WJ. Clinical expression of plakophilin-2 mutations in familial arrhythmogenic right ventricular cardiomyopathy. Circulation. 2006 Jan 24;113(3):356–364. DOI:10.1161/CIRCULATIONAHA.105.561654.

[23] Kannankeril PJ, Bhuiyan ZA, Darbar D, Mannens MM, Wilde AA, Roden DM. Arrhythmogenic right ventricular cardiomyopathy due to a novel plakophilin 2 mutation: wide spectrum of disease in mutation carriers within a family. Heart Rhythm. 2006;3:939–944. DOI:10.1016/j.hrthm.2006.04.028.

[24] van der Zwaag PA, Cox MG, van der Werf C, Wiesfeld AC, Jongbloed JD, Dooijes D, Bikker H, Jongbloed R, Suurmeijer AJ, van den Berg MP, Hofstra RM, Hauer RN, Wilde AA, van Tintelen JP. Recurrent and founder mutations in the Netherlands: plakophilin-2 p.Arg79X mutation causing arrhythmogenic right ventricular cardiomyopathy/dysplasia. Neth Heart J. 2010 Dec;18(12):583–591. DOI:10.1007/s12471-010-0839-5.

[25] Li Mura IE, Bauce B, Nava A, Fanciulli M, Vazza G, Mazzotti E, Rigato I, De Bortoli M, Beffagna G, Lorenzon A, Calore M, Dazzo E, Nobile C, Mostacciuolo ML, Corrado D, Basso C, Daliento L, Thiene G, Rampazzo A. Identification of a PKP2 gene deletion in a family with arrhythmogenic right ventricular cardiomyopathy. Eur J Hum Genet. 2013 Nov;21(11):1226–1231. DOI:10.1038/ejhg.2013.39.

[26] Zhou X, Chen M, Song H, Wang B, Chen H, Wang J, Wang W, Feng S, Zhang F, Ju W, Li M, Gu K, Cao K, Wang DW, Yang B. Comprehensive analysis of desmosomal gene mutations in Han Chinese patients with arrhythmogenic right ventricular cardiomyopathy. Eur J Med Genet. 2015 Apr;58(4):258–265. DOI:10.1016/j.ejmg.2015.02.009.

[27] van Tintelen JP, Entius MM, Bhuiyan ZA, Jongbloed R, Wiesfeld AC, Wilde AA, van der Smagt J, Boven LG, Mannens MM, van Langen IM, Hofstra RM, Otterspoor LC, Doevendans PA, Rodriguez LM, van Gelder IC, Hauer RN. Plakophilin-2 mutations are the major determinant of familial arrhythmogenic right ventricular dysplasia/cardiomyopathy. Circulation. 2006 Apr 4;113(13):1650–1658. DOI:10.1161/CIRCULA-TIONAHA.105.609719.

[28] Groeneweg JA, van der Zwaag PA, Olde Nordkamp LR, Bikker H, Jongbloed JD, Jongbloed R, Wiesfeld AC, Cox MG, van der Heijden JF, Atsma DE, de Boer K, Doevendans PA, Vink A, van Veen TA, Dooijes D, van den Berg MP, Wilde AA, van Tintelen JP, Hauer RN. Arrhythmogenic right ventricular dysplasia/cardiomyopathy according to revised 2010 task force criteria with inclusion of non-desmosomal phospholamban mutation carriers. Am J Cardiol. 2013 Oct 15;112(8):1197–206. DOI:10.1016/j.amjcard.2013.06.017.

[29] Al-Ghamdi B, Alhassnan Z, Al-Fayyadh M, Shafquat A, Manea W, Alhadeq F, Rababh M, Mallawi Y. Clinical and genetic characteristics of arrhythmogenic right ventricular cardiomyopathy/dysplasia patients in Saudi Arabia: a single centre experience. In: Cardiostim-EHRA Europace; 8–11 June 2016; Nice, France: Europace. June 2016;16:Supp 1.

[30] Antoniades L, Tsatsopoulou A, Anastasakis A, Syrris P, Asimaki A, Panagiotakos D, Zambartas C, Stefanadis C, McKenna WJ, Protonotarios N. Arrhythmogenic right ventricular cardiomyopathy caused by deletions in plakophilin-2 and plakoglobin (Naxos disease) in families from Greece and Cyprus: genotype-phenotype relations, diagnostic features and prognosis. Eur Heart J. 2006 Sep;27(18):2208–2216. DOI:10.1093/eurheartj/ehl184.

[31] Cox MG, van der Zwaag PA, van der Werf C, van der Smagt JJ, Noorman M, Bhuiyan ZA, Wiesfeld AC, Volders PG, van Langen IM, Atsma DE, Dooijes D, van den Wijngaard A, Houweling AC, Jongbloed JD, Jordaens L, Cramer MJ, Doevendans PA, de Bakker JM, Wilde AA, van Tintelen JP, Hauer RN.Arrhythmogenic right ventricular dysplasia/cardiomyopathy: pathogenic desmosome mutations in index-patients predict outcome of family screening: Dutch arrhythmogenic right ventricular dysplasia/cardiomyopathy genotype-phenotype follow-up study. Circulation. 2011 Jun 14;123(23):2690–2700. DOI:10.1161/CIRCULATIONAHA.110.988287.

[32] Lahtinen AM, Lehtonen E, Marjamaa A, Kaartinen M, Heliö T, Porthan K, Oikarinen L, Toivonen L, Swan H, Jula A, Peltonen L, Palotie A, Salomaa V, Kontula K. Population-prevalent desmosomal mutations predisposing to arrhythmogenic right ventricular

cardiomyopathy. Heart Rhythm. 2011 Aug;8(8):1214–1221. DOI:10.1016/j.hrthm. 2011.03.015.

[33] Sen-Chowdhry S, Syrris P, Ward D, Asimaki A, Sevdalis E, McKenna WJ. Clinical and genetic characterization of families with arrhythmogenic right ventricular dysplasia/ cardiomyopathy provides novel insights into patterns of disease expression. Circulation. 2007 Apr 3;115(13):1710–1720. DOI:10.1161/CIRCULATIONAHA.106.660241.

[34] van Tintelen JP, Hofstra RM, Wiesfeld AC, van den Berg MP, Hauer RN, Jongbloed JD. Molecular genetics of arrhythmogenic right ventricular cardiomyopathy: emerging horizon? Curr Opin Cardiol. 2007 May;22(3):185–192. DOI:10.1097/HCO. 0b013e3280d942c4.

[35] Awad MM, Calkins H, Judge DP. Mechanisms of disease: molecular genetics of arrhythmogenic right ventricular dysplasia/cardiomyopathy. Nat Clin Pract Cardiovasc Med. 2008 May;5(5):258–267. DOI:10.1038/ncpcardio1182.

[36] den Haan AD, Tan BY, Zikusoka MN, Lladó LI, Jain R, Daly A, Tichnell C, James C, Amat-Alarcon N, Abraham T, Russell SD, Bluemke DA, Calkins H, Dalal D, Judge DP. Comprehensive desmosome mutation analysis in North Americans with arrhythmogenic right ventricular dysplasia/cardiomyopathy. Circ Cardiovasc Genet. 2009 Oct; 2(5):428–435. DOI:10.1161/CIRCGENETICS.109.858217.

[37] Bauce B, Nava A, Beffagna G, Basso C, Lorenzon A, Smaniotto G, De Bortoli M, Rigato I, Mazzotti E, Steriotis A, Marra MP, Towbin JA, Thiene G, Danieli GA, Rampazzo A. Multiple mutations in desmosomal proteins encoding genes in arrhythmogenic right ventricular cardiomyopathy/dysplasia. Heart Rhythm. 2010 Jan;7(1):22–29. DOI: 10.1016/j.hrthm.2009.09.070.

[38] Fressart V, Duthoit G, Donal E, Probst V, Deharo JC, Chevalier P, Klug D, Dubourg O, Delacretaz E, Cosnay P, Scanu P, Extramiana F, Keller D, Hidden-Lucet F, Simon F, Bessirard V, Roux-Buisson N, Hebert JL, Azarine A, Casset-Senon D, Rouzet F, Lecarpentier Y, Fontaine G, Coirault C, Frank R, Hainque B, Charron P. Desmosomal gene analysis in arrhythmogenic right ventricular dysplasia/cardiomyopathy: spectrum of mutations and clinical impact in practice. Europace. 2010 Jun;12(6):861–868. DOI: 10.1093/europace/euq104.

[39] Gerull B. Skin-heart connection: what can the epidermis tell us about the myocardium in arrhythmogenic cardiomyopathy? Circ Cardiovasc Genet. 2014 Jun;7(3):225–227. DOI:10.1161/CIRCGENETICS.114.000647.

[40] Brun F, Barnes CV, Sinagra G, Slavov D, Barbati G, Zhu X, Graw SL, Spezzacatene A, Pinamonti B, Merlo M, Salcedo EE, Sauer WH, Taylor MR, Mestroni L. Titin and desmosomal genes in the natural history of arrhythmogenic right ventricular cardiomyopathy. J Med Genet. 2014 Oct;51(10):669–676. DOI: 10.1136/jmedgenet-2014-102591.

[41] Cerrone M, Lin X, Zhang M, Agullo-Pascual E, Pfenniger A, Chkourko Gusky H, Novelli V, Kim C, Tirasawadichai T, Judge DP, Rothenberg E, Chen HS, Napolitano C,

Priori SG, Delmar M. Missense mutations in plakophilin-2 cause sodium current deficit and associate with a Brugada syndrome phenotype. Circulation. 2014 Mar 11;129(10): 1092–103. DOI:10.1161/CIRCULATIONAHA.113.003077.

[42] Cerrone M, Delmar M. Desmosomes and the sodium channel complex: implications for arrhythmogenic cardiomyopathy and Brugada syndrome. Trends Cardiovasc Med. 2014 Jul;24(5):184–190. DOI:10.1016/j.tcm.2014.02.001

[43] Arnemann J, Spurr NK, Wheeler GN, Parker AE, Buxton RS. Chromosomal assignment of the human genes coding for the major proteins of the desmosome junction, desmo-glein DGI (DSG), desmocollins DGII/III (DSC), desmoplakins DPI/II (DSP), and plakoglobin DPIII (JUP). Genomics. 1991 Oct;10(3):640–645. DOI:10.1016/0888-7543(91)90446-L.

[44] Bornslaeger EA, Corcoran CM, Stappenbeck TS, Green KJ. Breaking the connection: displacement of the desmosomal plaque protein desmoplakin from cell-cell interfaces disrupts anchorage of intermediate filament bundles and alters intercellular junction assembly. J Cell Biol. 1996 Aug;134(4):985–1001. DOI:10.1083/jcb.134.4.985.

[45] Carvajal-Huerta L. Epidermolytic palmoplantar keratoderma with woolly hair and dilated cardiomyopathy. J Am Acad Dermatol. 1998 Sep;39(3):418–421. DOI:10.1016/s0190-9622(98)70317-2.

[46] Rampazzo A, Nava A, Malacrida S, Beffagna G, Bauce B, Rossi V, Zimbello R, Simionati B, Basso C, Thiene G, Towbin JA, Danieli GA. Mutation in human desmoplakin domain binding to plakoglobin causes a dominant form of arrhythmogenic right ventricular cardiomyopathy. Am J Hum Genet. 2002 Nov;71(5):1200–1206. DOI:10.1086/344208.

[47] Alcalai R, Metzger S, Rosenheck S, Meiner V, Chajek-Shaul T. A recessive mutation in desmoplakin causes arrhythmogenic right ventricular dysplasia, skin disorder, and woolly hair. J Am Coll Cardiol. 2003 Jul 16;42(2):319–327. DOI:10.1016/s0735-1097(03)00628-4.

[48] Uzumcu A, Norgett EE, Dindar A, Uyguner O, Nisli K, Kayserili H, Sahin SE, Dupont E, Severs NJ, Leigh IM, Yuksel-Apak M, Kelsell DP, Wollnik B. Loss of desmoplakin isoform I causes early onset cardiomyopathy and heart failure in a Naxos-like syn-drome. J Med Genet. 2006 Feb;43(2):e5. DOI:10.1136/jmg.2005.032904.

[49] van der Zwaag PA, Jongbloed JD, van den Berg MP, van der Smagt JJ, Jongbloed R, Bikker H, Hofstra RM, van Tintelen JP. A genetic variants database for arrhythmogenic right ventricular dysplasia/cardiomyopathy. Hum Mutat. 2009 Sep;30(9):1278–1283. DOI:10.1002/humu.21064.

[50] Al-Jassar C, Knowles T, Jeeves M, Kami K, Behr E, Bikker H, Overduin M, Chidgey M. The nonlinear structure of the desmoplakin plakin domain and the effects of cardio-myopathy-linked mutations. J Mol Biol. 2011 Sep 2;411(5):1049–1061. DOI:10.1016/j.jmb.2011.06.047.

[51] Whittock NV, Ashton GH, Dopping-Hepenstal PJ, Gratian MJ, Keane FM, Eady RA, McGrath JA. Striate palmoplantar keratoderma resulting from desmoplakin haploin-sufficiency. J Invest Dermatol. 1999 Dec;113(6):940–946. DOI:10.1046/j.1523-1747.1999.00783.x.

[52] Arnemann J, Spurr NK, Magee AI, Buxton RS. The human gene (DSG2) coding for HDGC, a second member of the desmoglein subfamily of the desmosomal cadherins, is, like DSG1 coding for desmoglein DGI, assigned to chromosome 18. Genomics. 1992 Jun;13(2):484–446. DOI:10.1016/0888-7543(92)90280-6.

[53] Pilichou K, Nava A, Basso C, Beffagna G, Bauce B, Lorenzon A, Frigo G, Vettori A, Valente M, Towbin J, Thiene G, Danieli GA, Rampazzo A. Mutations in desmoglein-2 gene are associated with arrhythmogenic right ventricular cardiomyopathy. Circulation. 2006 Mar;113(9):1171–1179. DOI:10.1161/CIRCULATIONAHA.105.583674.

[54] Posch MG, Posch MJ, Geier C, Erdmann B, Mueller W, Richter A, Ruppert V, Pankuweit S, Maisch B, Perrot A, Buttgereit J, Dietz R, Haverkamp W, Ozcelik C. A missense variant in desmoglein-2 predisposes to dilated cardiomyopathy. Mol Genet Metab. 2008 Sep-Oct;95(1-2):74–80. DOI:10.1016/j.ymgme.2008.06.005.

[55] Amagai M, Wang Y, Minoshima S, Kawamura K, Green KJ, Nishikawa T, Shimizu N. Assignment of the human genes for desmocollin 3 (DSC3) and desmocollin 4 (DSC4) to chromosome 18q12. Genomics. 1995 Jan;25(1):330–332. DOI:10.1016/0888-7543(95)80154-E.

[56] Syrris P, Ward D, Evans A, Asimaki A, Gandjbakhch E, Sen-Chowdhry S, McKenna WJ. Arrhythmogenic right ventricular dysplasia/cardiomyopathy associated with muta-tions in the desmosomal gene desmocollin-2. Am J Hum Genet. 2006 Nov;79(5):978–984. DOI:10.1086/509122.

[57] Heuser A, Plovie ER, Ellinor PT, Grossmann KS, Shin JT, Wichter T, Basson CT, Lerman BB, Sasse-Klaassen S, Thierfelder L, MacRae CA, Gerull B. Mutant desmocollin-2 causes arrhythmogenic right ventricular cardiomyopathy. Am J Hum Genet. 2006 Dec;79(6): 1081–1088. DOI:10.1086/509044.

[58] Groeneweg JA, van der Zwaag PA, Jongbloed JD, Cox MG, Vreeker A, de Boer RA, van der Heijden JF, van Veen TA, McKenna WJ, van Tintelen JP, Dooijes D, Hauer RN. Left-dominant arrhythmogenic cardiomyopathy in a large family: associated desmosomal or nondesmosomal genotype? Heart Rhythm. 2013 Apr;10(4):548–559. DOI:10.1016/j.hrthm.2012.12.020.

[59] Asimaki A, Syrris P, Wichter T, Matthias P, Saffitz JE, McKenna WJ. A novel dominant mutation in plakoglobin causes arrhythmogenic right ventricular cardiomyopathy. Am J Hum Genet. 2007 Nov;81(5):964–973. DOI:10.1086/521633.

[60] Protonotarios N, Tsatsopoulou A, Patsourakos P. Cardiac abnormalities in familial palmoplantar keratosis. Br Heart J. 1986 Oct;56(4):321–326.

[61] Protonotarios N, Tsatsopoulou A, Fontaine G. Naxos disease: keratoderma, scalp modifications, and cardiomyopathy. J Am Acad Dermatol. 2001 Feb;44(2):309–311. DOI: 10.1067/mjd.2001.110648.

[62] Marian AJ. On the diagnostic utility of junction plakoglobin in arrhythmogenic right ventricular cardiomyopathy. Cardiovasc Pathol. 2013 Sep-Oct;22(5):309–311. DOI: 10.1016/j.carpath.2013.05.002.

[63] McNally E, MacLeod H, Dellefave-Castillo L. Arrhythmogenic right ventricular dysplasia/cardiomyopathy. In: Pagon RA, Adam MP, Ardinger HH, Wallace SE, Amemiya A, Bean LJH, Bird TD, Fong CT, Mefford HC, Smith RJH, Stephens K, editors. GeneReviews® [Internet]. Seattle, WA: University of Washington, Seattle; 1993–2016. 2005 Apr 18 [Updated 2014 Jan 9]. Available from: http://www.ncbi.nlm.nih.gov/books/ NBK1131/ [Accessed: 2016-07-20]

[64] Sen-Chowdhry S, Syrris P, McKenna WJ. Role of genetic analysis in the management of patients with arrhythmogenic right ventricular dysplasia/cardiomyopathy. J Am Coll Cardiol. 2007 Nov 6;50(19):1813–1821.DOI:10.1016/j.jacc.2007.08.008.

[65] Tiso N, Stephan DA, Nava A, Bagattin A, Devaney JM, Stanchi F, Larderet G, Brahmb-hatt B, Brown K, Bauce B, Muriago M, Basso C, Thiene G, Danieli GA, Rampazzo A. Identification of mutations in the cardiac ryanodine receptor gene in families affected with arrhythmogenic right ventricular cardiomyopathy type 2 (ARVD2). Hum Mol Genet. 2001 Feb 1;10(3):189–194. DOI:10.1093/hmg/10.3.189.

[66] Bauce B, Rampazzo A, Basso C, Bagattin A, Daliento L, Tiso N, Turrini P, Thiene G, Danieli GA, Nava A. Screening for ryanodine receptor type 2 mutations in families with effort-induced polymorphic ventricular arrhythmias and sudden death: early diagno-sis of asymptomatic carriers. J Am Coll Cardiol. 2002 Jul 17;40(2):341–349. DOI:10.1016/ S0735-1097(02)01946-0.

[67] Priori SG, Napolitano C, Tiso N, Memmi M, Vignati G, Bloise R, Sorrentino V, Danieli GA. Mutations in the cardiac ryanodine receptor gene (hRyR2) underlie catecholami-nergic polymorphic ventricular tachycardia. Circulation. 2001 Jan 16;103(2):196–200. DOI:10.1161/01.CIR.103.2.196.

[68] Priori SG, Napolitano C, Memmi M, Colombi B, Drago F, Gasparini M, DeSimone L, Coltorti F, Bloise R, Keegan R, Cruz Filho FE, Vignati G, Benatar A, DeLogu A. Clinical and molecular characterization of patients with catecholaminergic polymorphic ventricular tachycardia. Circulation. 2002 Jul 2;106(1):69–74. DOI:10.1161/01.CIR. 0000020013.73106.D8.

[69] Laitinen PJ, Brown KM, Piippo K, Swan H, Devaney JM, Brahmbhatt B, Donarum EA, Marino M, Tiso N, Viitasalo M, Toivonen L, Stephan DA, Kontula K. Mutations of the cardiac ryanodine receptor (RyR2) gene in familial polymorphic ventricular tachycar-dia. Circulation. 2001 Jan 30;103(4):485–490. DOI:10.1161/01.CIR.103.4.485.

[70] Laitinen PJ, Swan H, Kontula K. Molecular genetics of exercise-induced polymorphic ventricular tachycardia: identification of three novel cardiac ryanodine receptor

mutations and two common calsequestrin 2 amino-acid polymorphisms. Eur J Hum Genet. 2003 Nov;11(11):888–891. DOI:10.1038/sj.ejhg.5201061.

[71] Leask A, Abraham DJ. TGF-beta signaling and the fibrotic response. FASEB J. 2004 May; 18(7):816–827. DOI:10.1096/fj.03-1273rev.

[72] Beffagna G, Occhi G, Nava A, Vitiello L, Ditadi A, Basso C, Bauce B, Carraro G, Thiene G, Towbin JA, Danieli GA, Rampazzo A. Regulatory mutations in transforming growth factor-beta3 gene cause arrhythmogenic right ventricular cardiomyopathy type 1. Cardiovasc Res. 2005 Feb 1;65(2):366–373. DOI:10.1016/j.cardiores.2004.10.005.

[73] Rampazzo A. Genetic bases of arrhythmogenic right ventricular cardiomyopathy. Heart Int. 2006;2(1):17. DOI:10.4081/hi.2006.17.

[74] Wiemann S, Weil B, Wellenreuther R, Gassenhuber J, Glassl S, Ansorge W, Böcher M, Blöcker H, Bauersachs S, Blum H, Lauber J, Düsterhöft A, Beyer A, Köhrer K, Strack N, Mewes HW, Ottenwälder B, Obermaier B, Tampe J, Heubner D, Wambutt R, Korn B, Klein M, Poustka A. Toward a catalog of human genes and proteins: sequencing and analysis of 500 novel complete protein coding human cDNAs. Genome Res. 2001 Mar; 11(3):422–435. DOI:10.1101/gr.154701.

[75] Merner ND, Hodgkinson KA, Haywood AF, Connors S, French VM, Drenckhahn JD, Kupprion C, Ramadanova K, Thierfelder L, McKenna W, Gallagher B, Morris-Larkin L, Bassett AS, Parfrey PS, Young TL. Arrhythmogenic right ventricular cardiomyopathy type 5 is a fully penetrant, lethal arrhythmic disorder caused by a missense mutation in the TMEM43 gene. Am J Hum Genet. 2008 Apr;82(4):809–821. DOI:10.1016/j.ajhg. 2008.01.010.

[76] Christensen AH, Andersen CB, Tybjaerg-Hansen A, Haunso S, Svendsen JH. Mutation analysis and evaluation of the cardiac localization of TMEM43 in arrhythmogenic right ventricular cardiomyopathy. Clin Genet. 2011 Sep;80(3):256–264. DOI:10.1111/j.1399-0004.2011.01623.x.

[77] Haywood AF, Merner ND, Hodgkinson KA, Houston J, Syrris P, Booth V, Connors S, Pantazis A, Quarta G, Elliott P, McKenna W, Young TL. Recurrent missense mutations in TMEM43 (ARVD5) due to founder effects cause arrhythmogenic cardiomyopathies in the UK and Canada. Eur Heart J. 2013 Apr;34(13):1002–1011. DOI:10.1093/eurheartj/ehs383.

[78] Baskin B, Skinner JR, Sanatani S, Terespolsky D, Krahn AD, Ray PN, Scherer SW, Hamilton RM. TMEM43 mutations associated with arrhythmogenic right ventricular cardiomyopathy in non-Newfoundland populations. Hum Genet. 2013 Nov;132(11): 1245–1252. DOI:10.1007/s00439-013-1323-2.

[79] Pilichou K, Thiene G, Bauce B, Rigato I, Lazzarini E, Migliore F, Perazzolo Marra M, Rizzo S, Zorzi A, Daliento L, Corrado D, Basso C. Arrhythmogenic cardiomyopathy. Orphanet J Rare Dis. 2016;11:33. DOI:10.1186/s13023-016-0407-1.

[80] Mallat Z, Tedgui A, Fontaliran F, Frank R, Durigon M, Fontaine G. Evidence of apoptosis in arrhythmogenic right ventricular dysplasia. N Engl J Med. 1996 Oct 17;335(16):1190–1196. DOI:10.1056/NEJM199610173351604.

[81] Fontaine G, Fontaliran F, Lascault G, Frank R, Tonet J, Chomette G, Grosgogeat Y. Congenital and acquired right ventricular dysplasia [Article in French]. Arch Mal Coeur Vaiss. 1990 Jun;83(7):915–920.

[82] Chimenti C, Pieroni M, Maseri A, Frustaci A. Histologic findings in patients with clinical and instrumental diagnosis of sporadic arrhythmogenic right ventricular dysplasia. J Am Coll Cardiol. 2004 Jun 16;43(12):2305–2313. DOI:10.1016/j.jacc.2003.12.056.

[83] d'Amati G, di Gioia CR, Giordano C, Gallo P. Myocyte transdifferentiation: a possible pathogenetic mechanism for arrhythmogenic right ventricular cardiomyopathy. Arch Pathol Lab Med. 2000 Feb;124(2):287–290. DOI:10.1043/0003-9985(2000)124<0287:MT>2.0.CO;2.

[84] Huber O. Structure and function of desmosomal proteins and their role in development and disease. Cell Mol Life Sci. 2003 Sep;60(9):1872–1890. DOI:10.1007/s00018-003-3050-7.

[85] Garrod D, Chidgey M. Desmosome structure, composition and function. Biochim Biophys Acta. 2008 Mar;1778(3):572–587. DOI:10.1016/j.bbamem.2007.07.014.

[86] Green KJ, Gaudry CA. Are desmosomes more than tethers for intermediate filaments? Nat Rev Mol Cell Biol. 2000 Dec;1(3):208-16. DOI:10.1038/35043032.

[87] Guiraudon CM. Histological diagnosis of right ventricular dysplasia: a role for electron microscopy? Eur Heart J. 1989 Sep;10(Suppl D):95–96. DOI:10.1093/eurheartj/10.suppl_D.95.

[88] Basso C, Czarnowska E, Della Barbera M, Bauce B, Beffagna G, Wlodarska EK, Pilichou K, Ramondo A, Lorenzon A, Wozniek O, Corrado D, Daliento L, Danieli GA, Valente M, Nava A, Thiene G, Rampazzo A. Ultrastructural evidence of intercalated disc remodelling in arrhythmogenic right ventricular cardiomyopathy: an electron microscopy investigation on endomyocardial biopsies. Eur Heart J. 2006 Aug;27(15):1847–1854. DOI:10.1093/eurheartj/ehl095.

[89] Sato PY, Coombs W, Lin X, Nekrasova O, Green KJ, Isom LL, Taffet SM, Delmar M. Interactions between ankyrin-G, Plakophilin-2, and Connexin43 at the cardiac intercalated disc. Circ Res. 2011 Jul 8;109(2):193–201. DOI:10.1161/CIRCRESAHA.111.247023.

[90] Hariharan V, Asimaki A, Michaelson JE, Plovie E, MacRae CA, Saffitz JE, Huang H. Arrhythmogenic right ventricular cardiomyopathy mutations alter shear response without changes in cell-cell adhesion. Cardiovasc Res. 2014 Nov 1;104(2):280–289. DOI:10.1093/cvr/cvu212.

[91] Asimaki A, Tandri H, Huang H, Halushka MK, Gautam S, Basso C, Thiene G, Tsatsopoulou A, Protonotarios N, McKenna WJ, Calkins H, Saffitz JE. A new diagnostic test

for arrhythmogenic right ventricular cardiomyopathy. N Engl J Med. 2009 Mar 12;360(11):1075–1084. DOI:10.1056/NEJMoa0808138.

[92] Garcia-Gras E, Lombardi R, Giocondo MJ, Willerson JT, Schneider MD, Khoury DS, Marian AJ. Suppression of canonical Wnt/beta-catenin signaling by nuclear plakoglobin recapitulates phenotype of arrhythmogenic right ventricular cardiomyopathy. J Clin Invest. 2006 Jul;116(7):2012–2021. DOI:10.1172/JCI27751.

[93] Swope D, Li J, Muller EJ, Radice GL. Analysis of a Jup hypomorphic allele reveals a critical threshold for postnatal viability. Genesis. 2012 Oct;50(10):717–727. DOI:10.1002/dvg.22034.

[94] Simcha I, Shtutman M, Salomon D, Zhurinsky J, Sadot E, Geiger B, Ben-Ze'ev A. Differential nuclear translocation and transactivation potential of beta-catenin and plakoglobin. J Cell Biol. 1998 Jun 15;141(6):1433–1448. DOI:10.1083/jcb.141.6.1433.

[95] Ross SE, Hemati N, Longo KA, Bennett CN, Lucas PC, Erickson RL, MacDougald OA. Inhibition of adipogenesis by Wnt signaling. Science. 2000 Aug 11;289(5481):950–953. DOI:10.1126/science.289.5481.950.

[96] Chen SN, Gurha P, Lombardi R, Ruggiero A, Willerson JT, Marian AJ. The hippo pathway is activated and is a causal mechanism for adipogenesis in arrhythmogenic cardiomyopathy. Circ Res. 2014 Jan 31;114(3):454–468. DOI:10.1161/CIRCRESAHA.114.302810.

[97] Basso C, Bauce B, Corrado D, Thiene G. Pathophysiology of arrhythmogenic cardiomyopathy. Nat Rev Cardiol. 2011 Nov 29;9(4):223–233. DOI:10.1038/nrcardio.2011.173.

[98] Kaplan SR, Gard JJ, Protonotarios N, Tsatsopoulou A, Spiliopoulou C, Anastasakis A, Squarcioni CP, McKenna WJ, Thiene G, Basso C, Brousse N, Fontaine G, Saffitz JE. Remodeling of myocyte gap junctions in arrhythmogenic right ventricular cardiomyopathy due to a deletion in plakoglobin (Naxos disease). Heart Rhythm. 2004 May;1(1): 3–11. DOI:10.1016/j.hrthm.2004.01.001.

[99] Fidler LM, Wilson GJ, Liu F, Cui X, Scherer SW, Taylor GP, Hamilton RM. Abnormal connexin43 in arrhythmogenic right ventricular cardiomyopathy caused by plakophilin-2 mutations. J Cell Mol Med. 2009 Oct;13(10):4219–4228. DOI:10.1111/j.1582-4934.2008.00438.x.

[100] Rizzo S, Lodder EM, Verkerk AO, Wolswinkel R, Beekman L, Pilichou K, Basso C, Remme CA, Thiene G, Bezzina CR. Intercalated disc abnormalities, reduced Na(+) current density, and conduction slowing in desmoglein-2 mutant mice prior to cardiomyopathic changes. Cardiovasc Res. 2012 Sep 1;95(4):409–418. DOI:10.1093/cvr/cvs219.

[101] Cerrone M, Noorman M, Lin X, Chkourko H, Liang FX, van der Nagel R, Hund T, Birchmeier W, Mohler P, van Veen TA, van Rijen HV, Delmar M. Sodium current deficit

and arrhythmogenesis in a murine model of plakophilin-2 haploinsufficiency. Cardio-vasc Res. 2012 Sep 1;95(4):460–468. DOI:10.1093/cvr/cvs218.

[102] Zhang Q, Deng C, Rao F, Modi RM, Zhu J, Liu X, Mai L, Tan H, Yu X, Lin Q, Xiao D, Kuang S, Wu S. Silencing of desmoplakin decreases connexin43/Nav1.5 expression and sodium current in HL-1 cardiomyocytes. Mol Med Rep. 2013 Sep;8(3):780–786. DOI: 10.3892/mmr.2013.1594.

[103] Noorman M, Hakim S, Kessler E, Groeneweg JA, Cox MG, Asimaki A, van Rijen HV, van Stuijvenberg L, Chkourko H, van der Heyden MA, Vos MA, de Jonge N, van der Smagt JJ, Dooijes D, Vink A, de Weger RA, Varro A, de Bakker JM, Saffitz JE, Hund TJ, Mohler PJ, Delmar M, Hauer RN, van Veen TA. Remodeling of the cardiac sodium channel, connexin43, and plakoglobin at the intercalated disk in patients with arrhyth-mogenic cardiomyopathy. Heart Rhythm. 2013 Mar;10(3):412–419. DOI:10.1016/j.hrthm.2012.11.018.

[104] Asimaki A, Kapoor S, Plovie E, Karin Arndt A, Adams E, Liu Z, James CA, Judge DP, Calkins H, Churko J, Wu JC, MacRae CA, Kléber AG, Saffitz JE. Identification of a new modulator of the intercalated disc in a zebrafish model of arrhythmogenic cardiomy-opathy. Sci Transl Med. 2014 Jun 11;6(240):240ra74. DOI:10.1126/scitranslmed.3008008.

[105] Protonotarios N, Tsatsopoulou A. Arrhythmogenic right ventricular cardiomyopathy: clinical forms of the disease. Hellenic J Cardiol. 1998;39(Suppl A):78–80.

[106] Protonotarios N, Tsatsopoulou A. Naxos disease and Carvajal syndrome: cardiocuta-neous disorders that highlight the pathogenesis and broaden the spectrum of arrhyth-mogenic right ventricular cardiomyopathy. Cardiovasc Pathol. 2004 Jul-Aug;13(4):185-94. DOI:10.1016/j.carpath.2004.03.609

[107] Bukhari I, Juma'a N. Naxos disease in Saudi Arabia. J Eur Acad Dermatol Venereol. 2004 Sep;18(5):614-6. DOI:10.1111/j.1468-3083.2004.01010.x.

[108] Protonotarios N, Tsatsopoulou A. Naxos disease: cardiocutaneous syndrome due to cell adhesion defect. Orphanet J Rare Dis. 2006 Mar 13;1:4. DOI:10.1186/1750-1172-1-4

[109] Coonar AS, Protonotarios N, Tsatsopoulou A, Needham EW, Houlston RS, Cliff S, Otter MI, Murday VA, Mattu RK, McKenna WJ. Gene for arrhythmogenic right ventricular cardiomyopathy with diffuse nonepidermolytic palmoplantar keratoderma and woolly hair (Naxos disease) maps to 17q21. Circulation. 1998 May 26;97(20):2049-58.

[110] Protonotarios N, Tsatsopoulou A, Anastasakis A, Sevdalis E, McKoy G, Stratos K, Gatzoulis K, Tentolouris K, Spiliopoulou C, Panagiotakos D, McKenna W, Toutouzas P. Genotype-phenotype assessment in autosomal recessive arrhythmogenic right ventricular cardiomyopathy (Naxos disease) caused by a deletion in plakoglobin. J Am Coll Cardiol. 2001 Nov 1;38(5):1477-84. DOI:10.1016/S0735-1097(01)01568-6

[111] Rao BH, Reddy IS, Chandra KS. Familial occurrence of a rare combination of dilated cardiomyopathy with palmoplantar keratoderma and curly hair. Indian Heart J. 1996 Mar-Apr;48(2):161-2.

[112] Kaplan SR, Gard JJ, Carvajal-Huerta L, Ruiz-Cabezas JC, Thiene G, Saffitz JE. Structural and molecular pathology of the heart in Carvajal syndrome. Cardiovasc Pathol. 2004 Jan-Feb;13(1):26-32. DOI:10.1016/S1054-8807(03)00107-8.

[113] De Pasquale CG, Heddle WF. Left sided arrhythmogenic ventricular dysplasia in siblings. Heart 2001;86:128-130 DOI:10.1136/heart.86.2.128

[114] Collett BA, Davis GJ, Rohr WB. Extensive fibrofatty infiltration of the left ventricle in two cases of sudden cardiac death. J Forensic Sci. 1994 Sep;39(5):1182-7. DOI:10.1520/JFS13703J.

[115] Michalodimitrakis M, Papadomanolakis A, Stiakakis J, Kanaki K. Left side right ventricular cardiomyopathy. Med Sci Law. 2002 Oct;42(4):313-7. DOI:10.1177/00258 0240204200406

[116] Gallo P, d'Amati G, Pelliccia F. Pathologic evidence of extensive left ventricular involvement in arrhythmogenic right ventricular cardiomyopathy. Hum Pathol. 1992 Aug;23(8):948-52.

[117] Sen-Chowdhry S, Syrris P, Prasad SK, Hughes SE, Merrifield R, Ward D, Pennell DJ, McKenna WJ. Left-dominant arrhythmogenic cardiomyopathy: an under-recognized clinical entity. J Am Coll Cardiol. 2008 Dec 16;52(25):2175-87. DOI:10.1016/j.jacc. 2008.09.019.

[118] McKenna WJ, Thiene G, Nava A, Fontaliran F, Blomstrom-Lundqvist C, Fontaine G, and Camerini F. Diagnosis of arrhythmogenic right ventricular dysplasia/cardiomy-opathy. Task Force of the Working Group Myocardial and Pericardial Disease of the European Society of Cardiology and of the Scientific Council on Cardiomyopathies of the International Society and Federation of Cardiology. Br Heart J. 1994 Mar;71(3):215–218.

[119] Marcus FI, McKenna WJ, Sherrill D, Basso C, Bauce B, Bluemke DA, Calkins H, Corrado D, Cox MG, Daubert JP, Fontaine G, Gear K, Hauer R, Nava A, Picard MH, Protonotarios N, Saffitz JE, Sanborn DM, Steinberg JS, Tandri H, Thiene G, Towbin JA, Tsatsopoulou A, Wichter T, Zareba W. Diagnosis of arrhythmogenic right ventricular cardiomyopathy/dysplasia: proposed modification of the task force criteria. Circulation. 2010;121(13):1533-41. DOI:10.1161/CIRCU-LATIONAHA.108.840827. Eur Heart J. 2010 Apr;31(7):806-14. DOI:10.1093/eurheartj/ehq025.

[120] White JB, Razmi R, Nath H, Kay GN, Plumb VJ, Epstein AE. Relative utility of magnetic resonance imaging and right ventricular angiography to diagnose arrhythmogenic right ventricular cardiomyopathy. J Interv Card Electrophysiol. 2004 Feb;10(1):19-26. DOI:10.1023/B:JICE.0000011480.66948.c3

[121] Lindstrom L, Wilkenshoff U, Larsson H, Wranne B. Echocardiographic assessment of arrhythmogenic right ventricular cardiomyopathy. Heart 2001;86:31-38 DOI:10.1136/heart.86.1.31

[122] Marcus FI, Fontaine G. Arrhythmogenic right ventricular dysplasia/cardiomyopathy: a review. Pacing Clin Electrophysiol. 1995 Jun;18(6):1298-314. DOI:10.1111/j.1540-8159.1995.tb06971.x.

[123] Yoerger DM, Marcus F, Sherrill D, Calkins H, Towbin JA, Zareba W, Picard MH. Multidisciplinary Study of Right Ventricular Dysplasia Investigators. Echocardiographic findings in patients meeting task force criteria for arrhythmogenic right ventricular dysplasia: new insights from the multidisciplinary study of right ventricular dysplasia. J Am Coll Cardiol. 2005 Mar 15;45(6):860-5. DOI:10.1016/j.jacc.2004.10.070

[124] Mast TP, Teske AJ, Doevendans PA, Cramer MJ. Current and future role of echocardiography in arrhythmogenic right ventricular dysplasia/cardiomyopathy. Cardiol J. 2015;22(4):362-74. DOI:10.5603/CJ.a2015.0018.

[125] Tandri H, Calkins H, Nasir K, Bomma C, Castillo E, Rutberg J, Tichnell C, Lima JA, Bluemke DA. Magnetic resonance imaging findings in patients meeting task force criteria for arrhythmogenic right ventricular dysplasia. J Cardiovasc Electrophysiol. 2003 May;14(5):476-82. DOI:10.1046/j.1540-8167.2003.02560.x.

[126] American College of Cardiology Foundation Task Force on Expert Consensus Documents, Hundley WG, Bluemke DA, Finn JP, Flamm SD, Fogel MA, Friedrich MG, Ho VB, Jerosch-Herold M, Kramer CM, Manning WJ, Patel M, Pohost GM, Stillman AE, White RD, Woodard PK. ACCF/ACR/AHA/NASCI/SCMR 2010 Expert Consensus Document on Cardiovascular Magnetic Resonance: A Report of the American College of Cardiology Foundation Task Force on Expert Consensus Documents. J Am Coll Cardiol. 2010 Jun 8;55(23):2614-62. DOI:10.1016/j.jacc.2009.11.011.

[127] Tandri H, Friedrich MG, Calkins H, Bluemke DA. MRI of arrhythmogenic right ventricular cardiomyopathy/dysplasia. J Cardiovasc Magn Reson. 2004;6(2):557-63. DOI:10.1081/JCMR-120030583

[128] Van der Wall EE, Kayser HW, Bootsma MM, de Roos A, Schalij MJ. Arrhythmogenic right ventricular dysplasia: MRI findings. Herz. 2000 Jun;25(4):356-64.

[129] Jain A, Tandri H, Calkins H, Bluemke DA. Role of cardiovascular magnetic resonance imaging in arrhythmogenic right ventricular dysplasia. J Cardiovasc Magn Reson. 2008;10(1):32. DOI:10.1186/1532-429X-10-32

[130] Tandri H, Castillo E, Ferrari VA, Nasir K, Dalal D, Bomma C, Calkins H, Bluemke DA. Magnetic resonance imaging of arrhythmogenic right ventricular dysplasia: sensitivity, specificity, and observer variability of fat detection versus functional analysis of the

right ventricle. J Am Coll Cardiol. 2006 Dec 5;48(11):2277-84. DOI:10.1016/j.jacc. 2006.07.051

[131] Corrado D, Basso C, Thiene G. Arrhythmogenic right ventricular cardiomyopathy: diagnosis, prognosis, and treatment. Heart. 2000 May;83(5):588–595. DOI: 10.1136/ heart.83.5.588

[132] Basso C, Ronco F, Marcus F, Abudureheman A, Rizzo S, Frigo AC, Bauce B, Maddalena F, Nava A, Corrado D, Grigoletto F, Thiene G. Quantitative assessment of endomyo-cardial biopsy in arrhythmogenic right ventricular cardiomyopathy/dysplasia: an in vitro validation of diagnostic criteria. Eur Heart J. 2008 Nov;29(22):2760-71. DOI: 10.1093/eurheartj/ehn415.

[133] Fontaine G, Umemura J, Di Donna P, Tsezana R, Cannat JJ, Frank R. Duration of QRS complexes in arrhythmogenic right ventricular dysplasia. A new noninvasive diag-nostic marker [Article in French]. Ann Cardiol Angeiol (Paris). 1993 Oct;42(8):399-405.

[134] Peters S, Trümmel M. Diagnosis of arrhythmogenic right ventricular dysplasia-cardiomyopathy: value of standard ECG revisited. Ann Noninvasive Electrocardiol. 2003 Jul;8(3):238-45. DOI:10.1046/j.1542-474X.2003.08312.x.

[135] Pinamonti B, Sinagra G, Salvi A, Di Lenarda A, Morgera T, Silvestri F, Bussani R, Camerini F. Left ventricular involvement in right ventricular dysplasia. Am Heart J. 1992 Mar;123(3):711-24. DOI:10.1016/0002-8703(92)90511-S.

[136] Cox MG, Nelen MR, Wilde AA, Wiesfeld AC, van der Smagt JJ, Loh P, Cramer MJ, Doevendans PA, van Tintelen JP, de Bakker JM, Hauer RN. Activation delay and VT parameters in arrhythmogenic right ventricular dysplasia/cardiomyopathy: toward improvement of diagnostic ECG criteria. J Cardiovasc Electrophysiol. 2008 Aug;19(8): 775-81. DOI:10.1111/j.1540-8167.2008.01140.x.

[137] Nasir K, Rutberg J, Tandri H, Berger R, Tomaselli G, Calkins H. Utility of SAECG in arrhythmogenic right ventricle dysplasia. Ann Noninvasive Electrocardiol. 2003 Apr; 8(2):112-20. DOI:10.1046/j.1542-474X.2003.08204.x.

[138] Oselladore L, Nava A, Buja G, Turini P, Daliento L, Livolsi B, Thiene G. Signal-averaged electrocardiography in familial form of arrhythmogenic right ventricular cardiomyop-athy. Am J Cardiol. 1995 May 15;75(15):1038-41. DOI:10.1016/S0002-9149(99)80720-6

[139] Turrini P, Angelini A, Thiene G, Buja G, Daliento L, Rizzoli G, Nava A. Late potentials and ventricular arrhythmias in arrhythmogenic right ventricular cardiomyopathy. Am J Cardiol. 1999 Apr 15;83(8):1214-9. DOI:10.1016/S0002-9149(99)00062-4

[140] Nava A, Bauce B, Basso C, Muriago M, Rampazzo A, Villanova C, Daliento L, Buja G, Corrado D, Danieli GA, Thiene G. Clinical profile and long-term follow-up of 37 families with arrhythmogenic right ventricular cardiomyopathy. J Am Coll Cardiol. 2000 Dec;36(7):2226-33. DOI:10.1016/S0735-1097(00)00997-9

[141]   Zareba W, Piotrowicz K, Turrini P. Electrocardiographic manifestations. In: Marcus FI, Nava A, Thiene G, editors. Arrhythmogenic Right Ventricular Dysplasia/Cardiomyopathy, Recent Advances. Milano: Springer Verlag; 2007. p. 121-8.

[142]   Lerman BB, Stein KM, Markowitz SM. Idiopathic right ventricular outflow tract tachycardia: a clinical approach. Pacing Clin Electrophysiol. 1996 Dec;19(12 Pt 1):2120-37. DOI:10.1111/j.1540-8159.1996.tb03287.x.

[143]   Markowitz SM, Litvak BL, Ramirez de Arellano EA, Markisz JA, Stein KM, Lerman BB. Adenosine-sensitive ventricular tachycardia, right ventricular abnormalities delineated by magnetic resonance imaging. Circulation. 1997 Aug 19;96(4):1192-200. DOI: 10.1161/01.CIR.96.4.1192

[144]   Chapelon C, Piette JC, Uzzan B, Coche E, Herson S, Ziza JM, Godeau P. The advantages of histological samples in sarcoidosis. Retrospective multicenter analysis of 618 biopsies performed on 416 patients. Rev Med Interne. 1987 Mar-Apr;8(2):181-5.

[145]   Ladyjanskaia GA, Basso C, Hobbelink MG, Kirkels JH, Lahpor JR, Cramer MJ, Thiene G, Hauer RN, Oosterhout MF V. Sarcoid myocarditis with ventricular tachycardia mimicking ARVD/C. J Cardiovasc Electrophysiol. 2010 Jan;21(1):94-8. DOI:10.1111/j.1540-8167.2009.01479.x.

[146]   Gerlis LM, Schmidt-Ott SC, Ho SY, Anderson RH. Dysplastic conditions of the right ventricular myocardium: Uhl's anomaly vs. arrhythmogenic right ventricular dysplasia. Br Heart J. 1993 Feb;69(2):142–150.

[147]   Corrado D, Wichter T, Link MS, Hauer RN, Marchlinski FE, Anastasakis A, Bauce B, Basso C, Brunckhorst C, Tsatsopoulou A, Tandri H, Paul M, Schmied C, Pelliccia A, Duru F, Protonotarios N, Estes NM 3rd, McKenna WJ, Thiene G, Marcus FI, Calkins H. Treatment of arrhythmogenic right ventricular cardiomyopathy/dysplasia. Circulation. 2015 Aug 4;132(5):441-53. DOI:10.1161/CIRCULATIONAHA.115.017944.

[148]   Dalal D, Jain R, Tandri H, Dong J, Eid SM, Prakasa K, Tichnell C, James C, Abraham T, Russell SD, Sinha S, Judge DP, Bluemke DA, Marine JE, Calkins H. Long-term efficacy of catheter ablation of ventricular tachycardia in patients with arrhythmogenic right ventricular dysplasia/cardiomyopathy. J Am Coll Cardiol. 2007 Jul 31;50(5):432-40. DOI: 10.1016/j.jacc.2007.03.049

[149]   Satomi K, Kurita T, Suyama K, Noda T, Okamura H, Otomo K, Shimizu W, Aihara N, Kamakura S. Catheter ablation of stable and unstable ventricular tachycardias in patients with arrhythmogenic right ventricular dysplasia. J Cardiovasc Electrophysiol. 2006 May;17(5):469-76. DOI:10.1111/j.1540-8167.2006.00434.x.

[150]   Verma A, Kilicaslan F, Schweikert RA, Tomassoni G, Rossillo A, Marrouche NF, Ozduran V, Wazni OM, Elayi SC, Saenz LC, Minor S, Cummings JE, Burkhardt JD, Hao S, Beheiry S, Tchou PJ, Natale A. Short- and long-term success of substrate-based mapping and ablation of ventricular tachycardia in arrhythmogenic right ventricular

dysplasia. Circulation. 2005 Jun 21;111(24):3209-16. DOI:10.1161/CIRCULATIONAHA.104.510503

[151] Reithmann C, Hahnefeld A, Remp T, Dorwarth U, Dugas M, Steinbeck G, Hoffmann E. Electroanatomic mapping of endocardial right ventricular activation as a guide for catheter ablation in patients with arrhythmogenic right ventricular dysplasia. Pacing Clin Electrophysiol. 2003 Jun;26(6):1308-16. DOI:10.1046/j.1460-9592.2003.t01-1-00188.x.

[152] Ellison KE, Friedman PL, Ganz LI, Stevenson WG. Entrainment mapping and radio-frequency catheter ablation of ventricular tachycardia in right ventricular dysplasia. J Am Coll Cardiol. 1998 Sep;32(3):724-8. DOI:10.1016/S0735-1097(98)00292-7

[153] Corrado D, Basso C, Pavei A, Michieli P, Schiavon M, Thiene G. Trends in sudden cardiovascular death in young competitive athletes after implementation of a preparticipation screening program. JAMA. 2006 Oct 4;296(13):1593-601. DOI:10.1001/jama.296.13.1593

[154] Corrado D, Thiene G, Nava A, Rossi L, Pennelli N. Sudden death in young competitive athletes: clinicopathologic correlations in 22 cases. Am J Med. 1990 Nov;89(5):588-96. DOI:10.1016/0002-9343(90)90176-E.

[155] Corrado D, Basso C, Rizzoli G, Schiavon M, Thiene G. Does sports activity enhance the risk of sudden death in adolescents and young adults? J Am Coll Cardiol. 2003 Dec 3;42(11):1959-63. DOI:10.1016/j.jacc.2003.03.002

[156] James CA, Bhonsale A, Tichnell C, Murray B, Russell SD, Tandri H, Tedford RJ, Judge DP, Calkins H. Exercise increases age-related penetrance and arrhythmic risk in arrhythmogenic right ventricular dysplasia/cardiomyopathy-associated desmosomal mutation carriers. J Am Coll Cardiol. 2013 Oct 1;62(14):1290-7. DOI:10.1016/j.jacc.2013.06.033.

[157] Saberniak J, Hasselberg NE, Borgquist R, Platonov PG, Sarvari SI, Smith HJ, Ribe M, Holst AG, Edvardsen T, Haugaa KH. Vigorous physical activity impairs myocardial function in patients with arrhythmogenic right ventricular cardiomyopathy and in mutation positive family members. Eur J Heart Fail. 2014 Dec;16(12):1337-44. DOI:10.1002/ejhf.181.

[158] Wichter T, Hindricks G, Lerch H, Bartenstein P, Borggrefe M, Schober O, Breithardt G. Regional myocardial sympathetic dysinnervation in arrhythmogenic right ventricular cardiomyopathy. An analysis using ^{123}I-metaiodobenzylguanidine scintigraphy. Circulation. 1994 Feb;89(2):667–683. DOI:10.1161/01.CIR.89.2.667

[159] Wichter T, Schäfers M, Rhodes CG, Borggrefe M, Lerch H, Lammertsma AA, Hermansen F, Schober O, Breithardt G, Camici PG. Abnormalities of cardiac sympathetic innervation in arrhythmogenic right ventricular cardiomyopathy: quantitative assessment of presynaptic norepinephrine reuptake and postsynaptic beta-adrenergic

receptor density with positron emission tomography. Circulation. 2000 Apr 4;101(13): 1552-8. DOI:10.1161/01.CIR.101.13.1552

[160] Wlodarska EK, Wozniak O, Konka M, Rydlewska-Sadowska W, Biederman A, Hoffman P. Thromboembolic complications in patients with arrhythmogenic right ventricular dysplasia/cardiomyopathy. Europace. 2006 Aug;8(8):596-600. DOI:10.1093/europace/eul053

[161] Ermakov S, Scheinman M. Arrhythmogenic right ventricular cardiomyopathy – antiarrhythmic therapy. Arrhythm Electrophysiol Rev. 2015 Aug;4(2):86-9. DOI: 10.15420/aer.2015.04.02.86.

[162] Nogami A, Sugiyasu A, Tada H, Kurosaki K, Sakamaki M, Kowase S, Oginosawa Y, Kubota S, Usui T, Naito S. Changes in the isolated delayed component as an endpoint of catheter ablation in arrhythmogenic right ventricular cardiomyopathy: predictor for long-term success. J Cardiovasc Electrophysiol. 2008 Jul;19(7):681-8. DOI:10.1111/j.1540-8167.2008.01104.x.

[163] Breithardt G, Wichter T, Haverkamp W, Borggrefe M, Block M, Hammel D, Scheld HH. Implantable cardioverter defibrillator therapy in patients with arrhythmogenic right ventricular cardiomyopathy, long QT syndrome, or no structural heart disease. Am Heart J. 1994 Apr;127(4 Pt 2):1151-8.DOI:10.1016/0002-8703(94)90103-1

[164] Wichter T, Borggrefe M, Haverkamp W, Chen X, Breithardt G. Efficacy of antiarrhythmic drugs in patients with arrhythmogenic right ventricular disease. Results in patients with inducible and noninducible ventricular tachycardia. Circulation. 1992 Jul;86(1): 29-37. DOI:10.1161/01.CIR.86.1.29

[165] Wichter T, Borggrefe M, Bocker D. Prevention of sudden cardiac death in arrhythmogenic right ventricular cardiomyopathy. In: Aliot E, Clementy J, Prystowsky EN, editors. Fighting Sudden Cardiac Death: A Worldwide Challenge. New York: Futura Publishing Company. 2000. p. 275–95.

[166] Marcus GM, Glidden DV, Polonsky B, Zareba W, Smith LM, Cannom DS, Estes NA 3rd, Marcus F, Scheinman MM; Multidisciplinary Study of Right Ventricular Dysplasia Investigators. Efficacy of antiarrhythmic drugs in arrhythmogenic right ventricular cardiomyopathy: a report from the North American ARVC Registry. J Am Coll Cardiol. 2009 Aug 11;54(7):609-15. DOI:10.1016/j.jacc.2009.04.052.

[167] Ermakov S, Hoffmayer KS, Gerstenfeld EP, Scheinman MM. Combination drug therapy for patients with intractable ventricular tachycardia associated with right ventricular cardiomyopathy. Pacing Clin Electrophysiol. 2014 Jan;37(1):90-4. DOI:10.1111/pace.12250.

[168] Leclercq JF, Coumel P. Characteristics, prognosis and treatment of the ventricular arrhythmias of right ventricular dysplasia. Eur Heart J. 1989 Sep;10 Suppl D:61-7. DOI: 10.1093/eurheartj/10.suppl_D.61

[169] Tonet J, Frank R, Fontaine G, Grosgogeat Y. Efficacy of the combination of low doses of beta-blockers and amiodarone in the treatment of refractory ventricular tachycardia [Article in French]. Arch Mal Coeur Vaiss. 1989 Sep;82(9):1511–1517.

[170] Bai R, Di Biase L, Shivkumar K, Mohanty P, Tung R, Santangeli P, Saenz LC, Vacca M, Verma A, Khaykin Y, Mohanty S, Burkhardt JD, Hongo R, Beheiry S, Dello Russo A, Casella M, Pelargonio G, Santarelli P, Sanchez J, Tondo C, Natale A. Ablation of ventricular arrhythmias in arrhythmogenic right ventricular dysplasia/cardiomyopathy: arrhythmia-free survival after endoepicardial substrate based mapping and ablation. Circ Arrhythm Electrophysiol 2011 Aug;4(4):478–485. DOI:10.1161/CIRCEP. 111.963066.

[171] Garcia FC, Bazan V, Zado ES, Ren JF, Marchlinski FE. Epicardial substrate and outcome with epicardial ablation of ventricular tachycardia in arrhythmogenic right ventricular cardiomyopathy/dysplasia. Circulation. 2009 Aug 4;120(5):366–375. DOI:10.1161/ CIRCULATIONAHA.108.834903.

[172] Sacher F, Roberts-Thomson K, Maury P, Tedrow U, Nault I, Steven D, Hocini M, Koplan B, Leroux L, Derval N, Seiler J, Wright MJ, Epstein L, Haissaguerre M, Jais P, Stevenson WG. Epicardial ventricular tachycardia ablation a multicenter safety study. J Am Coll Cardiol. 2010 May 25;55(21):2366–2372. DOI:10.1016/j.jacc.2009.10.084.

[173] Wichter T, Paul TM, Eckardt L, Gerdes P, Kirchhof P, Böcker D, Breithardt G. Arrhythmogenic right ventricular cardiomyopathy: antiarrhythmic drugs, catheter ablation, or ICD. Herz. 2005 Mar;30(2):91–101. DOI:10.1007/s00059-005-2677-6.

[174] Peters S, Peters H, Thierfelder L. Risk stratification of sudden cardiac death and malignant ventricular arrhythmias in right ventricular dysplasia-cardiomyopathy. Int J Cardiol. 1999 Dec 1;71(3):243–250. DOI:10.1016/S0167-5273(99)00142-4.

[175] Lemola K, Brunckhorst C, Helfenstein U, Oechslin E, Jenni R, Duru F. Predictors of adverse outcome in patients with arrhythmogenic right ventricular dysplasia/cardiomyopathy: long-term experience of a tertiary care centre. Heart. 2005 Sep;91(9):1167–1172. DOI:10.1136/hrt.2004.038620.

[176] Corrado D, Leoni L, Link MS, Della Bella P, Gaita F, Curnis A, Salerno JU, Igidbashian D, Raviele A, Disertori M, Zanotto G, Verlato R, Vergara G, Delise P, Turrini P, Basso C, Naccarella F, Maddalena F, Estes NA 3rd, Buja G, Thiene G. Implantable cardioverter defibrillator therapy for prevention of sudden death in patients with arrhythmogenic right ventricular cardiomyopathy/dysplasia. Circulation. 2003 Dec 23;108(25):3084–3091. DOI:10.1161/01.CIR.0000103130.33451.D2.

[177] Schinkel AF. Implantable cardioverter defibrillators in arrhythmogenic right ventricular dysplasia/cardiomyopathy: patient outcomes, incidence of appropriate and inappropriate interventions, and complications. Circ Arrhythm Electrophysiol. 2013 Jun;6(3):562–568. DOI:10.1161/CIRCEP.113.000392.

[178] Groeneweg JA, Bhonsale A, James CA, te Riele AS, Dooijes D, Tichnell C, Murray B, Wiesfeld AC, Sawant AC, Kassamali B, Atsma DE, Volders PG, de

Groot NM, de Boer K, Zimmerman SL, Kamel IR, van der Heijden JF, Russell SD, Jan Cramer M, Tedford RJ, Doevendans PA, van Veen TA, Tandri H, Wilde AA, Judge DP, van Tintelen JP, Hauer RN. Calkins H. Clinical presentation, long-term follow-up, and outcomes of 1001 arrhythmogenic right ventricular dysplasia/cardiomyopathy patients and family members. Circ Cardiovasc Genet. 2015 Jun;8(3):437–446. DOI:10.1161/CIRCGENETICS.114.001003.

[179] European Heart Rhythm Association; Heart Rhythm Society, Zipes DP, Camm AJ, Borggrefe M, Buxton AE, Chaitman B, Fromer M, Gregoratos G, Klein G, Moss AJ, Myerburg RJ, Priori SG, Quinones MA, Roden DM, Silka MJ, Tracy C, Smith SC Jr, Jacobs AK, Adams CD, Antman EM, Anderson JL, Hunt SA, Halperin JL, Nishimura R, Ornato JP, Page RL, Riegel B, Priori SG, Blanc JJ, Budaj A, Camm AJ, Dean V, Deckers JW, Despres C, Dickstein K, Lekakis J, McGregor K, Metra M, Morais J, Osterspey A, Tamargo JL, Zamorano JL; American College of Cardiology; American Heart Association Task Force; European Society of Cardiology Committee for Practice Guidelines. ACC/AHA/ESC 2006 guidelines for management of patients with ventricular arrhythmias and the prevention of sudden cardiac death: a report of the American College of Cardiology/American Heart Association Task Force and the European Society of Cardiology Committee for Practice Guidelines (Writing Committee to Develop Guidelines for Management of Patients With Ventricular Arrhythmias and the Prevention of Sudden Cardiac Death). J Am Coll Cardiol. 2006 Sep 5;48(5):e247–346. DOI: 10.1016/j.jacc.2006.07.010.

[180] Tedford RJ, James C, Judge DP, Tichnell C, Murray B, Bhonsale A, Philips B, Abraham T, Dalal D, Halushka MK, Tandri H, Calkins H, Russell SD. Cardiac transplantation in arrhythmogenic right ventricular dysplasia/cardiomyopathy. J Am Coll Cardiol. 2012 Jan 17;59(3):289–290. DOI:10.1016/j.jacc.2011.09.051.

[181] Bakir I, Brugada P, Sarkozy A, Vandepitte C, Wellens F. A novel treatment strategy for therapy refractory ventricular arrhythmias in the setting of arrhythmogenic right ventricular dysplasia. Europace. 2007 May;9(5):267–269. DOI:10.1093/europace/eum029.

[182] Zacharias J, Forty J, DOIg JC, Bourke JP, Hilton CJ. Right ventricular disarticulation. An 18-year single centre experience. Eur J Cardiothorac Surg. 2005 Jun;27(6):1000–1004. DOI:10.1016/j.ejcts.2005.02.020.

[183] Chachques JC, Argyriadis PG, Fontaine G, Hebert JL, Frank RA, D'Attellis N, Fabiani JN, Carpentier AF. Right ventricular cardiomyoplasty: 10-year follow-up. Ann Thorac Surg. 2003 May;75(5):1464–1468. DOI:10.1016/S0003-4975(02)04823-3.

[184] Coleman MA, Bos JM, Johnson JN, Owen HJ, Deschamps C, Moir C, Ackerman MJ. Videoscopic left cardiac sympathetic denervation for patients with recurrent ventricular fibrillation/malignant ventricular arrhythmia syndromes besides congenital long-QT syndrome. Circ Arrhythm Electrophysiol. 2012 Aug 1;5(4):782–788. DOI:10.1161/CIRCEP.112.971754.

[185] Te Riele AS, James CA, Groeneweg JA, Sawant AC, Kammers K, Murray B, Tichnell C, van der Heijden JF, Judge DP, Dooijes D, van Tintelen JP, Hauer RN, Calkins H, Tandri H. Approach to family screening in arrhythmogenic right ventricular dysplasia/cardiomyopathy. Eur Heart J. 2016 Mar 1;37(9):755–763. DOI:10.1093/eurheartj/ehv387.

[186] Que D, Yang P, Song X, Liu L. Traditional vs. genetic pathogenesis of arrhythmogenic right ventricular cardiomyopathy. Europace Apr 2015.

[187] Thiene G, Corrado and D, Basso C. Arrhythmogenic right ventricular cardiomyopathy/dysplasia. Orphanet J Rare Dis. 2007. 2:45 DOI:10.1186/1750-1172-2-45.

5

Pathophysiology in Heart Failure

Kaan Kırali, Tanıl Özer and Mustafa Mert Özgür

Abstract

Heart failure syndrome is defined as the inability of the heart to deliver adequate blood to the body to meet end-organ metabolic needs and oxygenation at rest or during mild exercise. Myocardial dysfunction can be defined as systolic and/or diastolic, acute or chronic, compensated or uncompensated, or uni- or biventricular. Several counter-regulatory mechanisms are activated depending on the duration of the heart failure. Neurohormonal reflexes such as sympathetic adrenergic system, renin-angiotensin cascade, and renal and peripheral alterations attempt to restore both cardiac output and end-tissue perfusion. An adequate stroke volume cannot be ejected from the left ventricle, which shifts the whole pressure-volume relationship to the right (systolic failure). Adequate filling cannot be realized due to diastolic stiffness, which shifts the diastolic pressure-volume curve upward without affecting the systolic pressure-volume curve (diastolic failure). Left ventricular heart failure is the dominant picture of heart failure syndrome, but the right heart can develop isolated failure as well. Biventricular failure is mostly an end-stage clinical situation of the heart failure syndrome. More recently, the rise in the incidence of right ventricular failure can be seen after the implantation of a left ventricular assist device. This chapter clarifies and presents pathophysiologic alterations in heart failure syndrome.

Keywords: heart failure, systolic dysfunction, diastolic dysfunction, myocardial stiffness, ventricular dilatation, neurohormonal, renin-angiotensin, norepinephrine

Heart failure is an epidemic contributing considerably to the overall cost of health care in developed and also developing countries. Heart failure syndrome (HFS) is the currently accepted term describing a systemic disease affecting several organs, creating high morbidity and mortality rates due to the heart's inability to supply oxygenated blood, including metabolites, to end organs and peripheral tissues (**Table 1**) [1]. Acute event or acute refractory form of chronic heart failure can be fatal, whereas chronic prognosis is characterized by terminal congestive heart failure symptoms. The failing heart strives to balance "preload" and "afterload" for compensation of impaired contractility and to deter the development of congestion using a myriad of mechanisms.

---

(1) Activated feedback signals from peripheral reflex circuit

   a. Inflammation

   b. Anabolic blunting (proteolysis)

   c. Insulin resistance (>50% reducing normal anabolic responses)

   d. Oxygen radical accumulation

(2) Global metabolic imbalance (increased catabolic/anabolic imbalance)

(3) Systemic dysregulation of several hormonal pathways

(4) Multi-organ dysfunction (hyperbilirubinemia, uremia, anemia, hypoalbuminemia, etc.)

(5) Development of sarcopenia and cachexia

Table 1. Heart failure syndrome as a multisystem disease.

1. Left heart failure

Left heart failure (LHF), with any structural and/or functional cardiac abnormalities, is a complex clinical state characterized by left ventricular pump dysfunction and related clinical symptoms (dyspnea, fatigue, exercise intolerance, etc.), including signs of volume overload (pulmonary crackles, peripheral edema, etc.) [2]. All steps of energy extraction, transfer, and utilization are affected, with metabolic failure being the important underlying pathophysiologic mechanism causing first myocardial and then systemic decompensation [3]. The pathophysiologic state perpetuates the progression of the failure, regardless of the precipitating event via several compensatory mechanisms. Compensatory mechanisms exist on every level of this scenario to restrain the clinical symptoms via correction of the global imbalance between the catabolic and anabolic status; however, they can lead to further myocardial deterioration and worsening HFS.

The most important classification of LHF is dependent on whether the left ventricular ejection fraction (LVEF) is reduced or preserved. The standard relationship between intracavitary volume and pressure values is affected in heart failure, and left ventricular pressure-volume curves change according to the failure type (**Figure 1**). In systolic LHF, an adequate stroke volume cannot be sustained due to reduced ventricular systolic contractile function, which shifts the whole pressure-volume relationships to the right. In diastolic LHF, an adequate filling cannot be realized due to diastolic stiffness (poor ventricular compliance, impaired relaxation, worsened end-diastolic pressure), which shifts the diastolic pressure-volume curve upward; however, the systolic pressure-volume curve does not change.

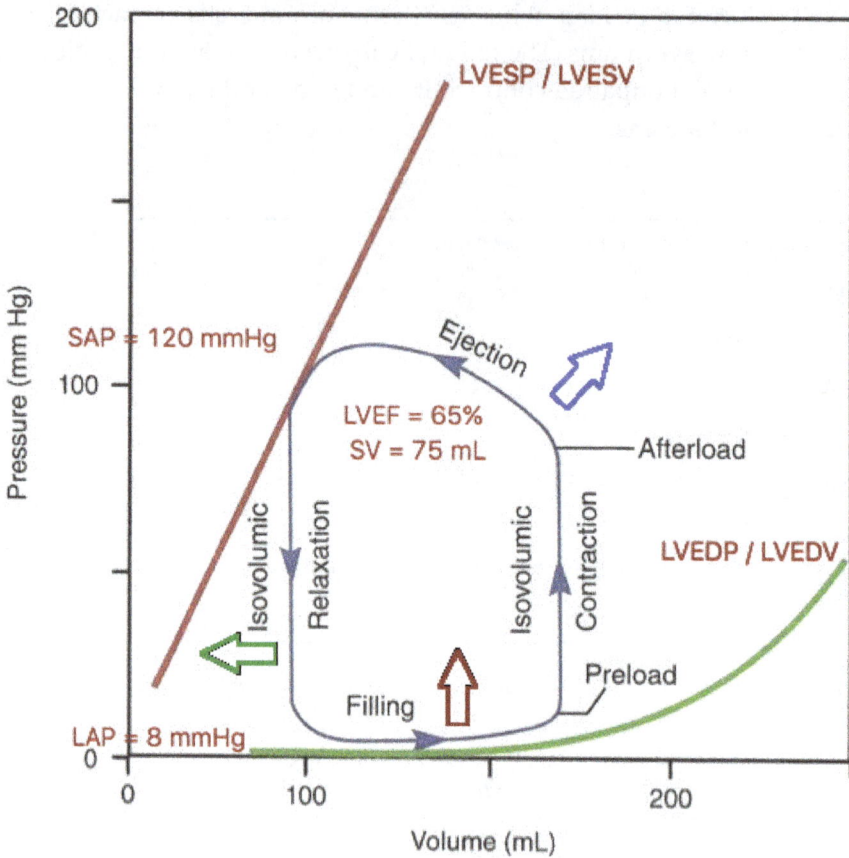

Figure 1. Left ventricular pressure-volume relationships: the green line represents the diastolic pressure-volume relationship, and the red line represents the end-systolic pressure-volume relationship. Both curves are shifted to the right in dilated CMP (blue arrow), to the left in hypertrophic CMP (green arrow), and only diastolic curve is shifted upward in restrictive CMP (red arrow). CMP, cardiomyopathy; LAP, left atrial pressure; LVEDP, left ventricular end-diastolic pressure; LVEDV, left ventricular end-diastolic volume; LVEF, left ventricular ejection fraction; LVESP, left ventricular end-systolic pressure; LVESV, left ventricular end-systolic volume; SAP, systolic aortic pressure; SV, stroke volume.

From asymptomatic to symptomatic stages, several counterregulatory mechanisms are activated (**Table 2**). First, inadequate stroke volume induces sympathetic nervous system activation, which increases cardiac contractile frequency and strength. This chronotropic effect leads to enhancement of total stroke volume per minute via increasing heart rate frequency, but this positive effect is reversed after tachycardia reaches a threshold of 140–150 beats/min (**Figure 2**). The next step is the augmentation of intravascular volume via neurohormonal system activation, which results in increasing intravascular volume, enlarging ventricular chambers, and improvement in myocardial fiber tension [4]. The inotropic effect via the Frank-Starling mechanism increases myocardial contraction power, but this positive effect reverses after the sarcomere length reaches the upper limit of 2.2 μm (**Figure 3**). At this stage, no physiologic mechanism can improve the contractility, stroke volume, and cardiac decompensation, and the left ventricle (LV) undergoes progressive alterations from reversible cellular to irreversible myocardial remodeling. The heart is a self-renewing organ, characterized by an increase in myocyte turnover rate during pathological stress, especially in heart failure. The turnover mechanism becomes overwhelmed by a faster loss of myocytes, and this unfavorable imbalance causes the progression of ventricular remodeling during heart failure.

(a) Activation of neurohormonal systems

(b) Increasing preload to help to sustain cardiac performance

(c) Myocardial cell regeneration and apoptosis

(d) Myocardial hypertrophy and/or ventricular dilatation

(e) Compensation of symptoms

(f) Irreversible myocardial remodeling

(g) Decompensation of clinic status

(h) End-stage multi-organ dysfunction

Table 2. Step-by-step counterregulatory actions during ventricular failure.

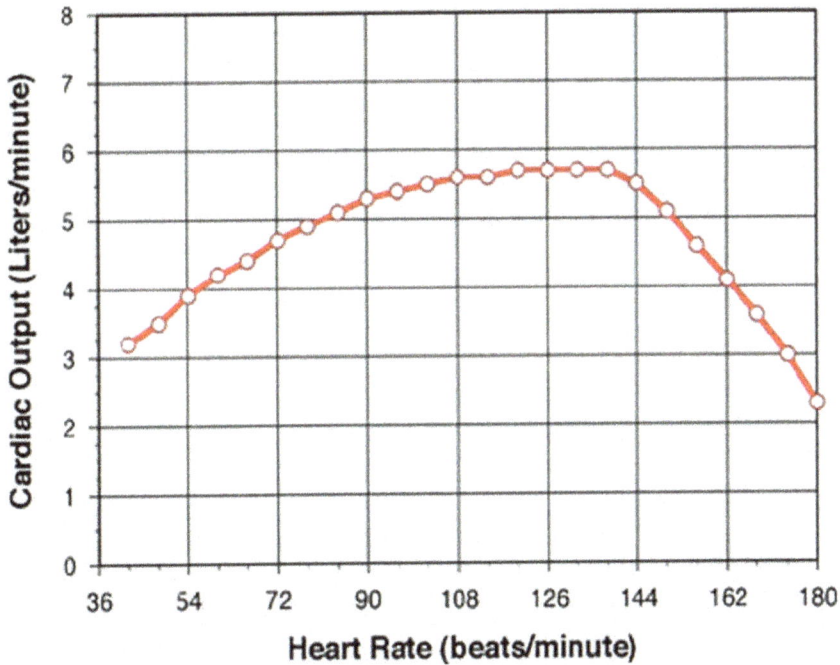

Figure 2. Relationship between cardiac output and heart rate (chronotropy; Bowditch effect).

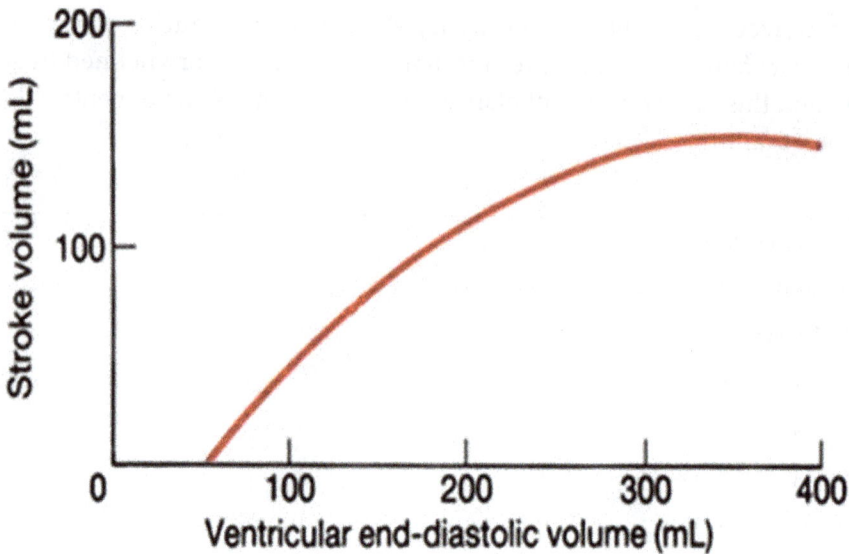

Figure 3. Relation between cardiac output and left ventricular filling (inotropy; Frank-Starling effect).

1.1. Morphological changes

Any of the cardiac pathology causing myocardial dysfunction results in abnormal myocyte growth, with a resultant cascade of gene activation stimulating cardiac remodeling. The hallmarks of cardiac remodeling are myocardial cell hypertrophy and cardiac dilatation with increased interstitial matrix formation. This compensatory mechanism to preserve contraction capability shifts to a maladaptive process after a cutoff level and contributes to the worsening of heart failure during myocardial degenerative progression. Progressive necrotic, apoptotic, or autophagic myocyte loss may contribute to worsening cardiac dysfunction and left ventricular remodeling. Changes within the extracellular matrix such as fibrillary collagen synthesis and degradation, loss of collagen struts, and collagen cross-linking characterize subsequent myocardial adaptation during cardiac remodeling. Cardiac fibroblasts are transformed into myofibroblasts and migrate into the area surrounding injured tissues to secrete collagen and restrict the injured site by scar formation (myocardial fibrosis).

Extracellular matrix requires myocytes to take appropriate position during the cardiac cycles and allows the opening of capillary vessels. Cardiac mitochondria are the main structure to generate energy, in the form of adenosine triphosphate (ATP), through oxidative phosphorylation and to continue cardiac function. Therefore, mitochondrial dysfunction is the major determinant for the development of heart failure via activation of cell death caused by excessive production of reactive oxygen radicals. In the early stage of left ventricular hypertrophy, the number of cardiac myocytes with preserved cellular organization increases; however, they are larger than normal due to the growing number of myofibrils and mitochondria, as well as the large size of the mitochondria and nuclei. Myocytes also increase autophagic activity in order to maintain ATP levels, to sustain contractile function during these demanding nutritional and energy-consuming phases. Mitophagy is a critical mitochondrial quality control mechanism in myocytes, whereas damaged mitochondria and autophagosomes are selectively sequestered and broken down. This process helps to prevent oxidative damage or myocardial stress under baseline conditions, whereas impaired or dysregulated mitophagy is a major contributor to the development and progression of heart failure [5]. Inhibiting autophagy reduces ATP levels and exacerbates remodeling, whereas enhancing autophagy mitigates remodeling and cardiac dysfunction. The hemodynamic and neurohormonal alterations cause an increase in cytosolic calcium entry, which augments myocardial contractility; on the other hand, it impairs the lusitropic effect and leads to increased myocardial energy consumption resulting in further reduction of cardiac function.

Long-standing hypertrophy disrupts cellular organization, such as enlarged nuclei with myofibril displacement. Additionally, some collagen lytic enzymes (matrix metalloproteinase) activated by neurohormonal substances can create progressive degradation of extracellular matrix. In late stages, the pathologic progress is characterized by myocytolysis, a disruption of sarcomeres and Z-bands. In the chronic phase, some components increase and cause myocyte death, creating perivascular fibrosis within intramuscular vessels. This process causes fibrillary collagen to fill the place of dead myocytes. Ultimately, the disruption of mechanical power by the damaged myocytes becomes detrimental, and the left ventricular wall becomes thinner and dilated.

1.2. Neuroendocrine changes

The pathophysiology of LHF is characterized by hemodynamic abnormalities resulting in autonomic nervous system imbalance and neurohormonal activation. Alterations in receptor activation cause an autonomic imbalance with increased sympathetic activity and diminished vagal activity, both of which may have profound effects on cardiac function and structure. Neurohormonal alterations act as a complex and combined compensatory mechanism to support and maintain tissue perfusion during the HFS (**Table 3**). However, these neurohormonal responses become maladaptive due to uncontrollable activation and promote progression of heart failure. The main sympathetic neurohormones are norepinephrine (noradrenaline) and angiotensin II, which act in an autocrine (myocardial synthesis) and paracrine (endocrine synthesis) manner.

1.2.1. Autonomic nervous system

Sympathetic (adrenergic) and parasympathetic (cholinergic) nerve systems are controlled by the central nervous system and are in balance in healthy individuals, where sympathetic activation is lower at rest, as well as in the normal heart [6]. Baroreceptors at the aortic arch and carotid sinuses, as well as mechanoreceptors at the cardiopulmonary tract, sense arterial wall tension and produce afferent signals resulting in a significant increase of excitatory (sympathetic) impulses via norepinephrine or inhibitory (parasympathetic) impulses via acetylcholine (**Figure 4**). Chemoreceptors at the peripheral vessels and metaboreceptors in the muscles sense acid-base balance and oxygenation of the blood and produce afferent signals resulting in a significant increase of sympathetic stimulation (the excitatory impulse). Mechanical and

chemical changes like hypoxia, hypotension, or acid-base imbalance are sensed by receptors, creating a feedback cascade to maintain cardiovascular homeostasis. In the case of heart
failure, the first response of sympathetic nervous system activation is the increasing release
and decreasing uptake of norepinephrine at the adrenergic nerve endings. In response, the
parasympathetic receptor activity becomes dysfunctional by the increased sympathetic stimulation, which in turn leads to increasing systemic vascular resistance and heart rate.

---

(1) Sympathetic nervous system

(2) Renin-angiotensin system

(3) Neurohormonal alterations of renal function

  (a) Arginine vasopressin

  (b) Natriuretic peptides

(4) Neurohormonal alterations in the peripheral vasculature

  (a) Vasoconstrictors

    (i) Endothelin

    (ii) Neuropeptide Y

    (iii) Urotensin II

    (iv) Thromboxane A_2

  (b) Vasodilators

    (i) Nitric oxide

    (ii) Bradykinin

    (iii) Adrenomedullin

    (iv) Prostaglandins (PGI_2 and PGE_2)

    (v) Adipokines

(5) Remodeling factors

  (a) Tumor necrosis factor

  (b) Soluble ST2

  (c) Growth differentiation factor (GDF)-15

  (d) Gelectin-3

(6) Interleukin activation

(7) Anabolic metabolism dysfunctions

  (a) Insulin resistance

  (b) Growth hormone resistance

  (c) Anabolic steroid resistance

Table 3. Neuroendocrine responses.

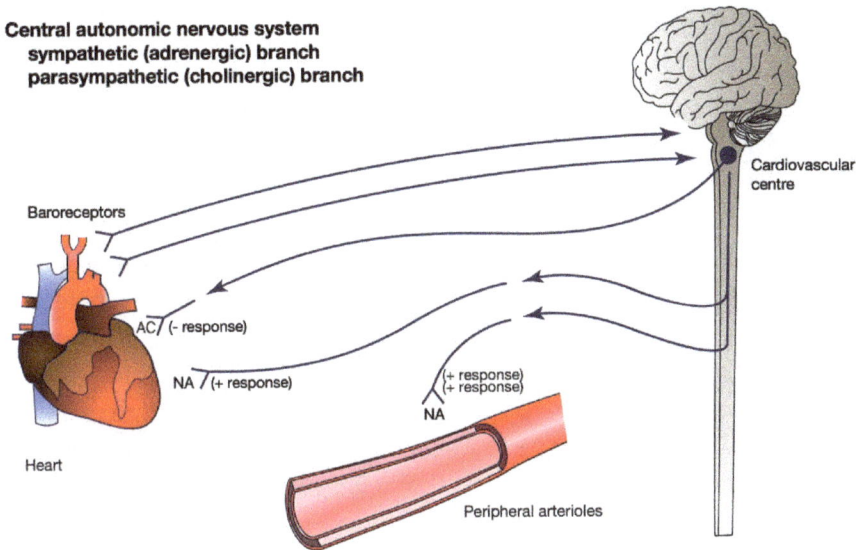

Figure 4. Autonomic nervous system function.

In the HFS, sympathetic stimulation affects several key organs to maintain cardiac output, especially the heart, the kidney, and the peripheral vasculature. Increased sympathetic activity (1) augments ventricular contractility and heart rate to sustain stroke volume, (2) stimulates efferent arteriole vasoconstriction and proximal tubular sodium reabsorption to improve ventricular preload, and (3) leads to systemic vasoconstriction and enhanced venous tone to increase systemic vascular resistance and blood pressure. Alternatively, alterations in autonomic function are broadly associated with both increased cardiovascular and, in many cases, all-cause mortality in humans. Norepinephrine is a potent adrenergic neurotransmitter and increases three to four times more than the normal level in HFS. This process has opposed effects: acute excretion or lower level of norepinephrine is associated with improvement of cardiac function; however, higher levels are associated with worsening of the HFS [7]. α-Adrenergic receptors are present in vascular smooth muscle much more so than in cardiac myocytes; however, only α^1-subtype receptors demonstrate significant density in myocardium, and their numbers increase modestly in heart failure, which leads to myocyte hypertrophy. Stimulation of these receptors in cardiac myocytes by norepinephrine induces myocyte growth and hypertrophy and reproduces fetal isoforms of contractile proteins. β-Adrenergic receptors consist of β^1 subtype and are present in more than 80% in the heart. This system plays a critical role in modulating cardiac performance, specifically inotropy, chronotropy, and lusitropy. However, chronically elevated stimulation of the sympathetic system has detrimental repercussions in HFS (cardiac β-adrenergic desensitization). Ongoing adrenergic stimulation reduces the β-adrenergic receptor, particularly β^1 concentrations in the myocardium (downregulation). This causes an increased expression of β-adrenergic receptor kinase inhibiting β-receptor (both β^1 and β^2) activation by phosphorylating them (functional desensitization).

1.2.2. Renin-angiotensin-aldosterone system

The renin-angiotensin-aldosterone system is a secondary compensatory mechanism that maintains intravascular volume and vascular resistance. This system is activated later in heart failure due to renal hypoperfusion, decreased sodium in the macula densa of the distal tubule, increased sympathetic stimulations (β^1 adrenergic activity), and diuretic therapy. The system is very sensitive and is activated with the extrication of renin from the juxtaglomerular apparatus. Renin is responsible for the conversion of angiotensinogen to angiotensin I (inactive decapeptide), and angiotensin I is then converted to angiotensin II (active octapeptide) by angiotensin-converting enzyme. The majority of angiotensin-converting enzyme (>90%) is found in tissues, with the rest located in the circulation. The activity of angiotensin-converting enzyme increases during heart failure with increased expression of myocardial form. Two opposing receptors are present; renin receptor type 1 and renin receptor type 2. Activation of type 1 receptors leads to cell growth, causing the release of norepinephrine from sympathetic nerves, either directly or indirectly. This in turn decreases lusitropy, increases afterload by inducing the release of aldosterone from the adrenal cortex indirectly and contributes to the increase of intravascular volume directly by promoting tubular reabsorption of sodium. Furthermore, this stimulates water intake by increasing thirst. The activation of type 2 receptors leads to the inhibition of cell growth, vasodilatation, and natriuresis. On the other hand, atrial natriuretic peptide (ANP) inhibits the release of renin.

Excessive production of angiotensin II can lead to fibrosis of several organs, especially the heart and kidneys, and can also induce cellular proliferation of cardiac fibroblasts and the rate of myocyte apoptosis. Aldosterone has similar actions with unfavorable effects of angiotensin II. Aldosterone provokes hypertrophy and fibrosis within the vasculature and myocardium, resulting in ventricular stiffness, endothelial cell and baroreceptor dysfunction, and the inhibition of norepinephrine uptake.

1.2.3. Renal neuroendocrine alterations

The most adverse outcome of HFS is increased salt and water retention by the kidneys, which results in the worsening of heart failure. Regulation of the fluid balance of the body is primarily managed by body fluid osmolality and changes in plasma volumes [8]. This is a normal pathway that is observed in non-failed hearts due to excessive intake of sodium, but it is a detrimental pathway in heart failure. Decreasing plasma volume or blood pressure is perceived as tissue hypoperfusion, which then stimulates specialized baroreceptors, and in turn activates several neurohormonal pathways that produce hypoperfusion of the tissues. Inadequate perfusion of the kidney and other organs results in adverse impulses that increase vasopressor response via angiotensin II, aldosterone, and norepinephrine production. This central response increases arginine vasopressin secretion, which regulates free water clearance and plasma osmolality. All of these responses try to prevent tissue hypoperfusion. Additionally, they can aggravate the process of heart failure and cause cardiac remodeling. Treatment modalities against any kind of heart failure syndrome can cause hyponatremia, which occurs as either depletional or delusional [9].

The natriuretic peptides provide the most important counterregulatory effect of the neurohormonal system via increasing excretion of sodium and water. Atrial (ANP) and B-type (BNP) natriuretic peptides are produced primarily in response to myocardial stretch due to pressure or volume overload: ANP from the atrial wall and BNP from the ventricular wall. Both peptides are responsible for vasodilatation, natriuresis, diuresis (inhibition of renin and aldosterone cascade), and inhibition of vascular smooth muscle proliferation. The third (C-type) natriuretic peptide released from endothelial cells results in vasodilatation and inhibits endothelin but does not promote natriuresis. These peptides increase during heart failure or decompensated situations, but they can also be used to guide heart failure therapy [10]. Both biomarkers are influenced by other factors such as obesity, arrhythmia, anemia, sepsis, pulmonary embolism, etc.

1.2.4. Peripheral neuroendocrine alterations

The main goal of the body is to preserve brain and cardiac circulation throughout the HFS via decreasing blood flow to peripheral tissues and visceral organs. The increased sympathetic adrenergic stimulation of the peripheral arteries causes arteriolar vasoconstriction for the maintenance of arterial pressure and vasoconstriction of the peripheral veins to increase venous return. Counterregulatory vasodilator responses result in vasodilatation of the peripheral vasculature to prevent aggressive overload of the circulatory system. Loss of the endothelium-mediated vasodilatory responsiveness in HFS causes the inability of counterregulatory and/or control of sympathetic adrenergic activation, which subsequently exacerbates heart failure, cardiac remodeling, and symptoms.

1.2.5. Anabolic metabolism alterations

Insulin is the strongest anabolic stimulatory signal via activation of transcription factor 4, which is complementary to the general amino acid control pathway. In heart failure, the anabolic efficiency of insulin decreases more than 50%. As a principal metabolic feature of heart failure, increased insulin resistance impairs functional capacity of the heart and muscles and worsens heart failure via impaired metabolic efficacy, tissue fibrosis, apoptosis, and lipotoxicity. Growth hormone or insulin-like growth factor 1 causes an anabolic signal rise; however, it cannot prevent cachexia. Anabolic steroid metabolism is also impaired in HFS.

Anabolic failure of the body occurring during long-standing heart failure appears with different clinical signs (**Table 4**). Skeletal muscle is the largest amino acid storage pool in the body, and its atrophy is the first clinical sign for cardiac cachexia (proteolysis). Adipose tissue is actively affected by different lipolytic signals, whereas insulin resistance blocks activation of lipogenic enzymes (lipolysis). Osteopenia or osteoporosis can develop in higher stages of the disease. This catabolic/anabolic imbalance leads to tissue wasting, weight loss, and ultimately cardiac cachexia (body weight loss > 6% in < 1 year), which is the worst and gravest prognosis of the HFS. Iron deficiency is another important metabolic dysfunction that occurs secondary to blood loss, malnutrition, inflammation (hepcidin dysfunction), and impaired synthesis of bioactive heme, and it impairs enzymatic electron transfer activities in the body with or without anemia.

1. Proteolysis

2. Lipolysis

3. Osteolysis

4. Cardiac cachexia

   a. Hypoalbuminemia

   b. Anemia

   c. Impaired glucose tolerance

   d. Inflammation

   e. Anorexia

5. Iron deficiency

6. Hyperuricemia

Table 4. Clinical presentation of imbalanced catabolic status in heart failure.

1.3. Left ventricular remodeling

Reversible or irreversible left ventricular failure (LVF) results in left ventricular remodeling via complex changes of cardiac myocytes and nonmyocyte components of the myocardium (**Table 5**) [11]. Treatment of reversible pathologies affecting the heart can reverse this process and maintain the anatomohistologic structure. Irreversible pathologies lead to progressive loss of myofilaments and contractile function, as well as alterations in excitation-contraction coupling, fatal arrhythmias, and desensitization of ß-adrenergic signaling. This type of left heart failure impacts the development of left ventricular hypertrophy, in that pressure overload or myocardial accumulation causes concentric hypertrophy with increased left ventricular wall stiffness, with or without left ventricular thickening. However, volume overload also causes eccentric hypertrophy with dilation of the left ventricular wall, with or without thinning. A progressive loss of connectivity of the collagen network causes progressive left ventricular dilatation, but it preserves the structural integrity of the heart. A change in left ventricular shape from an elliptical form to a spherical form creates increasing wall stress and mechanical energy, which results in left ventricular dilatation and wall thinning. This progressive dilatation causes pull-apart pathology of the papillary muscles resulting in significant mitral regurgitation from the inability of the valve leaflets to coapt. In addition, myocardial fibrosis results in arrhythmia and/or sudden death.

The heart anatomically consists of a single, intertwined muscle band. The muscle fibers, both inside and out, achieve maximum contractile performance by making a 60° angle from each other. This angle increases when a stretching occurs, as in heart failure, and the elliptical shape of the heart mutates into a spherical shape, which decreases stroke work and volume significantly. The oblique arrays of apical fibers create 60% LVEF with 15% fractional shortening, while transverse arrays can create just 15% LVEF. When the arrays of myocardial fibers are unbalanced from any cause, the contractile performance of the heart will be affected (**Table 6**). The enlargement of myocardial cells alters left ventricular shape and function.

Systolic dysfunction disrupts emptying of the ventricular chamber and decreases stroke volume, whereas volume overload increases left ventricular end-diastolic pressure. Diastolic dysfunction reduces the filling capacity of the LV due to myocardial stiffness, despite the relatively preserved contractile performance and ejection fraction. Each type of cardiomyopathy has one or both dysfunctional processes. Dilated cardiomyopathy is characterized by impaired systolic function, with enlargement of cardiac chambers, whereas hypertrophic cardiomyopathy is depicted by a smaller ventricular cavity due to a hypertrophic myocardium. Restrictive cardiomyopathy occurs secondarily from diastolic dysfunction and exhibits normal chamber size.

---

(1) Structural alterations

   (a) Ultrastructural remodeling

   (b) Mitochondrial remodeling

   (c) Extracellular matrix remodeling

   (d) Metabolic remodeling

(2) Electrophysiologic alterations

   (a) Action potential remodeling

   (b) Excitation-contraction coupling remodeling

   (c) Repolarization remodeling

(3) ß-Adrenergic receptor signaling alterations

Table 5. Myocardial remodeling.

(a) Myocardial infarction causes loss of contraction and subsequent to fibrosis of affected heart muscle, which breakdowns the array of myocardial fibers due to stretching of myocardial fibers

(b) Valvular and/or congenital heart diseases leading to biventricular volume overload derange the array of myocardial fibers due to ventricular dilatation

(c) Cardiomyopathies and the intrinsic disorders of the myocardium may cause a breakdown of the array of myocardial fibers due to both mechanisms

---

Table 6. Pathophysiologic changes in different etiologies.

2. Right heart failure

The right ventricle (RV) is not a mirror image of the LV and has its own anatomy, circulation, physiology, and hemodynamics. The RV consists of separated inlet (receives blood from the right atrium) and outlet (funnels blood into the pulmonary artery) portions and has a crescent-shaped structure with a concave free wall and convex interventricular septum (IVS) [12]. It is relatively thin walled with the muscle mass of the RV being relatively less than that of the LV (about 1/6). However, the RV can eject almost an equal stroke volume as the LV into a lower afterloaded (low pressure-low resistance) and highly compliant pulmonary circuit with a more complex contractile mechanism, but with lower stroke work than the LV (25% of the left ventricular stroke work). The dominant movements of the RV include longitudinal shortening, pressing of the free wall against the septum, contraction of the IVS, and a "wringing" action of the LV (**Table 7**). Right heart failure (RHF) is defined as persistent signs and symptoms of right ventricular dysfunction (RVD) in the absence of LVF, cardiac tamponade, ventricular arrhythmias, and/or pneumothorax.

1. Longitudinal/twisting motion (septal contraction)	80%
Interventricular septum shares fibers with both ventricles	
LV maintains 20–40% RV contractile function	
2. Transverse motion (free wall contraction)	20%
3. Traction of the RV free wall at the points of binding to the LV	

Table 7. Right ventricular contractile functions.

2.1. Pathophysiology of right heart failure

Right-sided heart failure has been accepted as an eventual consequence of left-sided heart failure (the LV as guilty and the RV as victim), and the RV has been largely ignored as a passive conduit or a bystander chamber for several decades [13]. The International Right Heart Foundation Working Group describes a comprehensive definition of RHF: "A clinical syndrome due to an alteration of structure and/or function of the right heart circulatory system that leads to suboptimal delivery of blood flow (high or low) to the pulmonary circulation and/or elevated venous pressures—at rest or with exercise" [14]. The definition of RHF represents a dysfunction of any components that constitute the right heart circulatory system, from systemic veins (post-systemic capillaries) to the pulmonary artery (pre-pulmonary capillaries). Right ventricular failure (RVF) can develop most commonly secondarily to left-sided HFS, but some specific etiologic pathologies result in isolated right-sided HFS (**Table 8**) [15]. The well-known etiologic reasons of RVF are pulmonary arterial hypertension (PAH) with or without LHF, LVF, or implantation of a left ventricular assist device (LVAD).

Pulmonary arterial hypertension (PAH) is seen in almost all RHF scenarios and occurs as a consequence of chronic left heart pathologies, chronic lung diseases, pulmonary embolism, or any pathology affecting the distal pulmonary vascular bed. Pressure overload caused by pre- or post-capillary dynamics starts the "RVD and RVF" vicious circle (**Figure 5**). The hemodynamic definition of PAH type is critical to determine the appropriate treatment modality. Pulmonary hypertension is a common complication of LHF and the diagnosis of PAH-related hemodynamic parameters (**Table 9**). The main differentiation between pre- and post-pulmonary types is pressure gradients between both sides of the pulmonary capillaries, whereas the diastolic pressure gradient has more prognostic value due to lesser dependence of stroke volume and loading conditions [16]. The threshold level of the transpulmonary pressure gradient (TPG) to discriminate between pre- and post-capillary PHT should be 12 mmHg. The diastolic pulmonary gradient (<5 mmHg) combined with the systemic blood pressure and cardiac output is superior to the TPG for determining the differential diagnosis between pulmonary vascular disease, high output or high left heart filling state, and sepsis.

---

1. Pressure overload

   a. Left-sided HFS (most common cause)

   b. Primary pulmonary hypertension

   c. Pulmonary embolism

   d. RVOT obstruction and/or peripheral pulmonary stenosis

2. Volume overload

   a. Tricuspid regurgitation

   b. Pulmonary regurgitation

   c. Atrial septal defect and/or anomalous pulmonary venous return

   d. Coronary artery fistula into right chambers

   e. Carcinoid syndrome

3. Ischemia and infarction

4. Intrinsic myocardial process

5. Arrhythmogenic RV dysplasia

6. Chronic lung diseases

Table 8. Etiology of right heart failure.

Right ventricular failure has a specific pathophysiologic algorithm (**Figure 6**). Increased afterload due to pressure overload of the pulmonary circulation prolongs the systolic contraction of the RV. On the other hand, the RV is able to tolerate an increased preload due to volume overload. In the early phase of RVF, wall thickening and enhanced contractility are the first important responses of pressure overload, which creates an adaptive remodeling with concentric hypertrophy and preserved right ventricular function. In chronic, higher afterload states even though myocardial contractility is advanced, the right pump functions decrease proportionally, and contractile dysfunction occurs later in the process. This remodeling process is sustained by the contribution of neurohormonal, genetic, and molecular components. Meanwhile, the RV dilates to provide adequate stroke volume, but this counter effect leads to tricuspid annular dilatation, valve coaptation defect, and eventually significant tricuspid regurgitation. This process triggers a maladaptive remodeling, which causes eccentric hypertrophy and deteriorated right ventricular function. In the beginning of diastole of the LV, the RV is contracting, and the IVS moves leftward causing ventricular dyssynchrony. Ventricular dyssynchrony accelerates right heart and biventricular failure with several fatal complications such as arrhythmia, hepatorenal failure, protein-losing enteropathy, and cardiac cachexia. Myocardial ischemia or infarction of the RV is not a significant factor for heart failure as it is in LVF, because the right ventricular free wall is supplied by a single coronary artery, whereas the IVS and the rest of the RV have the benefit of left-sided collateral blood flow, which protects the RV against ischemia.

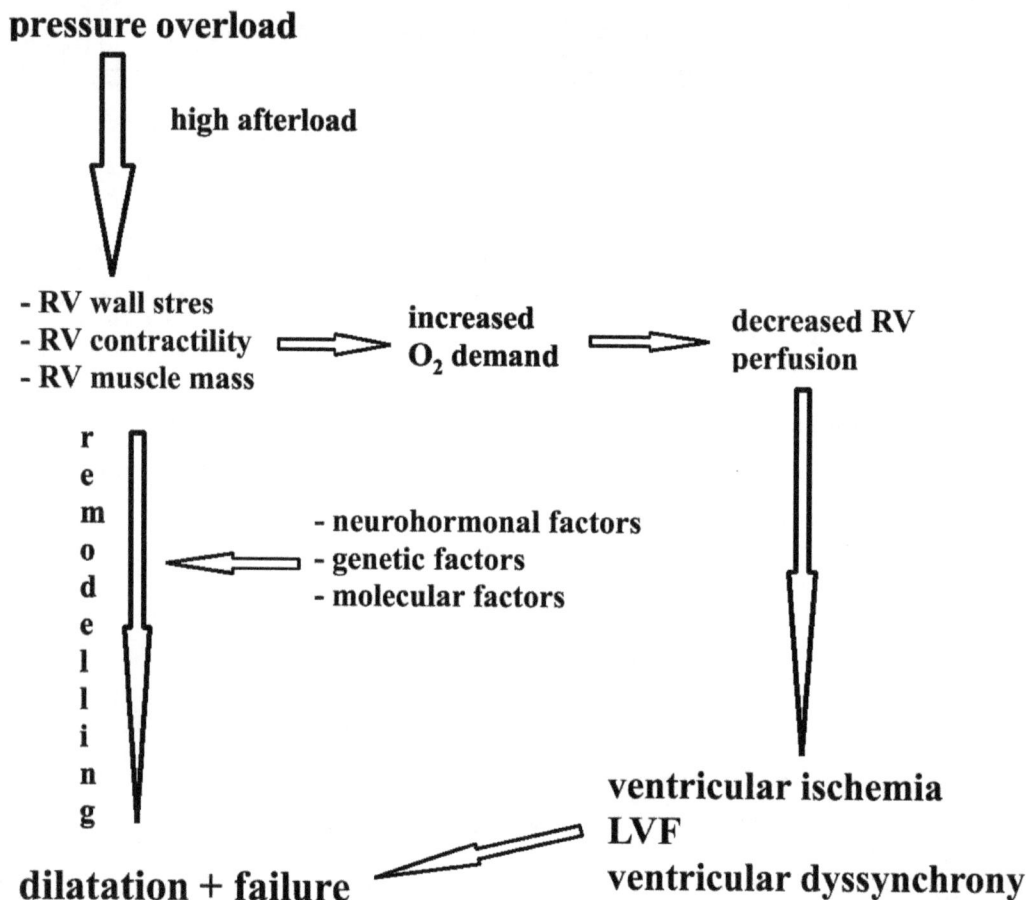

pressure overload

high afterload

- RV wall stres
- RV contractility   increased   decreased RV
- RV muscle mass   O₂ demand   perfusion

r
e
m
o   - neurohormonal factors
d   - genetic factors
e   - molecular factors
l
l
i
n   ventricular ischemia
g   LVF
dilatation + failure   ventricular dyssynchrony

Figure 5. Pathophysiological changes caused by pulmonary hypertension on the right heart.

2.2. Transition of left heart failure to right heart failure

The main cause of RHF is PAH related to an intolerable afterload increase in pulmonary circulation due to LHF and is associated with elevated left ventricular filling pressure, severe mitral regurgitation, and impaired left atrial compliance secondary to a dilated LV. Therefore, LHF is the most common (65–80%) reason for PAH (group 2 PAH) [17]. Sudden elevation of the left heart and consequently pulmonary circulatory pressure increases endothelial permeability causing fluid infiltration into alveolar and interstitial spaces. Pulmonary edema is one of the first signs of acute left HFS, although decreased permeability in the chronic stage of LHF does not cause pulmonary congestion. Significant overloading of the pulmonary arterial vasculature leads to mechanical, neurohormonal, and molecular changes in the pulmonary vasculature system. Destructive neurohormonal changes cause the desensitization of the pulmonary vascular bed against vasodilator agents (nitric oxide, natriuretic peptides, etc.) and excretion of vasoconstrictor agents (endothelin-1, etc.). Vasoconstriction is the net response of the pulmonary vasculature system to sustain and maintain the right heart stroke volume. If this process cannot be treated or resolved, long-standing PAH will cause reactive structural changes and interstitial fibrosis in the pulmonary vasculature, specifically in the small pulmonary resistance arteries, and will result in increasing pulmonary vascular resistance (PVR) [18]. The next step of this maladaptive process is pulmonary arteriolar remodeling, which includes thickening of the alveolar-capillary membrane, medial hypertrophy, intimal and adventitial fibrosis, and luminal occlusion in small pulmonary arterioles. Arterial resistance and compliance in the lung are determined by the small pulmonary resistance vessels, in contrast to the systemic circulation determined by the aorta. The last stage after irreversible PVR is remodeling of the right heart and organs behind the RV. Maladaptive remodeling of the RV is similar to that of the LV in that there is an increase in myocardial fibrosis, dilatation, wall thinning, tricuspid insufficiency, and contractile failure (**Figure 6**) [19]. Pulmonary hypertension associated with left heart disease is a significant predictor for rehospitalization and mortality [20].

	LVEF	RVEF	CVP (RAP)	mPAP	PCWP (LVEDP)	TPG	DPG	PVR
Normal	Normal	Normal	<10 mmHg	<15 mmHg	<10 mmHg	<10 mmHg	<5 mmHg	<2 WU
Precapillary (PVD)	Normal	Decreased	>15 mmHg	≥25 mmHg	≤15 mmHg	>12 mmHg	>7 mmHg	>3 WU
Post-capillary (LHF)	Decreased	Normal	>15 mmHg	≥25 mmHg	>15 mmHg	≤12 mmHg	<7 mmHg	<3 WU
Combined	Decreased	Decreased	>15 mmHg	≥25 mmHg	>15 mmHg	>12 mmHg	>7 mmHg	>3 WU
Irreversible PAH	Decreased	Decreased	>15 mmHg	≥25 mmHg	>15 mmHg	>15 mmHg	>10 mmHg	>6 WU

CVP, central venous pressure; DPG, diastolic pulmonary gradient; LHF, left heart failure; LVEDP, left ventricular end-diastolic pressure; LVEF, left ventricular ejection fraction; PAH, pulmonary arterial hypertension; mPAP, mean pulmonary artery pressure; PCWP, pulmonary capillary wedge pressure; PVD, pulmonary vascular disease; PVR, pulmonary vascular resistance; Rap, right atrial pressure; RVEF, right ventricular ejection fraction; TPG, transpulmonary gradient.

Table 9. Pulmonary hypertension types.

Increased filling pressure of the right heart chambers reflects back to the systemic venous system and affects visceral and peripheral tissues. The left HFS with low systemic perfusion pressure and elevated PVR contributes to this process and aggravates organ dysfunction. The liver is the most affected organ in RHF via congestive hepatopathy. Cardiac hepatopathy is a clinical entity with signs and symptoms of elevated hepatic biomarkers approximately twice the upper limit of normal: aspartate aminotransferase > 100 U/L, alkaline phosphatase > 200 U/L, and serum bilirubin > 2 mg/dL [21]. Increased elevation of the right atrial pressure and/or severe tricuspid regurgitation implies increased hepatic venous pressure causing hepatic circulatory failure, hepatic congestion, and hepatic ischemia. In the early phase, sinusoidal congestion with hemorrhagic necrosis and hepatocyte degeneration dominates the reversible silent clinical status. Chronically elevated right heart pressures disrupt hepatic venous return and consequently hepatic arterial circulation, so that decreased hepatic oxygen and nutrient delivery results in hepatocellular necrosis, fatty changes, and fibrosis. The congested and hypoxic liver cannot work properly, and, ultimately, cardiac cirrhosis develops, which is characterized by hepatic insufficiency such as portal hypertension, coagulation abnormality, biliary malfunctions, and other metabolic dysfunctions.

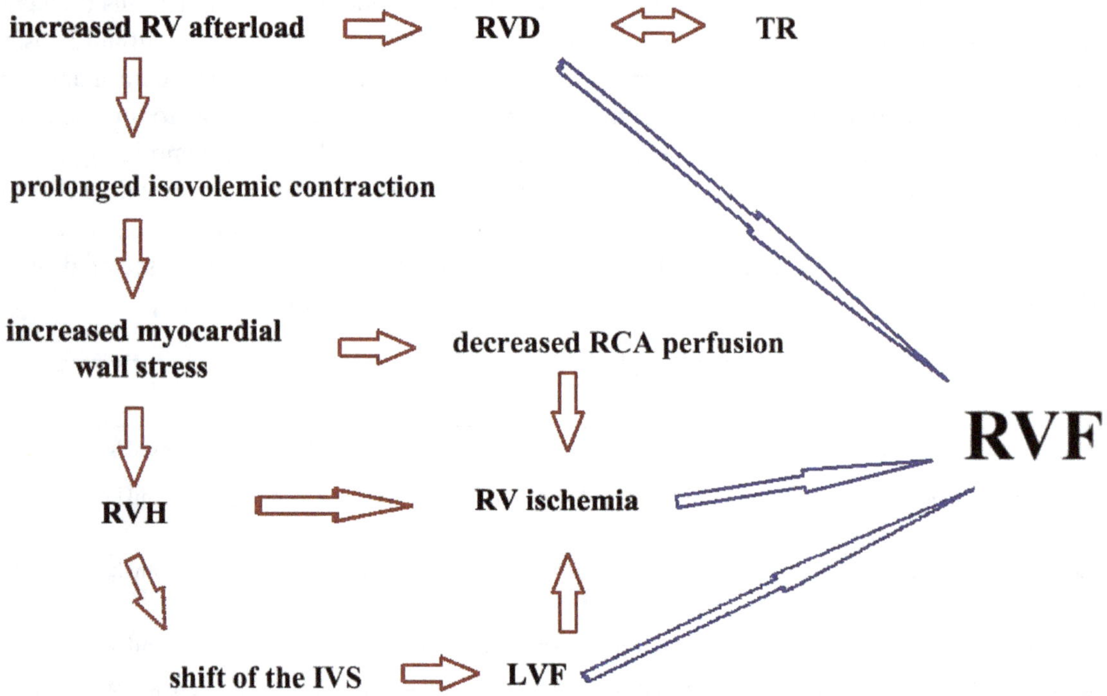

Figure 6. RVF pathophysiology. IVS, interventricular septum; LVF, left ventricular failure; RCA, right coronary artery; RV, right ventricle; RVD, right ventricular dysfunction; RVF, right ventricular failure; RVH, right ventricular hypertrophy; TR, tricuspid regurgitation.

3. Right ventricular failure after left ventricular assist device implantation

End-stage HFS requires mechanical uni- or biventricular circulatory support, but isolated LVAD implantation covers the majority (>90%) of treatments. Uni- or biventricular failure can be treated only by LVAD implantation. This therapy has several indications (**Table 10**). Currently, more LVADs have been implanted as destination therapy in advanced LVF with both advantages and disadvantages. The main intention of LVAD therapy is to provide support to the failing LV, allowing for improved stroke volume that ultimately promotes peripheral tissue perfusion. Furthermore, the LVAD improves right ventricular function due to unloading of the LV and consequently the RV [22]. The most serious complication of LVAD therapy can be a newly developed or continued deterioration of RVF as pathophysiologic sequela, which worsens postoperative mortality and morbidity, end-organ dysfunction due to severe congestion (coagulopathy, malnutrition, renal and hepatic dysfunctions, edema, ascites, etc.), hospitalization durations, and success of bridge to transplant therapy. The classification of RVF after LVAD implantation is described by The Interagency Registry for Mechanically Assisted Circulatory Support (INTERMACS) and is associated with increased perioperative mortality, prolonged length of stay, and worse survival even after cardiac transplantation (**Table 11**) [23]. The definition of serious RVF after LVAD implantation must be very clear, because it needs to be treated by heart transplantation or mechanical circulatory support (**Table 12**) [24]. Post-implant RVF can occur beyond the immediate postoperative period or later, and it significantly impacts survival after LVAD implantation because it is a progressive condition. Early post-implant RVF results in worse survival and is predicted by greater preoperative tricuspid incompetence [25]. Prolonged RVF for more than 2 weeks is associated with adverse outcomes, with the incidence of moderate or severe RVF necessitating right or biventricular ventricular assist device placement after LVAD implantation ranging between 10 and 40% [26].

---

1. Bridge to transplantation (BTT)

2. Bridge to candidacy for transplantation (BTC)

3. Destination therapy (DT)

4. Bridge to recovery (BTR)

Table 10. LVAD indications.

---

1. Mild

    a. Post-implant inotropes, inhaled nitric oxide, or intravenous vasodilators not continued beyond post-op Day 7 after LVAD implant

2. Moderate

    a. Post-implant inotropes, inhaled nitric oxide, or intravenous vasodilators continued beyond post-op Day 7 and up to post-op Day 14 after LVAD implant

    b. CVP or right atrial pressure >16 mm Hg

3. Severe

    a. Prolonged post-implant inotropes, inhaled nitric oxide, or intravenous vasodilators continued beyond post-op Day 14 after LVAD implant

    b. CVP or right atrial pressure >16 mmHg

    c. Need for RVAD at any time after LVAD implant

CVP, central venous pressure; INTERMACS, Interagency Registry for Mechanically Assisted Circulatory Support; LVAD, left ventricular assist device; RVAD, right ventricular assist device; RVF, right ventricular failure.

Table 11. INTERMACS definition of post-implant RVF (severity scale).

Right ventricular output determinants such as preload, afterload, and contractility are deranged in RVF after LVAD implantation (**Table 13**). Post-implant RVF is multifactorial and includes leftward shifting of the IVS, suboptimal RV afterload reduction, and RV myocardial dysfunction. Echocardiography is the primary imaging modality for monitoring cardiac function, filling and contraction behaviors, and device malfunctions [27].

1. Need for intravenous inotrope and pulmonary vasodilator therapy > 14 days

2. Need for RVAD implantation

3. Hemodynamic parameters

    a. CVP > 16 mmHg

    b. CVP/PCWP > 2/3

    c. PVR > 2 Wood units

    d. MAP < 55 mmHg

    e. CI < 2 L/min/m^2

    f. Inotropic support > 20 U

    g. MVS < 55%

    h. HR > 100 / min

4. Laboratory parameters

    a. Bilirubin > 2 mg/dL

    b. Creatinine > 2 mg/dL

    c. AST > 80 IU/L

    d. Albumin < 3 g/dL

5. Echocardiographic parameters

    a. TAPSE < 7.5 mm

    b. RAD > 5 cm

    c. RVEDD > 3.5 cm

    d. RVEF < 30%

AST, aspartate aminotransferase; CI, cardiac index; CVP, central venous pressure; HR, heart rate; MAP, mean arterial pressure; MVS, mixed venous oxygen saturation; PCWP, pulmonary capillary wedge pressure; PVR, pulmonary vascular resistance; RAD, right atrial diameter; RVAD, right ventricular assist device; RVEDD, right ventricular end-diastolic diameter; RVEF, right ventricular ejection fraction; RVF, right ventricular failure; TAPSE, tricuspid annular plane systolic excursion.

Table 12. Definition of serious RVF.

Increased preload (volume overload) causes the RV to fail due to the overstretching of the right ventricular myocardium. Improved left-sided forward flow with mechanical unloading in conjunction with perioperative transfusions of blood products suggests that increased venous return to the RV can be well tolerated. However, excessive fluid transfusions can aggravate RVF due to the effect of the Frank-Starling mechanism, exacerbation of tricuspid regurgitation, reduction of septal contribution, and ventriculo-arterial uncoupling. The main echocardiographic findings are a leftward shift of the interatrial septum, distension of the RV, worsening of tricuspid regurgitation, and plethora.

Despite the benefit of the LVAD decompressing the LV and reducing pulmonary overload significantly, it is not successful in every situation due to irreversibility of PAH, which is the main determinant for irreducible afterload. Reverse remodeling of the pulmonary vasculature can potentially occur with continued unloading, and, unlike heart transplantation, elevated PVR is not able to predict post-implant RVF. The second reason is continuity of preoperative significant mitral regurgitation due to untouched strategy, which cannot be improved and results pulmonary congestion though implantation of LVAD postoperatively. Because the RV has a very different myocardial structure than the left side and is very sensitive to acute change in afterload, any limited or huge failure of afterload decreasing causes significant post-implant RVF due to ineffectiveness of Frank-Starling mechanism on the right heart.

Improvement of right ventricular contractility after LVAD implantation is a predictor for positive outcomes; however, if the right ventricular systolic function does not improve, there are several risk-scoring algorithms that can be used to help predict the need for biventricular support [28]. Excessive leftward shift of the IVS due to volume overload and/or aggressive LV decompression may decrease septal contribution to right ventricular contraction causing mechanical dyssynchrony and elevation of right ventricular work. The main echocardiographic findings of post-implant RVF are decreased tricuspid annular plane systolic excursion (TAPSE < 7.5 mm), reduced right ventricular fractional area change (RVFAC < 35%), increased RV/LV ratio (>0.75), and septal akinesia. Severe unloading of the LV affects left ventricular contraction, depending on it right ventricular systolic function. In normal heart, the left ventricular contraction supplies roughly one half and septal contraction one quarter of the right ventricular ejection function. Prevention and treatment of RVF can be provided with the maintenance of the ejection function of the LV.

---

1. Preload

    a. Increased left ventricular output and venous return (approximately 100%)

    b. Excessive administration of blood products and fluids

2. Afterload

    a. Maintenance of pulmonary arterial hypertension

    b. Respiratory problems

3. Contractility

    a. Overstretched cardiac myofibrils (decreasing stroke volume)

    b. Aggravated annular dilatation and tricuspid regurgitation

    c. Impaired ventricular interdependence (left ventricular failure)

    d. Dyssynchronism of interventricular septum (noncontractible and/or leftward shift of the septum)

Table 13. Determinants leading to RVF after LVAD.

Author details

Kaan Kırali[1, 2*], Tanıl Özer[1] and Mustafa Mert Özgür[1]

*Address all correspondence to: imkbkirali@yahoo.com

1 Department of Cardiac Transplantation and Ventricular Assist Device, Kartal Koşuyolu YIEA Hospital, Istanbul, Turkey

2 Department of Cardiovascular Surgery, Faculty of Medicine, Sakarya University, Sakarya, Turkey

References

[1]   Warriner D, Sheridan P, Lawford P. Heart failure: Not a single organ disease but a multisystem syndrome. Br J Hosp Med 2015;76(6):330–336.

[2]   King M, Kingery J, Casey B. Diagnosis and evaluation of heart failure. Am Fam Physician 2012;85(12):1161–1168.

[3]   Doehner W, Frenneaux M, Anker SD. Metabolic impairment in heart failure. J Am Coll Cardiol 2014;64(13):1388–1400.

[4]   Gaggin HG, Januzzi JL Jr. Biomarkers and diagnostics in heart failure. Biochim Biophys Acta 2013;1832(12):2442–2450.

[5]   Shires ES, Gustafsson AB. Mitophagy and heart failure. J Mol Med 2015;93(3):253–262.

[6]   Florea VG, Cohn JN. The autonomic nervous system and heart failure. Circ Res 2014;114:1815–1826.

[7]   Joyner MJ. Preclinical and clinical evaluation of autonomic function in humans. J Physiol 2016;594(12):4009–4013.

[8]   Waldreus N, Hahn RG, Jaarsma T. Thirst in heart failure: A systematic literature review. Eur Heart J 2013;15(2):141–149.

[9]   Verbrugge FH, Steels P, Grieten L, Nijst P, Tang WHW, Mullens W. Hyponatremia in acute decompensated heart failure: Depletion versus dilution. J Am Coll Cardiol 2015;65(5):480–492.

[10] Troughton R, Felker GM, Januzzi JL Jr. Natriuretic peptide-guided heart failure management. Eur Heart J 2014;35:16–24.

[11] Gloschat CR, Koppel AC, Aras KK, Brennan JA, Holzem KM, Efimow IR. Arrhythmogenic and metabolic remodelling of failing human heart. J Physiol 2016;594(14):3963–3980.

[12] Kevin LG, Barnard M. Right ventricular failure. Contin Educ Anaesth Crit Care Pain 2007;7(3):89–94.

[13] Ryan JJ, Tedford RJ. Diagnosis and treating the failing right heart. Curr Open Cardiol 2015;30(3):292–300

[14] Mehra MR, Park MH, Landzberg MJ, Lala A, Waxman AB. Right heart failure: Toward a common language. Pulm Circ 2013;3(4):963–967. [Consensus statement from the International Right Heart Foundation Working Group includes a comprehensive definition of right heart failure.]

[15] Gerges M, Gerges C, Pistritto AM, Lang MB, Trip P, Jakowitsch J, Binder T, Lang IM. Pulmonary hypertension in heart failure. Epidemiology, right ventricular function, and survival. Am J Respir Crit Care Med 2015;192(10):1234–1246.

[16] Naeije R, Vachiery JL, Yerly P, Vanderpool R. The transpulmonary pressure gradient for the diagnosis of pulmonary vascular disease. Eur Respir J 2013;41(1):217–223.

[17] Rosenkranz S, Gibbs JSR, Wachter R, De Marco T, Vonk-Noordegraaf A, Vachiery JL. Left ventricular heart failure and pulmonary hypertension. Eur Heart J 2016;37(12):942–954.

[18] Vanderpool RR, Naeije R. Progress in pulmonary hypertension with left heart failure. beyond new definitions and acronyms. Am J Respir Crit Care Med 2015;192(10):1152–1154.

[19] Borgdorff MAJ, Dickinson MG, Berger RMF, Bartelds B. Right ventricular failure due to chronic pressure load: What have we learned in animal models since the NIH working group statement? Heart Fail Rev 2015;20(4):475–491.

[20] Dzudie A, Kengne AP, Thienemann F, Sliwa K. Predictors of hospitalisations for heart failure and mortality in patients with pulmonary hypertension associated with left heart disease: A systematic review. BMJ Open 2014;4(7):e004843.

[21] Megalla S, Holtzmann D, Aranow WS, Nazari R, Korenfeld S, Schwarcz A, Goldberg Y, Spevack DM. Predictors of cardiac hepatopathy in patients with right heart failure. Med Sci Monit 2011;17(10):537–541.

[22] Morgan JA, Paone G, Nemeh HW, Murthy R, Williams CT, Lanfear DE, Tita C, Brewer RJ. Impact of continuous-flow left ventricular assist device support on right ventricular function. J Heart Lung Transplant 2013;32:398–403.

[23] Lampert BC, Teuteberg JJ. Right ventricular failure after left ventricular assist devices. J Heart Lung Transplant 2015;34:1123–1130.

[24] Koprivanac M, Kelava M, Siric F, Cruz VB, Moazami N, Mihaljevic T. Predictors of right ventricular failure after left ventricular assist device implantation. Croat Med J 2014;55(6):587–595.

[25] Baumwol J, MacDonald PS, Keogh AM, Kotlyar E, Spratt P, JanszP Hawyard CS. Right heart failure and "failure to thrive" after left ventricular assist device: Clinical predictors and outcomes. J Heart Lung Transplant 2011;30(8):888–895.

[26] Fida N, Loebe M, Estep JD, Guha A. Predictors and management of right heart failure after left ventricular assist device implantation. Methodist DeBakey Cardiovasc J 2015;11(1):18–23.

[27] Argiriou M, Kolokotron SM, Sakellaridis T, Argiriou O, Charitos C, Zarogoulidis P, Katsikogiannis N, Kougioumtzi I, Machairiotis N, Tsiouda T, Tsakiridis K, Zarogoulidis K. Right heart failure post left ventricular assist device implantation. J Thorac Dis 2014;6(S1):S52–S59.

[28] Atluri P, Goldstone AB, Fairman AS, MacArthur JW, Shudo Y, Cohen JE, Acker AL, Hiesinger W, Howard JL, Acker MA, Woo YJ. Predicting right ventricular failure in the modern, continuous flow left ventricular assist device era. Ann Thorac Surg 2013;96(3):857–863.

6

Diabetic Cardiomyopathy: Focus on Oxidative Stress, Mitochondrial Dysfunction and Inflammation

Sara Nunes, Anabela Pinto Rolo,
Carlos Manuel Palmeira and Flávio Reis

Abstract

Diabetic cardiomyopathy (DCM) is an independent clinical entity defined as structural and functional changes in the myocardium because of metabolic and cellular abnormalities induced by diabetes, resulting in cardiac failure. Hyperglycemia has been seen as a major cause of DCM due to activation of different mechanisms leading to oxidative stress. Several body of evidence show that distinct pathways of oxygen and nitrogen reactive species formation contribute to myocardial impairment. Abnormal mitochondrial morphology and energetics, evoked by abnormal Ca^{2+} handling, metabolic changes and oxidative stress, are observed in DCM, suggesting a pivotal role of mitochondrial dynamics in disease pathogenesis. In addition, insulin resistance compromises myocardial glucose uptake due to cellular depletion of glucose transporter proteins, together with increased myocardial uptake of free fatty acids and augmented triglyceride levels, which cause cardiomyocyte lipotoxicity. Finally, the state of chronic low-grade inflammation, a feature of obese type 2 diabetes, seems to also play a major role in DCM progression, whose mechanisms have been progressively disclosed. In this book chapter, we review the cellular mechanism contributing to DCM development, focusing on oxidative stress, mitochondrial dysfunction and inflammation of cardiomyocytes, as well as on possible therapeutic strategies.

Keywords: diabetic cardiomyopathy, oxidative stress, mitochondrial dysfunction, inflammation, therapeutic strategies

1. Introduction

Type 2 diabetes mellitus (T2DM) is one of the most common endocrine deregulation worldwide, reaching pandemic proportions on a global scale [1]. In 2015, there were 415 million people with diabetes globally and an increase to 642 million by 2040 is estimated by the International Diabetes Federation [2]. In addition, T2DM is one of the leading causes of illness and premature death, with 5 million deaths in 2015, mainly affecting developed regions ("Occidental World"), as well as many countries in development, particularly due to unhealthy lifestyle habits, such as physical inactivity and high fat and sugar diets [1].

T2DM is a major risk factor for the development of cardiovascular diseases (CVD), which are responsible for up to 65% of all deaths in diabetic patients, as well as for substantial morbidity and loss of quality of life. As T2DM progresses, the heart and blood vessels undergo changes, leading to a number of different cardiovascular complications, including coronary artery disease (CAD), stroke, peripheral arterial disease, as well as diabetic cardiomyopathy (DCM) [2].

The original finding of Rubler et al. [3] of the existence of heart failure (HF) in postmortem diabetic patients free of detectable CAD was the basis of the first use of DCM terminology. Subsequent clinical and epidemiological studies have confirmed these observations [4, 5], suggesting that diabetes can damage the cardiac tissue independently of other cardiovascular risk factors. Such associations have provided a credible existence of DCM as a unique clinical entity, independent of hypertension, CAD, left ventricular hypertrophy (LVH), atrial fibrillation, or any other known cardiac diseases, leading to HF, caused by complex relationships between metabolic abnormalities that accompany diabetes and its cellular consequences [6].

Despite the development of asymptomatic DCM for a long period of time, the metabolic anomalies at the cardiac myocyte level progresses, leading to structural and functional abnormalities. Although hyperglycemia has been classically indicated as the primary responsible, other factors seem to be involved in the evolution of the disease and several substrates have been suggested [7]. During the last years, the structural, functional, pathological and molecular aspects of the disease have been increasingly investigated, but the issue is far to be elucidated and no specific markers and therapeutics have been found so far. Unravelling the molecular mechanisms underlying DCM development and progression is crucial to identify relevant therapeutic targets and generate novel therapies tailored to reduce the risk of HF in diabetic patients.

In this book chapter, we revisit some of the main features of DCM, focusing on pathophysiological mechanisms associated with cardiomyocyte oxidative stress, mitochondrial dysfunction and inflammation. We also indicate possible therapeutic strategies targeting those important cellular events that seem to play a major role in DCM development and progression.

2. Structural and functional cardiac changes

Increasing evidences from experimental, pathologic, epidemiologic and clinical studies have been shown that diabetes results in structural and functional cardiac changes. Anatomic changes in DCM, mainly assessed by echocardiography or magnetic resonance imaging, are essentially characterized by myocardial hypertrophy and fibrosis. In addition, although many studies have shown that diabetic patients have abnormal diastolic function but preserved systolic function, which might be due to the lower sensitivity to detect systolic dysfunction by some of the techniques used, the current knowledge points to the existence of a continuum of diastolic and systolic dysfunction in DCM.

2.1. Cardiac hypertrophy

One of the most important structural hallmarks of DCM is cardiac hypertrophy, which is a powerful predictor of cardiovascular events. Apoptotic and necrotic loss of cardiomyocytes causes compensatory hypertrophy of the remaining viable cardiomyocyte. Although the right ventricle can also become hypertrophic, LVH is more common and generally represents a more advanced stage of the disease. Even though the causes and mechanisms underlying LVH development in diabetic patients remain poorly understood, experimental and clinical studies have been suggesting that hyperinsulinemia, insulin resistance, hyperglycemia, and increased nonesterified fatty acids (NEFAs) may collectively play a major role. Insulin, in particular, is viewed as a growth factor in the myocardium, which is sustained by experimental findings that sustained hyperinsulinemia causes increased myocardial mass and decreased cardiac output in rats [8]. In addition, clinical and experimental data have been shown increased markers of cardiomyocyte hypertrophy, including augmented width and myofiber disarray of cardiomyocyte, as well overexpression of hypertrophic genes, namely β-myosin heavy chain, atrial natriuretic peptide (ANP) and brain natriuretic peptide (BNP) [9, 10].

2.2. Myocardial fibrosis, apoptosis and necrosis

Myocardial fibrosis has been indicated as another major mechanism contributing to cardiac alterations in DCM. This pathological feature of DCM that have been observed in diabetic patients without significant CAD and in animal models, results from the accumulation of interstitial glycoproteins and increased extracellular collagen matrix, which potentiates stiffening and inhibits ventricles relaxation [11, 12]. The echocardiographic features of increased left ventricular fibrosis appear in the form of impaired relaxation and diastolic dysfunction; consequently, alterations in collagen phenotype may play an important role in the impaired left ventricular diastolic filling that is typical of DCM [11]. It has been suggested that collagen is a major determinant of ventricular stiffness. In a study with rats, a correlation between increased extracellular collagen content and decrease in early mitral peak flow (decreased E/A ratio) was reported [12]. The cause for the accumulation of cardiac fibrosis in diabetes is believed to result from decreased degradation of glycosylated collagen by matrix metalloproteinases and, conversely, from excessive production of collagen by fibroblasts due to increased renin–angiotensin–aldosterone system (RAAS) activation [11]. Furthermore, increased formation in myocardial advanced glycation end-products (AGEs) has also been reported in diabetic patients, which has been attributed to hyperglycemia [13]. In fact, collagen cross-linked with AGEs causes myocardial stiffness and inhibits collagen degradation, which promotes additional collagen accumulation and fibrosis [11, 13]. This mechanism seems to be also a major contributor for the impaired left ventricular diastolic function observed in diabetic patients [13].

Finally, DCM is associated with increased myocyte cell death and apoptosis. Accelerated necrosis and apoptosis is caused by hyperglycemia, increased formation of ROS, overactivation of local RAAS system and of insulin-like growth factor-1 and transforming growth factor beta 1

(TGF-β1) [14]. While apoptosis does not cause scar formation or accumulation of interstitial collagen, because nuclear fragmentation and cell shrinkage is replaced by the surrounding cells, necrosis is able to promote the widening of extracellular compartments among myocytes and increased deposition of collagen, which causes replacement fibrosis and connective cell proliferation [15].

2.3. Diastolic dysfunction

In many cases, it has been found that abnormalities of diastolic function may advertise the subsequent progressive deterioration of cardiac function. Diastolic dysfunction is the basic hemodynamic feature and the earliest findings of DCM that can be detected using imaging techniques. The noninvasive assessment of diastolic dysfunction mainly relies on Doppler studies of diastolic transmitral inflow, flow velocities, flow patterns, isovolumic relaxation time and deceleration time, which are the most common criteria used in its evaluation. The criteria of the consensus statement on the diagnosis of heart failure with normal left ventricular ejection fraction by the Heart Failure and Echocardiography Associations of the European Society of Cardiology have been used to assess left ventricular diastolic dysfunction [16].

Diastolic dysfunction is characterized by an abnormal myocardial relaxation and filling. This condition is typically manifested by reduced early diastolic filling and increased atrial filling, by augmented isovolumetric relaxation and increased number of supraventricular premature beats, as well as by amplified left ventricular end-diastolic pressure and diminished left ventricular end-diastolic volume [17–19].

Diastolic dysfunction is found in several other cardiovascular diseases, such as hypertension, hypertrophic cardiomyopathy and CAD, even with intact systolic function. However, experimental and clinical studies have shown impaired diastolic function in the absence of manifestations of congestive HF, even in prediabetes or in early stages of diabetes [19], thus suggesting that could be a useful early marker for disease prognosis. Furthermore, left ventricular diastolic dysfunction may progress to a systolic dysfunction, causing reduced left ventricular ejection fraction (LVEF) in years. Therefore, it is very important to detect left ventricular diastolic dysfunction in diabetic patients, both for early diagnosis and treatment of DCM, as well as for prevention of further systolic dysfunction.

2.4. Systolic dysfunction

Systolic dysfunction, defined as impaired ability of the heart to pump arterial blood in the periphery, is typically associated with a reduced LVEF and cardiac output. In DCM, systolic dysfunction occurs late, often when patients have already developed significant diastolic dysfunction. The presence of systolic dysfunction in the early years of diabetes has been a controversial issue, while diastolic dysfunction is more easily detected by Doppler echocardiography. The controversy relies on the fact that current techniques used to assess systolic function are less sensitive than those used for diastolic dysfunction evaluation. For this reason, more sensitive and accurately techniques for systolic assessment have been developed, such as tissue Doppler imaging (TDI) and strain rate imaging techniques, which are able to estimate left ventricular function in longitudinal, radial and circumferential ways, thus allowing the detection of preclinical systolic abnormalities in diabetic patients. Currently, shortened left ventricular ejection time, decreased peak systolic velocity (S′), and smaller left ventricular fractional shortening can be the detectable parameters for identification of systolic dysfunction [20]. The prognosis in patients with depressed systolic dysfunction is poor with an annual mortality of 15–20%.

3. Overview of the molecular mechanisms involved in DCM development

The pathophysiological molecular mechanisms underlying the development and progression of DCM are multifactorial and complex and have been progressively disclosed. Some of the main features of DM are also pivotal elements in the pathogenesis of DCM, including hyperglycemia, hyperinsulinemia and insulin resistance, as well as hyperlipidemia (**Figure 1**).

Hyperglycemia has been seen as a major cause of DCM development due to activation of the classical oxidative stress pathways (polyol, hexosamine, AGEs and protein kinase C—PKC). These mechanisms cause increased production of mitochondrial reactive oxygen species (ROS), nonenzymatic glycation of proteins and glucose auto-oxidation, thus leading to cellular (cardiac) injury—glucotoxicity. Glucose and collagen interact to form Schiff bases and the fibrous network is reorganized with the so-called Amadori products, which can be transformed in AGEs. As above mentioned, the increased formation of AGEs is highly associated

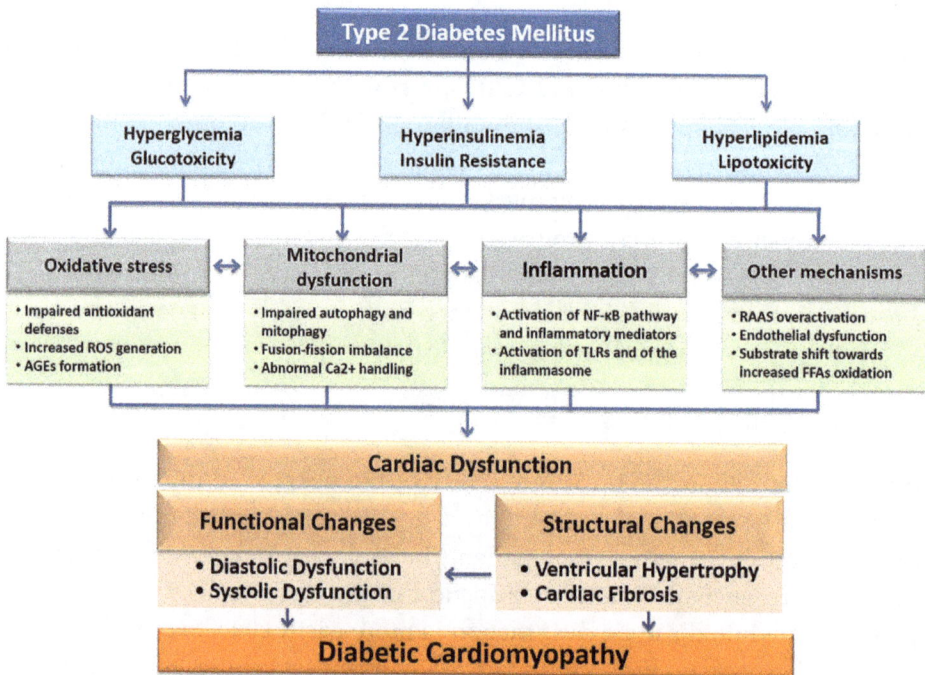

Figure 1. Metabolic abnormalities underlying T2DM that are considered the main triggers for the cellular and molecular pathways associated with structural and functional changes in DCM. Adapted with permission from Ref. [24]. *Abbreviations:* AGEs, advanced glycation end products; FFAs, free fatty acids, NF-κB, nuclear factor-κB; RAAS, renin–angiotensin–aldosterone system; ROS, reactive oxygen species; TLRs, Toll-like receptors.

with myocardial fibrosis in diabetic hearts by affecting the structural components of the extracellular matrix, such as collagen. This stable cross-linked collagen accumulate in vessel walls and in myocardial tissue, increasing diastolic stiffness of the heart and contributing to endothelial dysfunction, thus suggesting a key role of AGEs in DCM development.

Insulin resistance originates cellular depletion of glucose transporter proteins (GLUT-1 and GLUT-4) leading to reduced glucose uptake in the diabetic heart, which facilitates a substrate shift towards increased fatty acids (FAs) oxidation, resulting in reduced cardiac efficiency [21]. In brief, once inside the cardiomyocytes, the free fatty acids (FFAs) are converted into acetyl coenzyme A derivatives that will activate PKC isoforms responsible for blocking insulin cascade elevated levels of FFAs compete with glucose as energy substrate, with a shift in energy production from β-oxidation of FFAs. As a result, there is a reduced glucose utilization and oxidation, increased glucose and insulin levels, promoting insulin resistance.

Additionally, the increase concentration of FFAs and of its metabolism causes intracellular accumulation of toxic FA intermediates (such as ceramide and diacylglycerol) and formation of ROS. These mechanisms originates cardiac lipotoxicity by means of oxidative stress, cardiomyocyte apoptosis and increased myocardial consumption of oxygen, resulting in impaired contractility, mitochondrial uncoupling and decreased adenosine triphosphate (ATP) availability [22]. Intracellular deposition of FFAs is also responsible for the saturation of the mitochondrial capacity of oxidation, thus activating transcription factors, including the peroxisome proliferator-activated receptors (PPARs), which has been indicated as an inductor of cardiac lipotoxicity and dysfunction [23]. Several body of evidences show that distinct pathways of oxygen and nitrogen reactive species formation contribute to myocardial injury. Impaired mitochondrial morphology and energetics, evoked by abnormal Ca^{2+} handling, metabolic changes and oxidative stress, are observed in DCM, suggesting a pivotal role of mitochondrial dynamics in disease pathogenesis.

In addition, the state of chronic low-grade inflammation, a feature of obese T2DM, seems to also play a major role in DCM progression, whose mechanisms have been progressively disclosed [24]. The epicardial adipose tissue (EAT) that covers 80% of the heart surface and constitutes approximately 20% of the total heart weight have endocrine and paracrine properties that interfere with cardiac function, namely by the development of inflammation, insulin resistance and cardiac dysfunction [25].

As above mentioned, activation of the RAAS, locally and systemically, has been associated with the development of insulin resistance and the onset of T2DM. In addition, it has been associated with some of the hallmarks of DCM, such as increased fibrosis, oxidative damage, and cardiomyocyte and endothelial cell apoptosis and necrosis [26].

4. Oxidative stress and mitochondrial dysfunction

Mitochondria are dynamic organelles with a key role in energy transduction, signaling and cell death pathways. Consequently, mitochondrial dysfunction and oxidative stress are broadly relevant in the development of cardiovascular diseases, in both acquired and inherited disease [27]. Tissues with high aerobic metabolism demands, such as the heart muscle, are severely affected by a decline in mitochondrial efficiency such as in the context of diabetes, ischemia-reperfusion and aging [28, 29], associated with loss of calcium homeostasis and impaired contractile function. In fact, mitochondria comprise one-third of the volume of the heart and support the vast majority of ATP production derived from oxidation of fatty acids (FAs) and glucose, being FAs the preferred substrate in the normal adult myocardium, while failing human hearts shift to oxidizing glucose for energy production.

In the inner mitochondrial membrane, electrons deriving from the oxidation of NADH and FADH2 are funneled through the electron transport chain. This flow is coupled with the translocation of protons across the inner mitochondrial membrane to the intermembrane space, generating an electrochemical gradient. Under normal conditions, much of the energy of this gradient is used to generate ATP, as the collapse of the proton gradient through ATP synthase drives the ATP synthetic machinery. However, when the electrochemical potential difference generated by the electrochemical gradient is high (such as in high-fat or high-glucose states), or under conditions of inhibition of the ETC complexes, the life of superoxide-generating electron transport intermediates, such as ubisemiquinone radical, is prolonged [30], resulting in increased ROS generation. Although ROS are produced in multiple cell compartments, the majority of cellular ROS (approximately 90%) are mitochondrial, mainly at the level of complexes I and III of the ETC [31]. The activity of detoxifying enzymes and uncoupling proteins limits ROS generation. In the healthy myocardium, ROS concentration is tightly controlled to low steady-state level by superoxide dismutase (SOD) [32]. Superoxide anion is dismutated by mitochondrial manganese SOD into hydrogen peroxide, which is detoxified into water by the mitochondrial glutathione peroxidase (GPx), an action dependent on mitochondrial reduced glutathione (GSH) content. Mitochondrial catalase has a detoxifying effect against overproduction of hydrogen peroxide. An imbalance of antioxidant defenses that favors the accumulation of oxidants, expose mitochondria to oxidative stress, with ROS reacting with DNA, proteins and lipids, inactivating the ETC complexes and mitochondrial proteins, thus impairing both oxidative phosphorylation (OXPHOS) and inducing ROS accumulation. In the diabetic heart, increased FAs accumulation and metabolism is linked to oxidative stress [33]. Also, in the context of myocardial ischemia/reperfusion, oxidative stress is implicated in ATP depletion and cardiomyocyte death. At the onset of reperfusion, increased ROS and mitochondrial calcium influx favor induction of the mitochondrial permeability transition (MPT) and loss of mitochondrial inner membrane impermeability [34]. Recently, it has been shown that offspring of diabetic pregnancies are at risk of cardiovascular disease at birth and throughout life, with high-fat diet-exposed offspring exhibiting mitochondrial dysfunction and lipid peroxidation [35]. Each cell has normally several copies of mitochondrial DNA (mtDNA) which encodes ribosomal and transfer RNAs necessary for the synthesis of the mtDNA-encoded 13 OXPHOS polypeptides in the mitochondrial matrix [36]. The proximity to the inner membrane, the absence of protective histones, and incomplete repair mechanisms in mitochondria, renders mtDNA extremely sensitive to oxidative damage. The accumulation of mtDNA mutations due to oxidative damage results in further unbalanced ETC and increased ROS generation, perpetuating oxidative damage and enhancing inflammatory, hypertrophic, fibrotic, and cell death events in the myocardium [37]. Therefore, mechanisms able to eliminate dysfunctional mitochondria are essential to prevent the cytotoxic impact of ROS and thus maintain cellular homeostasis.

Autophagy is a tightly regulated cellular process which promotes the turnover of dysfunctional mitochondria along with the elimination of long-lived proteins and other damaged organelles, being essential for maintaining normal cardiac function [38]. Autophagy also maintains cell viability under stress conditions by supplying amino acids for de novo protein synthesis and providing substrates for the tricarboxylic acid cycle [39], as shown by myocardial survival promoted by activation of autophagy upon starvation or ischemia [40, 41]. Autophagy is redox-dependent due to redox regulation of metabolic alterations as well as ROS-mediated modification of autophagy-regulatory proteins. Disruption of ATG5, an autophagy-related gene, results in heart failure under basal and stress conditions [42]. In turn, autophagy regulates intracellular ROS by selective elimination of dysfunctional mitochondria (mitophagy) [43] and degradation of KEAP1 and activation of the nuclear factor erythroid 2-related factor 2 (NRF2), activating the expression of antioxidant genes such as glutathione peroxidase, superoxide dismutase and thioredoxin [44]. A decline in autophagy with aging, leading to increased levels of oxidative damage and the accumulation of dysfunctional mitochondria has been proposed as an underlying cause for the pathogenesis of cardiovascular diseases prevalent in late life [45].

Besides mitophagy, mitochondrial quality control is dependent on balanced fusion and fission events that continually alter mitochondrial morphology by undergoing fission to generate discrete fragmented mitochondria or fusion to form an interconnected elongated network. This dynamic behavior shapes mitochondria to adapt metabolism to the energetic needs of the cell, allows mixing of mtDNA, lipids, proteins and metabolites, enhances communication with the endoplasmic reticulum or segregates dysfunctional or depolarized mitochondria away from the healthy network, facilitating its clearance [46]. These two processes are under the control of mitochondrial fission and fusion proteins: mitofusins (MFN1 and MFN2) and optic atrophy 1 (OPA1) mediate mitochondrial fusion while dynamin-related protein 1 (DRP1) mediates mitochondrial fission by interaction with other fission mediators such as fission protein (FIS1) [47]. Changes on mitochondrial morphology, linked to altered expression of DRP1 and MFN2, are evident during stem cell differentiation into cardiomyocytes, transitioning from fragmented rounded mitochondria into an elongated network with well-developed cristae and an efficient OXPHOS system [48]. The essential role of MFN proteins is also shown by mitochondrial fragmentation, impaired mitochondrial function and development of heart failure in models of conditional cardiac ablation of MFN 1 and 2 [49]. In post-mitotic tissues with high metabolic demands, such as the heart, abnormal mitochondrial dynamics results in the development of cardiovascular disease, due to impaired mitochondrial turnover and accumulation of fragmented and depolarized mitochondria, sources of increased ROS generation [50]. Recently, it has also been shown that DRP1 ablation results in cardiomyocyte necrosis and dilated cardiomyopathy in mice, mitophagic mitochondrial depletion and favors MPT induction, probably linked to spatiotemporal alterations in calcium signaling [51]. When exposed to calcium overload, both neonatal and adult rat cardiomyocytes exhibited increased ROS generation and mitochondrial fragmentation, which suggested that activation of the fission machinery may be an event preceding ROS generation regulated by calcium signaling [52]. Giant or mega-mitochondria have been described in a variety of cardiomyopathies, including those associated with mtDNA mutations [53]. The observation of increased mtDNA content, induction of genes involved in mitochondrial biogenesis, fatty acid metabolism, and glucose transport, as well as uncoupling proteins and antioxidant enzymes in mitochondrial cardiomyopathies hearts, may indicate a compensatory response, although unable to prevent energy depletion and increased ROS generation [54].

Balanced fusion–fission events are essential for normal mitochondrial biogenesis, the process by which cells increase mitochondrial mass and copy number. Among the transcription factors involved in this process, peroxisome proliferator-activated receptor-γ coactivator-1, PGC-1α, is the master regulator. This inducible coactivator acts as a coactivator of the transcription factors involved in the expression of nuclear/mitochondrial genes and bioenergetic capacity, as well as regulates cardiac fuel selection and mitochondrial ATP-producing capacity [55]. An interplay between PGC-1α and MFN-2 has been shown as follows: MFN2 is critical for the stimulatory effect of PGC-1α on mitochondrial membrane potential while PGC-1α may regulate mitochondrial fusion/fission events [56]. Besides stimulating mitochondrial biogenesis and OXPHOS, PGC-1α prevents oxidative stress by inducing ROS-detoxifying enzymes [57]. Sirtuin 3 (SIRT3) has been shown essential for the stimulatory effect of PGC-1α on both mitochondrial biogenesis and ROS-detoxifying enzymes [58]. Sirtuins (1–7) are a conserved family of NAD+-dependent lysine-modifying acylases that regulate a variety of cellular functions such as metabolic responses to diet and exercise [59]. The decline in NAD+ during aging decreases sirtuin activity thus impairing the transcription of mitochondrial OXPHOS genes which leads to cardiovascular disease, an event precipitated by SIRT1 deletion [60]. Cardiac SIRT1 is upregulated during nutrient starvation, exercise and ischemic preconditioning while downregulated during I/R [61]. SIRT3, which exhibits mitochondrial deacetylase activity, deacetylates and increases the activity of mitochondrial metabolic and antioxidant enzymes [62] as well as regulates mitochondrial fusion–fission dynamics [63]. By deacetylating and suppressing the activity of cyclophilin D, SIRT3 increases resistance to MPT induction, preventing cell death and cardiac hypertrophy [64].

5. Inflammation

Chronic low-grade inflammation is commonly associated with obesity and T2DM, and clear evidence has emerged to suggest that inflammatory process also contributes to the pathogenesis of DCM. The inflammatory signaling in cardiomyocytes usually occurs as an early response to myocardial injury and involves an increased formation of cytosolic and mainly mitochondrial ROS. Several molecular pathways have been classically associated with the inflammatory response in the cardiac tissue: increased activation of the proinflammatory nuclear transcription factor-κB (NF-κB), overexpression of cytokines [namely the tumor necrosis factor-α (TNFα), some interleukins (such as IL-1β and IL-6), chemokines (i.e., monocyte chemotactic protein-1: MCP-1), adhesion molecules (i.e., selectins and adhesion molecules (ICAM-1, VCAM-1)] and migration of leukocytes into the myocardium [24]. There is evidence that chronic progression of hypertrophy, fibrosis and ventricular dysfunction is correlated with a local increase in cytokines and activation of NF-κB [65]. Activation of NF-κB is associated with the increased release of cytokines, such as TNF-α and IL-6, which are often involved in cardiac damage (hypertrophy and fibrosis) and left ventricular dysfunction [65, 66]. Accumulating data have been demonstrated that increased IL-1β and TNF-α are implicated in DCM, increasing epicardial thickness, promoting myocyte contractile dysfunction, thus depressing myocardial function and contributing to HF [67]. The inflammatory stimuli in the diabetic heart include hyperglycemia, hyperlipidemia, ROS, angiotensin II and the activation of Toll-like receptors (TLRs). Hyperglycemia-induced oxidative stress and inflammation seem to be deeply correlated with development of DCM. In fact, hyperglycemia activates several oxidative stress-responsive/proinflammatory transcription factors, including NF-κB, which is able to induce collagen and fibronectin synthesis, as well as to stimulate the production of inflammatory cytokines. Hyperglycemia-evoked diastolic dysfunction may be mediated partly by the macrophage migration inhibitory factor, suggesting that the NF-κB pathways may be involved in this process [68].

RAAS overactivation seems to also play an important role in the modulation of inflammation associated with DCM. In fact, Ang II not only induces vasoconstriction, cell growth and oxidative stress but also stimulates inflammation, namely by inducting cytokines release, by stimulating the production of PAI-1 and pro-inflammatory transcription factors, such as NF-κB, which in turn regulate adhesion molecules (VCAM-1 and ICAM-1) and the expression of several cytokines [69].

Activation of TLRs and the inflammasome complex has been recently proposed to play a pivotal role in cardiac inflammation and likely in the pathogenesis of DCM [70]. Accumulating evidences support the hypothesis that hyperglycemia and FFA are able to stimulate TLRs, thus inducing proinflammatory pathways in DCM. In fact, TLR-dependent NF-κB and ROS seem to be able to regulate both the priming and the posttranslational pathways required for the assembly and activation of the inflammasome, thus opening new therapeutic opportunities to DCM treatment, as further discussed.

6. Therapeutic strategies

Despite a specific therapy for the treatment or prevention of DCM is still lacking, some therapeutic strategies could present potential benefits. The advances on the knowledge of DCM pathogenesis provides us with improved management options, including lifestyle measures, strategies to improve diabetic control, lipid lowering therapy, as well as agents directed to target some of the main molecular events and mechanisms underlying DCM development and progression, including fibrosis, hypertrophy, oxidative stress and inflammation.

6.1. Physical exercise

Regular physical activity (training) has been associated with improved glycemic control and insulin sensitivity, as well as with amelioration of the metabolism of glucose and fatty acids in heart muscle, thus improving left ventricular function and attenuating diabetes induced-cardiac alterations. Physical exercise has also greater anti-inflammatory effects by decreasing the release of inflammatory cytokines from the skeletal muscles endothelial cells and immune system, together with increasing the anti-inflammatory cytokines, such as adiponectin [71]. In an animal model of T2DM, the Zucker Diabetic Fatty (ZDF) rat regular aerobic exercise (training) was able to not only improve the glycemic control and attenuate dyslipidaemia, but also to promote an anti-inflammatory effect, viewed by the reduction in pro-inflammatory cytokines, such as TNF-α and CRP, and by the increment of adiponectin levels [72–74]. This effect occurred independently of weight loss and was not observed when an acute extenuating exercise was used [75].

6.2. Antidiabetic agents

Improvement of glycemic control has been shown to be associated with better outcomes in diabetic microvascular complications in many clinical trials. Even though the impact of strict glycemic control on macrovascular outcomes remains debatable, the recognized role of microvascular disease in DCM development suggests that a better glycemic control would benefit patients.

6.2.1. Insulin-sensitizing agents

Insulin resistance is a hallmark of T2DM and plays an important role in the pathogenesis of DCM. Accordingly, agents used to ameliorate insulin resistance might be useful to prevent DCM progression. The beneficial effects of insulin may rely not only on the improved glycemic control in some patients but also on cardioprotective anti-inflammatory properties. Several data show a reduction in adhesion molecules, such as ICAM-1 and E-selection, circulating CRP, IL-6 and PAI-1 due to insulin-sensitizing therapy [76]. Metformin, one of the most commonly prescribed anti-diabetic drugs and a known insulin-sensitizing agent, improves peripheral sensitivity to insulin and promotes intensive glucose control [77]. Besides, cardioprotective actions of metformin have been described, namely inhibition of hypertrophy and pro-authophagic and anti-inflammatory actions [78].

The possible beneficial effects of thiazolidinediones (TZDs) and PPAR agonists on the myocardium have been demonstrated in several studies. Pioglitazone was associated with improved diabetic cardiac function in animal models, by raising myocardial glucose uptake and improving myocardial fatty acid metabolism [79]. In addition, rosiglitazone showed an amelioration of myocardial diastolic function in T2DM patients, which was related to an antioxidant and anti-inflammatory effect [80]. Other factors involved in improved cardiac function with TZDs therapy include decreased collagen accumulation and fibrosis, as well as inhibition of cardiomyocyte hypertrophy [79, 81]. Pioglitazone and rosiglitazone stimulate the PPAR-γ, which regulates important genes for the metabolism of glucose and fat and enhance insulin sensitivity in skeletal muscle and adipose tissue [82]. Additionally, PPAR activators may have anti-inflammatory effects by inhibition of TNF-α expression at the transcriptional level due to attenuation of NF-κB activity in cardiomyocytes [83]. However, the effects of this therapy on cardiac function in patients with T2DM have not yet been fully elucidated. On the other hand, experimental studies using PPARα agonists suggested cardiac benefits related to apoptosis and hypertrophy [84]. However, further research is still required in order to fully understand the role of PPARα agonists, as well as TZDs, in DCM.

6.2.2. Incretin-based therapies

Glucagon-like peptide-1 (GLP-1), an incretin hormone rapidly released by the L-cells of the small intestine after a meal intake, presents several actions that contribute to glucose homeostasis, including stimulation of postprandial insulin secretion by pancreatic beta cells, thus improving insulin sensitivity. GLP-1 is metabolized by the enzyme dipeptidyl peptidase 4 (DPP-4), thus inactivating their insulinotropic activities. In diabetic patients, the incretin effect is partially blunted, which contributes to a poor glycemic control. The incretin-based therapies, a new class of antidiabetic drugs currently available for the treatment of diabetic patients, include DPP-4 inhibitors (such as sitagliptin) and GLP-1 receptor (GLP-1R) agonists (namely exenatide). GLP-1R and DPP-4 are expressed in several extra-pancreatic tissues, including the heart, which has encouraged studies concerning its role in cardiac physiology, as well putative cardiac and cardiovascular benefits of incretin-based therapies.

Several body of experimental and clinical data have suggested a considerable cardioprotective role of GLP-1 agonists in the myocardium. Myocardial ischemia-reperfusion injury was attenuated by GLP-1 in vitro rat hearts, showing cardioprotective and inotropic effects [85]. Furthermore, it has been shown that mice with genetic deletion of GLP-1 receptor display reduced heart rate, elevated left ventricular end-diastolic pressure and impaired left ventricular contractility and diastolic function after insulin administration. Furthermore, infusion of GLP-1 resulted in improved left ventricular function, hemodynamic status and efficiency, indicating a direct role of GLP-1 on the cardiac physiology [86]. Apart the clinical pharmacological effects on body weight reduction, amelioration of blood pressure and improvement of glycemic control and lipid profile, GLP-1R agonists have been experimentally shown to exert antioxidant, vasoprotective and anti-inflammatory properties. One of these studies showed that liraglutide exerts anti-inflammatory effect on vascular endothelial cells through increased NO production and suppressed NF-κB activation, which is at least partly mediated via AMPK activation [87]. In another study, liraglutide was able to ameliorate cardiac hypertrophy in mice [88]. However, further research is advisory to better understand the complete benefits of GLP-1R agonists in the treatment of DCM.

DPP-4 inhibitors are able to increase the endogenous contents of incretins, such as GLP-1. Besides their effect on glycemic control, beneficial actions on other tissues, including on the heart tissue, have been shown, which might be due to anti-inflammatory, antioxidant and anti-apoptotic properties [89–94]. DPP-IV inhibitors have the advantage of being available for oral administration and do not raise supra-physiological concentration of GLP-1. However, further research is needed to elucidate the effective relevance of DPP-IV inhibitors in DCM.

6.3. Other non-antidiabetic agents

6.3.1. Statins

Statins are primarily inhibitors of cholesterol biosynthesis and the control of hyperlipidemia will benefit T2DM patients. However, although the key benefits of statins were initially attributed to their lipid lowering effects, it is now known that they directly act through other cellular mechanisms, known as pleiotropic effects [95]. Statins increase the expression and activation of eNOS thus causing an increase in the bioavailability of nitric oxide (NO), which contribute to the reduction in blood thrombogenicity, of oxidative stress and of cell proliferation. In addition, statins may also exert anti-inflammatory effects by several pathways, including reduced activity of VCAM-1 and ICAM-1, decreased function and levels of MCP-1 and decreased CRP [96]. Atorvastatin have been associated with improved left ventricular function, reduced fibrosis and hypertrophy; the protective effects on cardiac remodeling have been attributed to its anti-inflammatory actions [97]. However, further studies should be conducted to better evaluate the possible beneficial effects in DCM.

6.3.2. RAAS inhibitors

Angiotensin converting enzyme inhibitors (ACEIs) and angiotensin receptor blockers (ARBs) are the most used drugs to block the RAAS, and there are numerous evidences suggesting that these antihypertensive agents reduce cardiovascular mortality in diabetic patients due to improvement of cardiac dysfunction [98]. ACEI and ARBs have been associated with several beneficial properties at cardiac level, including improved cardiac fibrosis, reduced collagen synthesis and deposition, amelioration of cardiomyocyte apoptosis and cardiac hypertrophy [98–100]. Experimental and clinical studies also suggest a beneficial effect on T2DM by ameliorating insulin sensitivity, enhancing glucose uptake, improving pancreatic and skeletal muscle blood flow and stimulating proliferation and differentiation of adipocytes, beyond the reduction in blood pressure [99]. Additionally, inhibition of Ang II production and/or action with ACEI and ARBs attenuate its pro-inflammatory actions. In fact, although further clinical evidences are still needed, several studies have showed beneficial effect on markers of inflammation (such as TNF-α, IL-6 and IFN-γ) in heart failure patients [100].

6.3.3. Modulators of mitochondrial function

Numerous studies have highlighted the pivotal importance of impaired mitochondrial metabolism and increased formation of ROS in the pathogenesis of cardiac dysfunction, as discussed previously. Therefore, strategies aiming at modulation of different aspects of mitochondria such as biogenesis, fusion and fission, mitophagy, MPT and ROS generation may lead to effective treatments for cardiomyopathies [101]. Modulation of sirtuins activity, exercise-induced PGC-1 activation, fission and fusion as well as autophagy/mitophagy [102–105] are examples. Interestingly, although increased ROS generation and consequent oxidative damage is associated with pathological processes, mild levels of mitochondrial-derived ROS have been proposed to induce a hormetic response. The concept of mitohormesis proposes that a mild increase in mitochondrial ROS may act as a sublethal trigger of cytoprotective long-lasting metabolic and biochemical changes against larger subsequent stresses [106]. This approach was addressed in mice as a pathway to stimulate mitochondrial energy metabolism and to induce antioxidant defenses, thus preventing cardiomyopathy induced by the cardiotoxic doxorubicin [107], an effect that was also triggered by exercise [108]. Moreover, it has been shown that the development of cardiomyopathy due to impaired mitophagy and consequent accumulation of damaged ROS-forming mitochondria can be surprisingly improved by ROS-dependent activation of compensatory autophagic pathways of mitochondrial quality control, preventing a vicious cycle of ROS formation and mitochondrial dysfunction [109].

7. Concluding remarks

Over the years, DCM has evolved from a nebulous concept to concrete reality and is now viewed as a specific clinical entity caused by the complex relationships between metabolic abnormalities that accompany diabetes, resulting in functional and structural changes in the myocardium that ultimately leads to HF. DCM involves the damage of the myocardium through several mechanisms, namely hypertrophy, fibrosis, apoptosis and necrosis of cardiomyocytes. Some of the main factors involved in diabetes pathogenesis are also pivotal in DCM development, including hyperglycemia-evoked oxidative stress and mitochondrial dysfunction (by impaired autophagy, mitophagy and fusion–fission balance), hyperlipidemia, accompanied by inflammation and a switch of substrate supply to FFAs, as well as insulin resistance. Increasing body of evidence suggests the existence of relevant links between some of these pathways, including between oxidative energy metabolism dysregulation, impaired mitochondrial morphology and energetics evoked by abnormal Ca^{2+} handling, metabolic changes and oxidative stress, as well as chronic low-grade inflammation. The improved knowledge regarding the molecular mechanisms underlying DCM development has contributed to identify novel putative targets and therapeutic opportunities for the management of DCM. Pharmacological options targeting hyperglycemia, insulin resistance and reduced sensitivity, hyperlipidemia, inflammation, oxidative stress and mitochondrial dysfunction have been increasingly investigated, and it is hoped that could significantly improve the ability to prevent and/or improve management of DCM.

Acknowledgements

Authors thank the financial support of Fundação para a Ciência e Tecnologia through (FCT) for the Sara Nunes PhD scholarship (SFRH/BD/109017/2015) and UID/NEU/04539/2013 (CNC.IBILI Consortium), as well as FEDER-COMPETE (FCOMP-01-0124-FEDER-028417 and POCI-01-0145-FEDER-007440).

Author details

Sara Nunes[1†], Anabela Pinto Rolo[2†], Carlos Manuel Palmeira[2]* and Flávio Reis[1]*

*Address all correspondence to: palmeira@uc.pt; freis@fmed.uc.pt

1 Laboratory of Pharmacology and Experimental Therapeutics, Institute for Biomedical Imaging and Life Sciences (IBILI), Faculty of Medicine and CNC.IBILI Consortium, University of Coimbra, Coimbra, Portugal

2 Department of Life Sciences and Center for Neurosciences and Cell Biology, University of Coimbra, Coimbra, Portugal

† These authors contributed equally for this work.

References

[1]   Hossain P, Kawar B, El Nahas M. Obesity and diabetes in the developing world: a growing challenge. N Engl J Med. 2007;**356**:213–5. doi:10.1056/NEJMp068177.

[2]   Tuomilehto J, Lindström J. The major diabetes prevention trials. Curr Diab Rep. 2003;**3**:115–22. doi:10.1007/s11892-003-0034-9.

[3]   Rubler S,Dlugash J, Yuceoglu YZ, Kumral T, Branwood AW, Grishman A. New type of cardiomyopathy associated with diabetic glomerulosclerosis. Am J Cardiol. 1972;**30**:595–602. doi:10.1016/0002-9149(72)90595-4.

[4]   Shrestha NR, Sharma SK, Karki P, Shrestha NK, Acharya P. Echocardiographic evaluation of diastolic function in asymptomatic type 2 diabetes. JNMA J Nepal Med Assoc. 2009;**48**:20–3.

[5]   Wilson Tang WH. Glycemic control and treatment patterns in patients with heart failure. Curr Cardiol Rep. 2007;**9**:242–7. doi:10.1007/BF02938357.

[6]   Letonja M, Petrovič D. Is diabetic cardiomyopathy a specific entity? World J Cardiol. 2014;**6**:8–13. doi:10.4330/wjc.v6.i1.8.

[7]   Boudina S, Abel ED. Diabetic cardiomyopathy, causes and effects. Rev Endocr Metab Disord. 2010;**11**:31–9. doi:10.1007/s11154-010-9131-7.

[8]   Karason K, Sjostrom L, Wallentin I, Peltonen M. Impact of blood pressure and insulin on the relationship between body fat and left ventricular structure. Eur Heart J. 2003;**24**:1500–5. [pii]:S0195668X03003129.

[9]   Rosenkranz AC, Hood SG, Woods RL, Dusting GJ, Ritchie RH. B-type natriuretic peptide prevents acute hypertrophic responses in the diabetic rat heart: importance of cyclic GMP. Diabetes. 2003;**52**:2389–95. doi:10.2337/diabetes.52.9.2389.

[10] Nunes S, Soares E, Fernandes J, Viana S, Carvalho E, Pereira FC, et al. Early cardiac changes in a rat model of prediabetes: brain natriuretic peptide overexpression seems to be the best marker. Cardiovasc Diabetol. 2013;**12**:44. doi:10.1186/1475-2840-12-44.

[11] van Heerebeek L, Hamdani N, Handoko ML, Falcao-Pires I, Musters RJ, Kupreishvili K, et al. Diastolic stiffness of the failing diabetic heart: importance of fibrosis, advanced glycation end products, and myocyte resting tension. Circulation. 2008;**117**:43–51. doi:10.1161/CIRCULATIONAHA.107.728550.

[12] Mizushige K, Yao L, Noma T, Kiyomoto H, Yu Y, Hosomi N, et al. Alteration in left ventricular diastolic filling and accumulation of myocardial collagen at insulin-resistant prediabetic stage of a type II diabetic rat model. Circulation. 2000;**101**:899–907. doi:10.1161/01.CIR.101.8.899.

[13] Aronson D. Cross-linking of glycated collagen in the pathogenesis of arterial and myocardial stiffening of aging and diabetes. J Hypertens. 2003;**21**:3–12. doi:10.1097/01. hjh.0000042892.24999.92.

[14] D'Souza A, Howarth FC, Yanni J, Dobrzynski H, Boyett MR, Adeghate E, et al. Chronic effects of mild hyperglycaemia on left ventricle transcriptional profile and structural remodelling in the spontaneously type 2 diabetic Goto-Kakizaki rat. Heart Fail Rev. 2014;**19**:65–74. doi:10.1007/s10741-013-9376-9.

[15] Eckhouse SR, Spinale FG. Changes in the myocardial interstitium and contribution to the progression of heart failure. Heart Fail Clin. 2012;**8**:7–20. doi:10.1016/j.hfc.2011.08.012.

[16] Paulus WJ, Tschöpe C, Sanderson JE, Rusconi C, Flachskampf FA, Rademakers FE, et al. How to diagnose diastolic heart failure: a consensus statement on the diagnosis of heart failure with normal left ventricular ejection fraction by the Heart Failure and Echocardiography Associations of the European Society of Cardiology. Eur Heart J. 2007;**28**:2539–50. doi:10.1093/eurheartj/ehm037.

[17] Schannwell CM, Schneppenheim M, Perings S, Plehn G, Strauer BE. Left ventricular diastolic dysfunction as an early manifestation of diabetic cardiomyopathy. Cardiology. 2002;**98**:33–9. doi:64682.

[18] Hamblin M, Friedman DB, Hill S, Caprioli RM, Smith HM, Hill MF. Alterations in the diabetic myocardial proteome coupled with increased myocardial oxidative stress underlies diabetic cardiomyopathy. J Mol Cell Cardiol. 2007;**42**:884–95. doi:10.1016/j.yjmcc.2006.12.018.

[19] Von Bibra H, St John Sutton M. Diastolic dysfunction in diabetes and the metabolic syndrome: promising potential for diagnosis and prognosis. Diabetologia. 2010;**53**:1033–45. doi:10.1007/s00125-010-1682-3.

[20] Yilmaz S, Canpolat U, Aydogdu S, Abboud HE. Diabetic cardiomyopathy; summary of 41 years. Korean Circ J. 2015;**45**:266–72. doi:10.4070/kcj.2015.45.4.266.

[21] Jia G, DeMarco VG, Sowers JR. Insulin resistance and hyperinsulinaemia in diabetic cardiomyopathy. Nat Rev Endocrinol. 2016;**12**:144–53. doi:10.1038/nrendo.2015.216.

[22] Khullar M, Al-Shudiefat AA-RS, Ludke A, Binepal G, Singal PK. Oxidative stress: a key contributor to diabetic cardiomyopathy. Can J Physiol Pharmacol. 2010;**88**:233–40. doi:10.1139/Y10-016.

[23] Son NH, Park TS, Yamashita H, Yokoyama M, Huggins LA, Okajima K, et al. Cardiomyocyte expression of PPARgamma leads to cardiac dysfunction in mice. J Clin Invest. 2007;**117**:2791–801. doi:10.1172/JCI30335.

[24] Nunes S, Soares E, Pereira F, Reis F. The role of inflammation in diabetic cardiomyopathy. Int J Interf Cytokine Mediat Res. 2012;**4**:59. doi:10.2147/IJICMR.S21679.

[25] Iacobellis G, Sharma AM. Epicardial adipose tissue as new cardio-metabolic risk marker and potential therapeutic target in the metabolic syndrome. Curr Pharm Des. 2007;**13**:2180–4.

[26] Singh VP, Le B, Khode R, Baker KM, Kumar R. Intracellular angiotensin II production in diabetic rats is correlated with cardiomyocyte apoptosis, oxidative stress, and cardiac fibrosis. Diabetes. 2008;**57**:3297–306. doi:10.2337/db08-0805.

[27] Dorn GW, Vega RB, Kelly DP. Mitochondrial biogenesis and dynamics in the developing and diseased heart. Genes Dev. 2015;**29**:1981–91. doi:10.1101/gad.269894.115.

[28] Huss JM, Kelly DP. Mitochondrial energy metabolism in heart failure: a question of balance. J Clin Invest. 2005;**115**:547–55. doi:10.1172/JCI200524405.

[29] Lesnefsky EJ, Chen Q, Hoppel CL. Mitochondrial metabolism in aging heart. Circ Res. 2016;**118**:1593–611. doi:10.1161/CIRCRESAHA.116.307505.

[30] Korshunov SS, Skulachev VP, Starkov AA. High protonic potential actuates a mechanism of production of reactive oxygen species in mitochondria. FEBS Lett. 1997;**416**:15–8. doi:10.1016/S0014-5793(97)01159-9.

[31] Turrens JF. Mitochondrial formation of reactive oxygen species. J Physiol. 2003;**552**:335–44. doi:10.1113/jphysiol.2003.049478.

[32] Giordano FJ. Oxygen, oxidative stress, hypoxia, and heart failure. J Clin Invest. 2005;**115**:500–8. doi:10.1172/JCI200524408.

[33] Di Filippo C, Cuzzocrea S, Rossi F, Marfella R, D'Amico M. Oxidative stress as the leading cause of acute myocardial infarction in diabetics. Cardiovasc Drug Rev. 2006;**24**:77–87. doi:10.1111/j.1527-3466.2006.00077.x.

[34] Halestrap AP. Mitochondria and reperfusion injury of the heart—A holey death but not beyond salvation. J Bioenerg Biomembr. 2009;**41**:113–21. doi:10.1007/s10863-009-9206-x.

[35] Mdaki KS, Larsen TD, Wachal AL, Schimelpfenig MD, Weaver LJ, Dooyema SDR, et al. Maternal high-fat diet impairs cardiac function in offspring of diabetic pregnancy through metabolic stress and mitochondrial dysfunction. Am J Physiol Heart Circ Physiol. 2016:ajpheart.00795.2015. doi:10.1152/ajpheart.00795.2015.

[36] Wallace DC, Fan W. Energetics, epigenetics, mitochondrial genetics. Mitochondrion 2010;**10**:12–31. doi:10.1016/j.mito.2009.09.006.

[37] Ricci C, Pastukh V, Leonard J, Turrens J, Wilson G, Schaffer D, et al. Mitochondrial DNA damage triggers mitochondrial-superoxide generation and apoptosis. Am J Physiol Cell Physiol. 2008;**294**:C413–22. doi:10.1152/ajpcell.00362.2007.

[38] Filomeni G, Zio D De, Cecconi F, De Zio D, Cecconi F. Oxidative stress and autophagy: the clash between damage and metabolic needs. Cell Death Differ. 2015;**22**:377–88. doi:10.1038/cdd.2014.150.

[39] Rabinowitz JD, White E. Autophagy and metabolism. Science. 2010;**330**:1344–8. doi:10.1126/science.1193497.

[40] Yan L, Vatner DE, Kim SJ, Ge H, Masurekar M, Massover WH, et al. Autophagy in chronically ischemic myocardium. Proc Natl Acad Sci USA. 2005;**102**:13807–12. doi:10.1073/pnas.0506843102.

[41] Matsui Y, Takagi H, Qu X, Abdellatif M, Sakoda H, Asano T, et al. Distinct roles of autophagy in the heart during ischemia and reperfusion: roles of AMP-activated protein

kinase and beclin 1 in mediating autophagy. Circ Res. 2007;**100**:914–22. doi:10.1161/01. RES.0000261924.76669.36.

[42] Nakai A, Yamaguchi O, Takeda T, Higuchi Y, Hikoso S, Taniike M, et al. The role of autophagy in cardiomyocytes in the basal state and in response to hemodynamic stress. Nat Med. 2007;**13**:619–24. doi: 10.1038/nm1574. pii:nm1574.

[43] Wang K, Klionsky DJ. Mitochondria removal by autophagy. Autophagy. 2011;**7**:297–300. doi:10.4161/auto.7.3.14502.

[44] Komatsu M, Kurokawa H, Waguri S, Taguchi K, Kobayashi A, Ichimura Y, et al. The selective autophagy substrate p62 activates the stress responsive transcription factor Nrf2 through inactivation of Keap1. Nat Cell Biol. 2010;**12**:213–23. doi:10.1038/ncb2021.

[45] Wohlgemuth SE, Calvani R, Marzetti E. The interplay between autophagy and mitochondrial dysfunction in oxidative stress-induced cardiac aging and pathology. J Mol Cell Cardiol. 2014;**71**:62–70. doi:10.1016/j.yjmcc.2014.03.007.

[46] Liesa M, Palacín M, Zorzano A. Mitochondrial dynamics in mammalian health and disease. Physiol Rev. 2009;**89**:799–845. doi:10.1152/physrev.00030.2008.

[47] Lee Y, Jeong S-Y, Karbowski M, Smith CL, Youle RJ. Roles of the mammalian mitochondrial fission and fusion mediators Fis1, Drp1, and Opa1 in apoptosis. Mol Biol Cell. 2004;**15**:5001–11. doi:10.1091/mbc.E04-04-0294.

[48] Papanicolaou KN, Kikuchi R, Ngoh GA, Coughlan KA, Dominguez I, Stanley WC, et al. Mitofusins 1 and 2 are essential for postnatal metabolic remodeling in heart. Circ Res. 2012;**111**:1012–26. doi:10.1161/CIRCRESAHA.112.274142.

[49] Chen Y, Liu Y, Dorn GW. Mitochondrial fusion is essential for organelle function and cardiac homeostasis. Circ Res. 2011;**109**:1327–31. doi:10.1161/CIRCRESAHA.111.258723.

[50] Ong S-B, Hausenloy DJ. Mitochondrial morphology and cardiovascular disease. Cardiovasc Res. 2010;**88**:16–29. doi:10.1093/cvr/cvq237.

[51] Song M, Mihara K, Chen Y, Scorrano L, Dorn GW. Mitochondrial fission and fusion factors reciprocally orchestrate mitophagic culling in mouse hearts and cultured fibroblasts. Cell Metab. 2015;**21**:273–85. doi:10.1016/j.cmet.2014.12.011.

[52] Hom J, Yu T, Yoon Y, Porter G, Sheu S-S. Regulation of mitochondrial fission by intracellular Ca(2+) in rat ventricular myocytes. Biochim Biophys Acta. 2010;**1797**:913–21. doi:10.1016/j.bbabio.2010.03.018.

[53] Tandler B, Dunlap M, Hoppel CL, Hassan M. Giant mitochondria in a cardiomyopathic heart. Ultrastruct Pathol. 2002;**26**:177–83. doi:10.1080/01913120290076847.

[54] Sebastiani M, Giordano C, Nediani C, Travaglini C, Borchi E, Zani M, et al. Induction of mitochondrial biogenesis is a maladaptive mechanism in mitochondrial cardiomyopathies. J Am Coll Cardiol. 2007;**50**:1362–9. doi:10.1016/j.jacc.2007.06.035.

[55] Kelly DP, Scarpulla RC. Transcriptional regulatory circuits controlling mitochondrial biogenesis and function. Genes Dev. 2004;**18**:357–68. doi:10.1101/gad.1177604.

[56] Soriano FX, Liesa M, Bach D, Chan DC, Palacín M, Zorzano A. Evidence for a mitochondrial regulatory pathway defined by peroxisome proliferator-activated receptor-gamma coactivator-1 alpha, estrogen-related receptor-alpha, and mitofusin 2. Diabetes. 2006;**55**:1783–91. doi:10.2337/db05-0509.

[57] St-Pierre J, Drori S, Uldry M, Silvaggi JM, Rhee J, Jäger S, et al. Suppression of reactive oxygen species and neurodegeneration by the PGC-1 transcriptional coactivators. Cell. 2006;**127**:397–408. doi:10.1016/j.cell.2006.09.024.

[58] Kong X, Wang R, Xue Y, Liu X, Zhang H, Chen Y, et al. Sirtuin 3, a new target of PGC-1alpha, plays an important role in the suppression of ROS and mitochondrial biogenesis. PLoS One. 2010;**5**:e11707. doi:10.1371/journal.pone.0011707.

[59] Haigis MC, Sinclair DA. Mammalian sirtuins: biological insights and disease relevance. Annu Rev Pathol. 2010;**5**:253–95. doi:10.1146/annurev.pathol.4.110807.092250.

[60] Gomes AP, Price NL, Ling AJY, Moslehi JJ, Montgomery MK, Rajman L, et al. Declining NAD+ induces a pseudohypoxic state disrupting nuclear-mitochondrial communication during aging. Cell. 2013;**155**:1624–38. doi:10.1016/j.cell.2013.11.037.

[61] Matsushima S, Sadoshima J. The role of sirtuins in cardiac disease. Am J Physiol Hear Circ Physiol. 2015;**1**:ajpheart.00053.2015. doi:10.1152/ajpheart.00053.2015.

[62] Horton JL, Martin OJ, Lai L, Riley NM, Richards AL, Vega RB, et al. Mitochondrial protein hyperacetylation in the failing heart. JCI Insight. 2016;1. doi:10.1172/jci.insight.84897.

[63] Samant S a, Zhang HJ, Hong Z, Pillai VB, Sundaresan NR, Wolfgeher D, et al. SIRT3 deacetylates and activates OPA1 to regulate mitochondrial dynamics during stress. Mol Cell Biol. 2014;**34**:807–19. doi:10.1128/MCB.01483-13.

[64] Hafner A V, Dai J, Gomes AP, Xiao CY, Palmeira CM, Rosenzweig A, et al. Regulation of the mPTP by SIRT3-mediated deacetylation of CypD at lysine 166 suppresses age-related cardiac hypertrophy. Aging (Albany NY). 2010;**2**:914–23. doi:10.18632/aging.100252.

[65] Lorenzo O, Picatoste B, Ares-Carrasco S, Ramírez E, Egido J, Tuñón J. Potential role of nuclear factor-kb in diabetic cardiomyopathy. Mediators Inflamm. 2011;2011. doi:10.1155/2011/652097.

[66] Sun M, Dawood F, Wen WH, Chen M, Dixon I, Kirshenbaum LA, et al. Excessive tumor necrosis factor activation after infarction contributes to susceptibility of myocardial rupture and left ventricular dysfunction. Circulation. 2004;**110**:3221–8. doi:10.1161/01. CIR.0000147233.10318.23.

[67] Westermann D, Rutschow S, Van Linthout S, Linderer A, Bücker-Gärtner C, Sobirey M, et al. Inhibition of p38 mitogen-activated protein kinase attenuates left ventricular dysfunction by mediating pro-inflammatory cardiac cytokine levels in a mouse model of diabetes mellitus. Diabetologia. 2006;**49**:2507–13. doi:10.1007/s00125-006-0385-2.

[68] Yu X-Y, Chen H-M, Liang J-L, Lin Q-X, Tan H-H, Fu Y-H, et al. Hyperglycemic myocardial damage is mediated by proinflammatory cytokine: macrophage migration inhibitory factor. PLoS One. 2011;**6**:e16239. doi:10.1371/journal.pone.0016239.

[69] Schieffer B, Luchtefeld M, Braun S, Hilfiker a, Hilfiker-Kleiner D, Drexler H. Role of NAD(P)H oxidase in angiotensin II-induced JAK/STAT signaling and cytokine induction. Circ Res. 2000;**87**:1195–201. doi:10.1161/01.RES.87.12.1195.

[70] Fuentes-Antrás J, Ioan AM, Tuñón J, Egido J, Lorenzo O. Activation of toll-like receptors and inflammasome complexes in the diabetic cardiomyopathy-associated inflammation. Int J Endocrinol. 2014;2014:847827. doi:10.1155/2014/847827.

[71] Hopps E, Canino B, Caimi G. Effects of exercise on inflammation markers in type 2 diabetic subjects. Acta Diabetol. 2011;**48**:183–9. doi:10.1007/s00592-011-0278-9.

[72] de Lemos ET, Reis F, Baptista S, Pinto R, Sepodes B, Vala H, et al. Exercise training is associated with improved levels of C-reactive protein and adiponectin in ZDF (type 2) diabetic rats. Med Sci Monit. 2007;**13**:BR168–74.

[73] Teixeira de Lemos E, Reis F, Baptista S, Pinto R, Sepodes B, Vala H, et al. Exercise training decreases proinflammatory profile in Zucker diabetic (type 2) fatty rats. Nutrition. 2009;**25**:330–9. doi:10.1016/j.nut.2008.08.014.

[74] Teixeira-Lemos E, Nunes S, Teixeira F, Reis F. Regular physical exercise training assists in preventing type 2 diabetes development: focus on its antioxidant and anti-inflammatory properties. Cardiovasc Diabetol. 2011;**10**:12. doi:10.1186/1475-2840-10-12.

[75] Teixeira De Lemos E, Pinto R, Oliveira J, Garrido P, Sereno J, Mascarenhas-Melo F, et al. Differential effects of acute (extenuating) and chronic (training) exercise on inflammation and oxidative stress status in an animal model of type 2 diabetes mellitus. Mediators Inflamm. 2011;2011. doi:10.1155/2011/253061.

[76] Dandona P, Chaudhuri A, Ghanim H, Mohanty P. Insulin as an anti-inflammatory and antiatherogenic modulator. J Am Coll Cardiol. 2009;53. doi:10.1016/j.jacc.2008.10.038.

[77] Group UP. Effects of Intensive blood glucose control with metformin on complications in overweight patients with type 2 diabetes (UKPDS 34). Lancet. 1998;**352**:854–65.

[78] Gundewar S, Calvert JW, Jha S, Toedt-Pingel I, Ji SY, Nunez D, et al. Activation of AMP-activated protein kinase by metformin improves left ventricular function and survival in heart failure. Circ Res. 2009;**104**:403–11. doi:10.1161/CIRCRESAHA.108.190918.

[79] Tsuji T, Mizushige K, Noma T, Murakami K, Ohmori K, Miyatake A, et al. Pioglitazone improves left ventricular diastolic function and decreases collagen accumulation in prediabetic stage of a type II diabetic rat. J Cardiovasc Pharmacol. 2001;**38**:868–74. doi:10.1097/00005344-200112000-00008.

[80] von Bibra H, Diamant M, Scheffer PG, Siegmund T, Schumm-Draeger P-M. Rosiglitazone, but not glimepiride, improves myocardial diastolic function in association with reduction

in oxidative stress in type 2 diabetic patients without overt heart disease. Diabetes Vasc Dis Res. 2008;**5**:310–8. doi:10.3132/dvdr.2008.045.

[81] Terui G, Goto T, Katsuta M, Aoki I, Ito H. Effect of pioglitazone on left ventricular diastolic function and fibrosis of type III collagen in type 2 diabetic patients. J Cardiol. 2009;**54**:52–8. doi:10.1016/j.jjcc.2009.03.004.

[82] Hayat SA, Patel B, Khattar RS, Malik RA. Diabetic cardiomyopathy: mechanisms, diagnosis and treatment. Clin Sci (Lond). 2004;**107**:539–57. doi:10.1042/CS20040057.

[83] Takano H, Nagai T, Asakawa M, Toyozaki T, Oka T, Komuro I, et al. Peroxisome proliferator-activated receptor activators inhibit lipopolysaccharide-induced tumor necrosis factor-alpha expression in neonatal rat cardiac myocytes. Circ Res. 2000;**87**:596–602.

[84] Ares-Carrasco S, Picatoste B, Camafeita E, Carrasco-Navarro S, Zubiri I, Ortiz A, et al. Proteome changes in the myocardium of experimental chronic diabetes and hypertension. Role of PPARα in the associated hypertrophy. J Proteomics. 2012;**75**:1816–29. doi:10.1016/j.jprot.2011.12.023.

[85] Ossum A, van Deurs U, Engstrøm T, Jensen JS, Treiman M. The cardioprotective and inotropic components of the postconditioning effects of GLP-1 and GLP-1(9–36)a in an isolated rat heart. Pharmacol Res. 2009;**60**:411–7. doi:10.1016/j.phrs.2009.06.004.

[86] Hansotia T, Drucker DJ. GIP and GLP-1 as incretin hormones: lessons from single and double incretin receptor knockout mice. Regul Pept. 2005;**128**:125–34. doi:10.1016/j.regpep.2004.07.019.

[87] Hattori Y, Jojima T, Tomizawa A, Satoh H, Hattori S, Kasai K, et al. A glucagon-like peptide-1 (GLP-1) analogue, liraglutide, upregulates nitric oxide production and exerts anti-inflammatory action in endothelial cells. Diabetologia. 2010;**53**:2256–63. doi:10.1007/s00125-010-1831-8.

[88] Mells JE, Fu PP, Sharma S, Olson D, Cheng L, Handy J a., et al. Glp-1 analog, liraglutide, ameliorates hepatic steatosis and cardiac hypertrophy in C57BL/6J mice fed a Western diet. AJP Gastrointest Liver Physiol. 2012;**302**:G225–35. doi:10.1152/ajpgi.00274.2011.

[89] Ferreira L, Teixeira-De-Lemos E, Pinto F, Parada B, Mega C, Vala H, et al. Effects of sitagliptin treatment on dysmetabolism, inflammation, and oxidative stress in an animal model of type 2 diabetes (ZDF rat). Mediators Inflamm. 2010;2010. doi:10.1155/2010/592760.

[90] Mega C, Teixeira De Lemos E, Vala H, Fernandes R, Oliveira J, Mascarenhas-Melo F, et al. Diabetic nephropathy amelioration by a low-dose sitagliptin in an animal model of type 2 diabetes (Zucker diabetic fatty rat). Exp Diabetes Res. 2011;2011. doi:10.1155/2011/162092.

[91] Gonçalves A, Leal E, Paiva A, Teixeira Lemos E, Teixeira F, Ribeiro CF, et al. Protective effects of the dipeptidyl peptidase IV inhibitor sitagliptin in the blood-retinal

barrier in a type 2 diabetes animal model. Diabetes Obes Metab. 2012;14:454–63. doi:10.1111/j.1463-1326.2011.01548.x.

[92] Gonçalves A, Marques C, Leal E, Ribeiro CF, Reis F, Ambrósio AF, et al. Dipeptidyl peptidase-IV inhibition prevents blood-retinal barrier breakdown, inflammation and neuronal cell death in the retina of type 1 diabetic rats. Biochim Biophys Acta Mol Basis Dis. 2014;1842:1454–63. doi:10.1016/j.bbadis.2014.04.013.

[93] Marques C, Mega C, Gonçalves A, Rodrigues-Santos P, Teixeira-Lemos E, Teixeira F, et al. Sitagliptin prevents inflammation and apoptotic cell death in the kidney of type 2 diabetic animals. Mediators Inflamm. 2014;2014. doi:10.1155/2014/538737.

[94] Mega C, Vala H, Rodrigues-Santos P, Oliveira J, Teixeira F, Fernandes R, et al. Sitagliptin prevents aggravation of endocrine and exocrine pancreatic damage in the Zucker Diabetic Fatty rat—focus on amelioration of metabolic profile and tissue cytoprotective properties. Diabetol Metab Syndr. 2014;6:42. doi:10.1186/1758-5996-6-42.

[95] Davignon J. Beneficial cardiovascular pleiotropic effects of statins. Circulation. 2004;109:III39–43. doi:10.1161/01.CIR.0000131517.20177.5a.

[96] Blanco-Colio LM, Tuñón J, Martín-Ventura JL, Egido J. Anti-inflammatory and immunomodulatory effects of statins. Kidney Int. 2003;63:12–23. doi:10.1046/j.1523-1755.2003.00744.x.

[97] Sola S, Mir MQS, Lerakis S, Tandon N, Khan B V. Atorvastatin improves left ventricular systolic function and serum markers of inflammation in nonischemic heart failure. J Am Coll Cardiol. 2006;47:332–7. doi:10.1016/j.jacc.2005.06.088.

[98] Shekelle PG, Rich MW, Morton SC, Atkinson SW, Tu W, Maglione M, et al. Efficacy of angiotensin-converting enzyme inhibitors and beta-blockers in the management of left ventricular systolic dysfunction according to race, gender, and diabetic status: a meta-analysis of major clinical trials. J Am Coll Cardiol. 2003;41:1529–38. doi:10.1016/S0735-1097(03)00262-6.

[99] Scheen a J. Prevention of type 2 diabetes mellitus through inhibition of the renin-angiotensin system. Drugs. 2004;64:2537–65. doi:10.2165/00003495-200464220-00004.

[100] Proudfoot JM, Croft KD, Puddey IB, Beilin LJ. Angiotensin II type 1 receptor antagonists inhibit basal as well as low-density lipoprotein and platelet-activating factor-stimulated human monocyte chemoattractant protein-1. J Pharmacol Exp Ther. 2003;305:846–53. doi:10.1124/jpet.102.047795.

[101] Muntean DM, Sturza A, Dănilă MD, Borza C, Duicu OM, Mornoș C. The role of mitochondrial reactive oxygen species in cardiovascular injury and protective strategies. Oxid Med Cell Longev. 2016;2016:8254942. doi:10.1155/2016/8254942.

[102] Wu Y-T, Wu S-B, Wei Y-H. Roles of sirtuins in the regulation of antioxidant defense and bioenergetic function of mitochondria under oxidative stress. Free Radic Res. 2014;48:1070–84. doi:10.3109/10715762.2014.920956.

[103] Wang H, Bei Y, Lu Y, Sun W, Liu Q, Wang Y, et al. Exercise prevents cardiac injury and improves mitochondrial biogenesis in advanced diabetic cardiomyopathy with PGC-1α and Akt activation. Cell Physiol Biochem. 2015;**35**:2159–68. doi:10.1159/000374021.

[104] Hall AR, Burke N, Dongworth RK, Hausenloy DJ. Mitochondrial fusion and fission proteins: novel therapeutic targets for combating cardiovascular disease. Br J Pharmacol. 2014;**171**:1890–906. doi:10.1111/bph.12516.

[105] Disatnik MH, Hwang S, Ferreira JCB, Mochly-Rosen D. New therapeutics to modulate mitochondrial dynamics and mitophagy in cardiac diseases. J Mol Med. 2015;**93**:279–87. doi:10.1007/s00109-015-1256-4.

[106] Ristow M, Zarse K. How increased oxidative stress promotes longevity and metabolic health: the concept of mitochondrial hormesis (mitohormesis). Exp Gerontol. 2010;**45**:410–8. doi:10.1016/j.exger.2010.03.014.

[107] Schulz TJ, Westermann D, Isken F, Voigt A, Laube B, Thierbach R, et al. Activation of mitochondrial energy metabolism protects against cardiac failure. Aging (Albany NY). 2010;**2**:843–53.

[108] Marques-Aleixo I, Santos-Alves E, Mariani D, Rizo-Roca D, Padrão AI, Rocha-Rodrigues S, et al. Physical exercise prior and during treatment reduces sub-chronic doxorubicin-induced mitochondrial toxicity and oxidative stress. Mitochondrion. 2015;**20**:22–33. doi:10.1016/j.mito.2014.10.008.

[109] Song M, Chen Y, Gong G, Murphy E, Rabinovitch PS, Dorn GW. Super-suppression of mitochondrial reactive oxygen species signaling impairs compensatory autophagy in primary mitophagic cardiomyopathy. Circ Res. 2014;**115**:348–53. doi:10.1161/CIRCRESAHA.115.304384.

7

Cardiomyopathies in Sub-Saharan Africa: Hypertensive Heart Disease (Cardiomyopathy), Peripartum Cardiomyopathy and HIV-Associated Cardiomyopathy

Okechukwu S. Ogah and Ayodele O. Falase

Abstract

Cardiomyopathy is an important cause of cardiac-related morbidity and mortality in sub-Saharan Africa. Dilated cardiomyopathy is responsible for 20–30% of adult heart failure (HF) in the region. It is only second to hypertensive heart disease as etiological risk factor for HF in many parts of the continent. The aim of the chapter is to review the current epidemiology, clinical features, management, and prognosis of hypertensive heart disease, peripartum cardiomyopathy, and HIV-associated cardiomyopathy in sub-Saharan Africa.

Keywords: cardiomyopathy, heart muscle disease, hypertensive heart disease, peripartum cardiomyopathy, HIV-associated cardiomyopathy, heart failure

1. Introduction

Cardiomyopathies are common in Africa. Common causes of myocardial diseases in the region are hypertensive heart disease, endemic cardiomyopathies such as dilated cardiomyopathy, endomyocardial fibrosis, and peripartum cardiomyopathy and most recently heart diseases due to HIV/AIDS and ischemic cardiomyopathy. They are often associated with high morbidity and mortality due to late presentation, lack of modern day treatment available in high-income countries, as well poverty, which limits access to healthcare. **Figure 1** shows the common causes of heart failure (HF) in sub-Saharan Africa (SSA) based on a recent survey of acute HF in the region [1]. The chapter deals with hypertensive heart disease (hypertensive cardiomyopathy) peripartum cardiomyopathy and HIV-associated cardiomyopathy.

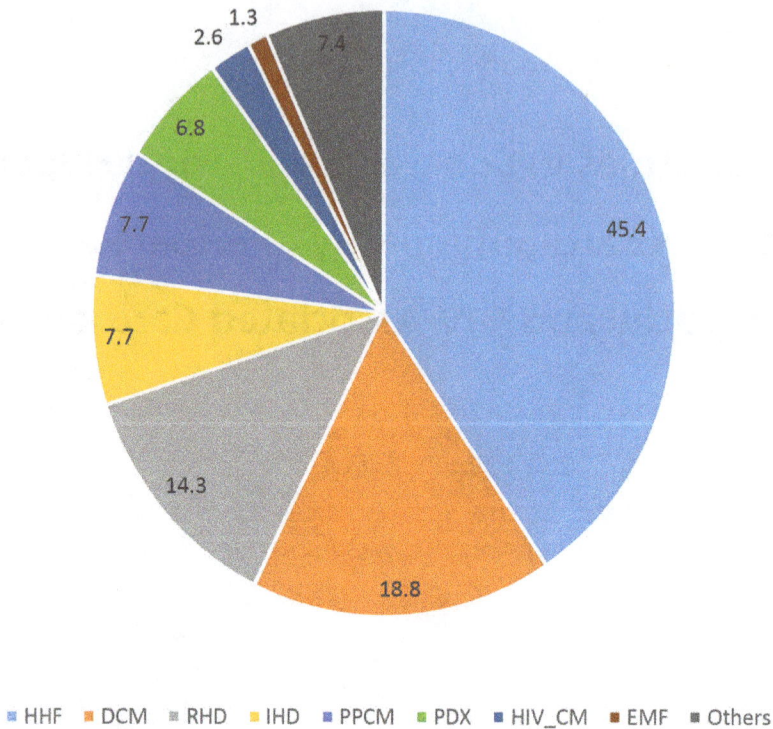

Figure 1. Etiological risk factors for heart failure in sub-Saharan Africa. (Adapted from Damasceno et al. HHF = Hypertensive heart failure, DCM = Dilated cardiomyopathy, RHD = Rheumatic heart disease, IHD = Ischemic heart disease, PPCM = Peripartum cardiomyopathy, PDX = Pericardial diseases, HIV_CM = HIV associated cardiomyopathy, EMF = Endomyocardial fibrosis.

2. Hypertensive heart disease (hypertensive cardiomyopathy)

2.1. Epidemiology

More than 30% of adults in SSA have hypertension. The prevalence rate is among the world highest. Worse still, the region has some of the world's lowest rates of hypertension aware-ness, treatment, and control. About 66% of the people are not aware, 82% are not treated and 93% are uncontrolled. In the year 2010, the age standardized prevalence of hypertension in adults aged 20-years and above was estimated as 36.9 and 36.3% for men and women, respectively (this is compared to 20.9 and 20.3%, 10 years earlier). This translates to 64.8 and 63.8 million men and women with elevated blood pressure in 2010 (compared to 25.5 and 24.9 million hypertensive men and women in the year 2000).

In a recent systematic analysis of population-based studies of hypertension in SSA, the pooled prevalence in the region rose from 19.7% in 1990 to 30.8% in 2010. It is estimated that there were about 54.6 million people with hypertension in Africa in 1990. This rose to 130.2 million cases in 2010. It is also projected that by the year 2030, there will be about 216.8 million cases of hypertension in the region [2].

Hypertension is the commonest and strongest risk factor for cardiovascular disease (CVD) in SSA [3]. It is also the commonest cause of disability and death from non-communicable diseases (NCDs) in the region [4]. The condition often manifests in young and middle aged adults in their productive years [4]. It is estimated to cause over 500,000 adult deaths annually and about 10-million years of life lost. Over 50% of heart disease and HF in the region is attributed to elevated blood pressure.

According to the African Union, hypertension is one of the greatest health challenges in adults in Africa after HIV/AIDS [4]. Recent data indicate that hypertension is rising in SSA at a faster rate compared to other regions of the world [5, 6]. This has been attributed to that adoption of western lifestyle, diet and culture, urbanization, urban migration from rural areas, ageing of the population, and increasing use of cigarettes and alcohol [3, 5–7].

It has been demonstrated that a chronic hyperadrenergic state is common among African hypertensives and may be responsible for the high prevalence of hypertension observed in Africans [8].

2.2. Clinical features

Heart disease secondary to elevated blood pressure (hypertensive heart disease), which may manifest in the following ways:

2.2.1. LV diastolic dysfunction

LV diastolic dysfunction is common in hypertensive subjects in the region [9–12]. About 62% of hypertensive individuals have various degrees of LV diastolic dysfunction compared to 12% of normal subjects [9, 13]. Diastolic dysfunction is worse in those with concentric LV geometry [9] as well as in individuals at risk of obstructive sleep apnea [14]. Diastolic dysfunction also occurs in offspring of hypertensive subjects [15–17].

2.2.2. RV diastolic dysfunction

Right ventricular systolic dysfunction has been reported in about 62% of a cohort of hypertensive patients [18, 19]. RV diastolic dysfunction may be an early clue to the development of hypertensive heart disease in Africans [19].

2.2.3. Atrial function and dysfunction

Absolute and indexed left atrial diameter, area, or volume is increased in African hypertensive subjects [20, 21]. Compared to their age- and sex-matched controls, hypertensive Africans show statistically significant left atrial structural and functional alterations [21].

2.3. Left ventricular hypertrophy

Electrocardiographic LVH occurs in 18–56% of hypertensive Africans depending on the criteria employed for the diagnosis. Sokolow-Lyon criteria appear to have the best sensitivity, while Estes score and Cornell criteria have the best specificity. Some workers in the region have proposed new criteria for ECG diagnosis of LVH in Africans especially in obese subjects [22–28]. ECG LVH with strain pattern is associated with worse LV structure and function in hypertensive Africans [29, 30].

The prevalence of echocardiographic LVH ranges from 30.9 to 74%. This, however, depends on the threshold used for the indexation of LV mass. Adebiyi et al. report 61–74% prevalence of abnormal LV geometry in hospital patients at the University College Hospital, Ibadan, Nigeria [31].

In a similar study in Northern Tanzania [32], 70% of the hypertensive subjects have abnormal LV geometry. The distribution of the abnormal LV geometric patterns is 19.8, 28.2, and 22% for concentric remodeling, concentric hypertrophy, and eccentric LVH, respectively. The best yield appears to be when LV mass is indexed to height raised to the power of 2.7 (allomeric growth rate of the heart). Age, systolic blood pressure, and duration of hypertension are independent predictors of LVH.

2.3.1. LV systolic dysfunction

LV systolic dysfunction (LVSD) occurs in 18.1% (9.6, 3.7, and 4.8% for mild, moderate, and severe LVSD, respectively) of hypertensive Africans [33]. The independent predictors of LVSD are LV mass, body mass index, and male gender. Ojji et al. [34] report LVSD in 6.7% (mild—3.5%, moderate—2.3%, and severe—0.9%) of 1943 hypertensive subjects and LV dysfunction is associated with older age, male sex, presence of diabetes mellitus, and some indices of the LV structure.

The Tei index (index of global myocardial performance) is significantly higher in hypertensive Africans compared to controls. The index increases with severity of LVSD. It is negatively related to the LVEF.

2.3.2. RV systolic dysfunction

RV systolic dysfunction occurs in about in 32% of hypertensive subjects seen in tertiary centers in the region [18, 35, 36]. RVSD is worse in subjects with eccentric LV geometry. LVEF appears to be the main determinant of RVSD. Recently, Ojji et al. [37] reported RVSD in 44.5% of 611 hypertensive subjects. RVSD estimated by TAPSE <15mm is associated with worse prognosis. LVEF and right atrial area are the main determinants of RVSD.

2.4. Hypertensive heart failure

Hypertensive HF (HHF) is a common and major form of presentation of HF in Africa. **Table 1** shows the contribution of hypertension in the etiology of HHF in SSA. In the Heart of Soweto study [38], 54% of hypertensive patients visit the hospital on account of this disorder. This devastating form of HHD is often associated with concurrent LVH, renal dysfunction, and anemia. In a study of 180 HHF patients in Ghana, the mean age of presentation is 63.6 years (range-24–88 years) and seen more often in women. The mean systolic blood pressure at presentation is 162.4 mmHg. Shortness of breath, easy fatigability, and palpitation are common symptoms while pulmonary edema and displaced apex beat are the common signs.

S. No.	Author/Publication Year	Country	HHF (%)
1	Damasceno [1], 2012	9 countries	45.4
2	Stewart [41], 2008	South Africa (Soweto)	33.3
3	Ojji [42], 2009	Nigeria(Abuja)	62.6
4	Ojji [43], 2013	Nigeria(Abuja)	60.6
5	Ogah [44], 2014	Nigeria(Abeokuta)	78.5
6	Karaye [45], 2008	Nigeria(Kano)	57
7	Laabes [46], 2008	Nigeria(Jos)	44.1
8	Onwuchekwa [47], 2009	Nigeria(Port-Harcourt)	56.3
9	Adewuya [48], 2006	Nigeria(Ile-Ife)	54
10	Yonga [49], 2010	Kenya	64
11	Kingue [50], 2005	Cameroon (Urban)	54.5
12	Tantchou [51], 2011	Cameroon (rural)	15
13	Soliman [52], 2008	Malawi	24
14	Kuule [53], 2009	Uganda	24.2
15	Okello [54], 2014	Uganda	9.1
17	Owusu [55], 2013	Ghana (Outpatients-Kumasi)	45
18	Owusu [56], 2006	Ghana (In-patients-Kumasi)	42.6
19	Soliman [52], 2011	Sudan	28
20	Habte [57], 2010	Ethiopia	24.2
21	Makubi [58], 2014	Tanzania	45

Table 1. Summary of contribution of hypertension to HF in recent SSA studies.

Cardiomegaly on chest radiography is present in 75.6%. ECG-LVH or ECHO-LVH occur in 75.6 and 83.3%, respectively. About 62% have heart failure with preserved ejection fraction HFpEF [39].

In Nigeria, HHF is more common in men (56%). The mean age of presentation is 58.4 and 60.6 years in men and women, respectively. Over 80% present in NYHA class III and IV. HFpEF is present in about 35% of cases. The median length of hospital stay is about 9-days while 3.4% die while on admission. A 30-, 90-, and 180-day mortality rates of 0.9, 3.5, and 11.7%, respectively have been reported. Renal dysfunction appears to be the main independent predictor of mortality [40].

Table 2 shows the characteristics of African patients with HHF compared with similar patients in other parts of the world.

2.5. Possible pathophysiologic mechanism of hypertensive heart disease in SSA

Hypertension is a common cause of pressure overload of the left ventricle. LVH develops as an adaptation to this overload. Hypertensive patient with ECG LVH has 10-fold higher risk

Characteristics	Ogah et al. [40] (n = 320)	Stewart et al. [41] (n = 281)	Nieminen et al. [59] (n = 200)	Spinar et al. [60] (n = 179)	Venskutonyte et al. [61] (n = 65)
Female (%)	42.5	61	39.6	65.4	33.3
Mean age (yrs)	59.3	61	69.8	74.8	65.5
Denovo HF (%)	85.6	NA	37.3	74.3	66.7
NYHA III+IV (%)	82.2	29	NA	34.0	NA
Previous history of hypertension (%)	90.6	100	94.6	94.3	100
Diabetes mellitus (%)	12.2	14	34.5	43.1	33.3
Previous MI or CAD (%)	0.3	1.0	53.8	26.4	46.7
COPD (%)	2.5	NA	18.0	17.8	26.7
Stroke or TIA in history (%)	0.3	12	16.0	26.4	20
Atrial fibrillation (%)	12.8	9	37.7	19.0	46.7
Mean systolic BP(mmHg)	144	140	NA	198	NA
Mean diastolic BP(mmHg)	91	80	NA	100	NA
Heart rate (beats/min)	96	NA	NA	93	NA
Body mass index (kg/m^2)	24.2	NA	NA	28.0	33.9
Hospitalization for HF within last 12 months (%)	82.2	NA	NA	45.1	46.6
Renal failure (%)	14.4	27	18.7	NA	NA
Anemia (%)	11.5	10	11.3	NA	NA
Infection (%)	63.4	NA	15.6	NA	13.3
Noncompliance with therapy (%)	74.1	NA	21.9	NA	66.7
ACE inhibitors (%)	99.1	NA	NA	71.3	NA
Beta-blockers (%)	2.7	NA	NA	77.0	NA
Calcium antagonists (%)	30.6	NA	NA	51.1	NA
Diuretics (%)	86.9	NA	NA	88.5	NA
Spironolactone (%)	81.3	NA	NA	36.2	NA
Digoxin (%)	73.1	NA	NS	13.8	NA
LVEDD (mm)	55	46	56	NA	50*
Mean ejection fraction	42.7	53	44	55	50.5
LA (mm)	47	NA	45	NA	42*
Mitral regurgitation (%)	79.1	7	77.6	NA	100
Tricuspid regurgitation (%)	60.8	6	53.7	NA	93.3
LOS days, median	9	NA	8	NA	13
Intrahospital mortality (%)	3.4	NA	1.5	2.2	6.6

Abbreviation: HOS = Heart of Soweto Study, EHFS II = European Heart Failure Survey II, AHEAD = Acute Heart Failure Database, HF = Heart Failure, NYHA = New York Heart Association, MI = Myocardial Infarction, CAD = Coronary Artery Disease, COPD = Chronic Obstructive Pulmonary Disease, TIA = Transient Ischemic Attack, BP = Blood Pressure, LVEDD = Left Ventricular End-Diastolic Diameter, LA = Left Atrium, LOS = Length of Hospital Stay

Table 2. Comparison of our findings with similar studies in other parts of the world.

of developing HF [41]. There is increased wall thickness at the expense of chamber volume in LVH due to hypertrophy of the myocyte and by a parallel alignment of the sarcomere [42]. Specific hypertensive cardiomyopathy has been proposed. This cardiomyopathy has been divided into four stages: in stage 1, there is diastolic dysfunction, which is present in 20–30% of patients. This is common in elderly women, hypertensive diabetics, and ischemic heart disease patients [43]. LV diastolic dysfunction precedes systolic HF and is therefore a more common mechanism of HF in hypertension. Stage 2 is hypertension with impaired LV relaxation abnormalities, while grade 4 is dilated cardiomyopathy with LV systolic dysfunction. It has been shown that apoptosis may be responsible for the reduction of myocyte mass that accompanies progression from compensated hypertrophy to HF.

Several theories have been proposed to explain the relationship between LVH and HF. This includes changes in the coronary microcirculation, which leads to poor myocardial perfusion, impaired cardiac function, loss of contractile protein, and thus reduced cardiac contractility [44]. The second theory is increased LV pressure overload, which leads to ventricular dilatation and reduced cardiac output [45].

Finally, LVH in hypertension is governed by different loading conditions, which involve both hormonal and paracrine factors such as the sympathetic nervous system and renin-angiotensin-aldosterone axis [46].

3. Peripartum cardiomyopathy (PPCM)

3.1. Definition

Peripartum cardiomyopathy (PPCM) is a form of heart disease characterized by "the development of HF in the last month of pregnancy or within the first 5 months postpartum in the absence of any other determinable cause for cardiac failure and in the absence of demonstrable heart disease before the last month of pregnancy, and bears echocardiographic evidence of left ventricular systolic dysfunction" [62]. In addition, the diagnosis of the condition requires evidence of impaired LV systolic function by echocardiography (LVEF < 45% or LVFS < 30%). LV dilation is common although in some patients, LV dimension may be normal but the LV systolic function is impaired [62, 63].

3.2. Epidemiology

In terms of epidemiology, PPCM is common in developing and poor communities. The incidence is 1/1000 in most parts of low- and middle-income countries [64]. However, very high incidence has been reported from Northern Nigeria (1/100 live births) [65–69] and Haiti (1/300 live births) [70, 71]. The incidence in high-income countries is in the range of 1/3000–1/4000 deliveries [64]. There has been an increase in the awareness of the disease worldwide with the establishment of a global registry.

PPCM is responsible for about 1.5% cases of HF in the Heart of Soweto study [41], 1.3% in the Abeokuta HF registry [44] and 3.2% in the Abuja Heart Study [42]. It is still the most prevalent form of cardiomyopathy (54.6%) in Northern Nigeria [45].

3.3. Risk factors

Risk factors for the development of this cardiac disorder include low socioeconomic status, women of African descent (although PPCM is a global disease), young pregnant women, multiparity, multiple pregnancy, and longer period of breast feeding [64]. However, recent prospectively collected data on PPCM do not support strong association with older age of pregnancy, multiparity, twin pregnancy, gestational hypertension, and the use of tocolytic agents [72].

3.4. Clinical features

Shortness of breath is common form of presentation. Other common clinical features include, cardiomegaly, tachycardia, pulmonary rales, high blood pressure and dysrhythmias. Dyspnea, cough, orthopnea, palpitation, hemoptysis, chest pain, and abdominal pain are other common features. Most patients in SSA present in NYHA class III/IV [68, 72]. Thromboembolic complications are common in the form of pulmonary embolism and stroke from mural thrombus [73, 74].

There are some differences between PPCM and hypertensive heart failure of pregnancy (HHFP). Patients with HHFP are more likely to present in the last trimester, while PPCM patients are more likely to present within the first month of the postpartum period. Family history of hypertension and history of hypertension in previous pregnancy is commoner in HHFP. Twin pregnancy and presence of leg edema are more common in PPCM. Blood pressures are generally higher in HHFP and they are also more likely to have basal rales. Furthermore, functional murmurs (tricuspid and mitral regurgitation) occur more often in PPCM compared to HHFP [75].

3.5. Laboratory findings

Arrhythmias are also common. In severe cases, anemia and renal dysfunction may be present. The liver enzymes may be normal or mildly raised from hepatic congestion. Some authors in Benin republic, Mali and Nigeria have reported the association of PPCM with micronutrient deficiencies, e.g., selenium, ceruloplasmin [76–78]. LV function and mortality in PPCM patients with HIV infection and those without have been found not to differ significantly [79].

The 12-leads ECG often show sinus rhythm, ST-T changes are common, which resolves after the postpartum. Ventricular arrhythmia occurs in about 20% [80–83].

Echocardiography is the diagnostic procedure of choice. Useful for the evaluation of LV systolic function ($EF < 45\%$), and diastolic function as well as assessment for presence of intramural thrombus formation. The mean LV internal dimension in diastole is often about 6 cm; however, some patients have nondilated LV. Where available in SSA, magnetic resonance imaging helps in the detection of myocardial fibrosis with late enhancement imaging. It also helps in the assessment function, shape, size, as well as contents. Immunohistochemistry of biopsy specimen from patient with PPCM is not different from that of idiopathic DCM. Similar viral particles, e.g., coxsackie, encephalomyelocarditis, parvovirus B19, adenoviruses, herpes simplex virus, Ebstein-Burr virus, and cytomegalovirus DNA. Inflammatory markers such as tumor necrosis factor alpha (TNF-alpha) and C-reactive protein levels are raised in both conditions and cannot be used to differentiate one from the other. However, peculiar to PPCM are some immune activation processes, e.g., elevated levels of marker of apoptosis-FAS/APO 1. This has been shown to predict prognosis [84].

3.6. Recent advances in the pathophysiology

More recently, Sliwa and her colleagues have shown the role of cleavage of prolactin in the pathogenesis of PPCM. A 16-KDa fragment of prolactin may induce myocardial damage [85]. This has provided a new option of blocking prolactin secretion with bromocriptine in the treatment of PPCM.

3.7. Prognosis

Full recovery of LV function occurs in about half of PPCM patients [72]. About 25% recover by the end of 6 months and around 10–15% die within 6 months. Long-term prospective follow-up studies show that overall recovery occurs in about 25% of patients and this mostly occurs in the first 18–24 months of diagnosis [79].

In recent time, there has been an increased awareness of this condition, and it has been recognized in the guidelines of the American College of Cardiology and European Society of Cardiology. Large global or continental registries of PPCM exist and many centers in SSA are participating. The European society of Cardiology has recently released a position paper on the disorder [62].

4. HIV-associated cardiomyopathy

4.1. Prevalence

SSA contributes about 69 and 90% of the global adult and childhood HIV/AIDS burden. HIV-associated cardiomyopathy is therefore a significant contributor to CVD morbidity and mortality in the region [86, 87].

The true prevalence of HIV-associated cardiomyopathy is unknown. The prevalence of HIV-associated cardiomyopathy in the pre-HAART era was about 50%. The incidence of any cardiac abnormality in HIV-infected individuals was 55% over a 7-year period [88–90]. It was common in young persons with CD4 count of <100 cells/mm^3, lower socioeconomic class, longer duration of the infection, higher viral load, and advanced stage of the disease [89, 91]. In-hospital mortality was 15% [89].

Because of the availability of HAART, the prevalence has reduced by about 50% in high-income countries [92]. However, in low-income countries (where most of the countries in SSA belong to), the prevalence of the condition has increased by 32% due to poor and limited access to HAART as well the impact of malnutrition [93].

Echocardiographic studies have reported prevalence ranging from 5% (in Nigeria) to 57% in Burkina Faso [89, 91, 94]. Differences may be due to study design and lack of common definition of the disorder [95].

In the Heart of Soweto study, about 9.7% of the cohort were HIV infected, 54% of who were on HAART [41, 81]. They were younger, had lower blood pressure and body mass index, and higher heart rate compared to the general cohort. HIV associated HF was the commonest diagnosis. The mean LVEF was 46% and common in women who were also about 6-years younger than the men. HIV patients who had HF had lower CD4 count compared to those who did not have. They were also more likely to have right-heart failure and valve dysfunction [96].

About 2.6% of HF cases in the THESU-HF survey were due to HIV infection. They were younger by 10–15 years and were less often smokers, hypertensive, or diabetic. They had larger LV dimensions but had similar LVEF compared to the general cohort [1]. The findings from the Heart of Soweto and the THESUS-HF survey are similar to more recent observational studies in the region. The prevalence is in the range of 1–5% [67, 73, 74]. It is often diagnosed in the third decade of life and more often in women. Both systolic and diastolic HF are common (about 30%).

4.2. Pathophysiologic mechanism

The proposed mechanism in the pathogenesis of HIV-associated cardiomyopathy include the direct myocardial invasion by the HIV, post-viral autoimmunity, immune system dysregulation, adverse effect of the viral protein, endothelial dysfunction, transcriptional activation of cellular genes, and beta-adrenergic dysregulation. Others include HIV-immunosuppression-related myocarditis due to opportunistic infection with toxoplasmosis, cryptococcus, and mycobacteria. Myocardial dysfunction as a result of systemic effects of sepsis may also play a role. Some of the anti-retroviral medications may play a role in the pathogenesis. Nucleoside reverse transcriptase inhibitors cause mitochondrial damage by inhibiting mitochondrial DNA polymerase. Zalcitabine is thought to exhibit the greatest toxicity among this group [97]. Zidovudine causes cardiac and skeletal myopathy [98].

Malnutrition especially selenium deficiency is another possible mechanism. Selenium has an antioxidant property and protects against endothelial dysfunction. Its deficiency is associated with cardiac dysfunction. Due to soil composition and agricultural practices in the region, selenium deficiency is common and 285 of the SSA population are at risk of selenium deficiency. Selenium deficiency has been demonstrated in HIV patients [99]. Selenium supplementation has also been shown to improve cardiac function in some studies [100].

Heavy alcohol use and smoking have also been implicated especially in high-income countries [101]. This was not demonstrated in a Rwandan study [101].

The role of genetic factor has not been demonstrated in Africa. " The mitochondrial DNA T16189C polymorphism, with a homopolymeric C-tract of 10-12 cystosines—a putative genetic risk factor for idiopathic dilated cardiomyopathy in the African and British populations—was not associated with HIV-associated cardiomyopathy in a South-African case control study" [102].

Author details

Okechukwu S. Ogah* and Ayodele O. Falase

*Address all correspondence to: osogah56156@gmail.com

Division of Cardiology, Department of Medicine, University College Hospital, Ibadan, Nigeria

References

[1] Damasceno A, Mayosi BM, Sani M, Ogah OS, Mondo C, Ojji D, et al. The causes, treatment, and outcome of acute heart failure in 1006 Africans from 9 countries: results of the sub-Saharan Africa survey of heart failure. Archives of Internal Medicine. 2012;172 (18):1386–94.

[2] Adeloye D, Basquill C. Estimating the prevalence and awareness rates of hypertension in Africa: a systematic analysis. PLoS One. 2014;9(8):e104300.

[3] Organization WH. A global brief on hypertension: silent killer, global public health crisis. World. 2016.

[4] WHO RO for Africa. The health of the people: the African regional health report. World Health Organization. 2006.

[5] Lawes CM, Vander Hoorn S, Law MR, Elliott P, MacMahon S, Rodgers A. Blood pressure and the global burden of disease 2000. Part 1: estimates of blood pressure levels. Journal of Hypertension. 2006;24(3):413–22.

[6] Lawes CM, Vander Hoorn S, Law MR, Elliott P, MacMahon S, Rodgers A. Blood pressure and the global burden of disease 2000. Part II: estimates of attributable burden. Journal of Hypertension. 2006;24(3):423–30.

[7] Beaglehole R, Bonita R, Alleyne G, Horton R, Li L, Lincoln P, et al. UN high-level meeting on non-communicable diseases: addressing four questions. The Lancet. 2011;378(9789):449–55.

[8] Adebiyi AA, Akinosun OM, Nwafor CE, Falase AO. Plasma catecholamines in Nigerians with primary hypertension. Ethnicity & Disease. 2011;21(2):158–62.

[9] Adamu UG, Kolo PM, Katibi IA, Opadijo GO, Omotosho AB, Araoye MA. Relationship between left ventricular diastolic function and geometric patterns in Nigerians with newly diagnosed systemic hypertension. Cardiovascular Journal of Africa. 2009;20(3):173–7.

[10] Adebiyi AA, Aje A, Ogah OS, Ojji DB, Oladapo OO, Falase AO. Left ventricular diastolic function parameters in hypertensives. Journal of the National Medical Association. 2005;97(1):41–5.

[11] Akintunde AA, Familoni OB, Akinwusi PO, Opadijo OG. Relationship between left ventricular geometric pattern and systolic and diastolic function in treated Nigerian hypertensives. Cardiovascular Journal of Africa. 2010;21(1):21–5.

[12] Ike SO, Onwubere JC. For the patient. Poor diastolic function and blood pressure in Blacks. Ethnicity & Disease. 2003;13(4):547.

[13] Adebayo AK, Oladapo OO, Adebiyi AA, Ogunleye OO, Ogah OS, Ojji DB, et al. Characterisation of left ventricular function by tissue Doppler imaging technique in newly diagnosed, untreated hypertensive subjects. Cardiovascular Journal of Africa. 2008;19(5):259–63.

[14] Akintunde A, Kareem L, Bakare A, Audu M. Impact of obstructive sleep apnea and snoring on left ventricular mass and diastolic function in hypertensive Nigerians. Annals of Medical and Health Sciences Research. 2014;4(3):350–4.

[15] Adeoye AM, Adebiyi AA, Oladapo OO, Ogah OS, Aje A, Ojji DB, et al. Early diastolic functional abnormalities in normotensive offspring of Nigerian hypertensives. Cardiovascular Journal of Africa. 2012;23(5):255–9.

[16] Kolo P, Sanya E, Ogunmodede J, Omotoso A, Soladoye A. Normotensive offspring of hypertensive Nigerians have increased left ventricular mass and abnormal geometric patterns. The Pan African Medical Journal. 2012;11:6.

[17] Kolo PM, Sanya EO, Omotoso AB, Soladoye A, Ogunmodede JA. Left ventricular hypertrophy is associated with diastolic filling alterations in normotensive offspring of hypertensive Nigerians. ISRN Cardiology. 2012;2012:256738.

[18] Karaye KM, Habib AG, Mohammed S, Rabiu M, Shehu MN. Assessment of right ventricular systolic function using tricuspid annular-plane systolic excursion in Nigerians with systemic hypertension. Cardiovascular Journal of Africa. 2010;21(4):186–90.

[19] Akintunde AA, Akinwusi PO, Familoni OB, Opadijo OG. Effect of systemic hypertension on right ventricular morphology and function: an echocardiographic study. Cardiovascular Journal of Africa. 2010;21(5):252–6.

[20] Adebiyi AA, Aje A, Ogah OS, Ojji DB, Dada A, Oladapo OO, et al. Correlates of left atrial size in Nigerian hypertensives. Cardiovascular Journal of South Africa: Official Journal for Southern Africa Cardiac Society [and] South African Society of Cardiac Practitioners. 2004;16(3):158–61.

[21] Adebayo AK, Oladapo OO, Adebiyi AA, Ogunleye OO, Ogah OS, Ojji DB, et al. Changes in left atrial dimension and function and left ventricular geometry in newly diagnosed untreated hypertensive subjects. Journal of Cardiovascular Medicine. 2008;9(6):561–9.

[22] Jaggy C, Perret F, Bovet P, van Melle G, Zerkiebel N, Madeleine G, et al. Performance of classic electrocardiographic criteria for left ventricular hypertrophy in an African population. Hypertension. 2000;36(1):54–61.

[23] Huston SL, Bunker CH, Ukoli FA, Rautaharju PM, Kuller LH. Electrocardiographic left ventricular hypertrophy by five criteria among civil servants in Benin City, Nigeria: prevalence and correlates. International Journal of Cardiology. 1999;70(1):1–14.

[24] Lodha SM, Makene WJ. Electrocardiographic changes in systemic hypertension. (A study of Tanzanian Africans). East African Medical Journal. 1976;53(8):424–34.

[25] Maunganidze F, Woodiwiss AJ, Libhaber CD, Maseko MJ, Majane OH, Norton GR. Left ventricular hypertrophy detection from simple clinical measures combined with electro-cardiographic criteria in a group of African ancestry. Clinical Research in Cardiology. 2014;103(11):921–9.

[26] Maunganidze F, Woodiwiss AJ, Libhaber CD, Maseko MJ, Majane OH, Norton GR. Obesity markedly attenuates the validity and performance of all electrocardiographic criteria for left ventricular hypertrophy detection in a group of black African ancestry. Journal of Hypertension. 2013;31(2):377–83.

[27] Sliwa K, Ojji D, Bachelier K, Bohm M, Damasceno A, Stewart S. Hypertension and hypertensive heart disease in African women. Clinical Research in Cardiology. 2014; 103(7):515–23.

[28] Robinson C, Woodiwiss AJ, Libhaber CD, Norton GR. Novel approach to the detection of left ventricular hypertrophy using body mass index–corrected electrocardiographic voltage criteria in a group of African ancestry. Clinical Cardiology. 2016;39(9):524–30.

[29] Ogah O, Oladapo O, Adebiyi A, Salako B, Falase A, Adebayo A, et al. Electrocardiographic left ventricular hypertrophy with strain pattern: prevalence, mechanisms and prognos-tic implications. Cardiovascular Journal of Africa. 2008;19(1):39.

[30] Ogah O, Adebiyi A, Oladapo O, Aje A, Ojji D, Adebayo A, et al. Association between electrocardiographic left ventricular hypertrophy with strain pattern and left ventricular structure and function. Cardiology. 2006;106(1):14–21.

[31] Adebiyi AA, Ogah OS, Aje A, Ojji DB, Adebayo AK, Oladapo OO, et al. Echocardiographic partition values and prevalence of left ventricular hypertrophy in hypertensive Nigerians. BMC Medical Imaging. 2006;6(1):1.

[32] Silangei LK, Maro VP, Diefenthal H, Kapanda G, Dewhurst M, Mwandolela H, et al. Assessment of left ventricular geometrical patterns and function among hypertensive patients at a tertiary hospital, Northern Tanzania. BMC Cardiovascular Disorders. 2012;12:109.

[33] Ogah OS, Akinyemi RO, Adegbite GD, Udofia OI, Udoh SB, Adesina JO, et al. Prevalence of asymptomatic left ventricular systolic dysfunction in hypertensive Nigerians: echocar-diographic study of 832 subjects. Cardiovascular Journal of Africa. 2011;22(6):297–302.

[34] Ojji D, Atherton J, Sliwa K, Alfa J, Ngabea M, Opie L. Left ventricular systolic dysfunc-tion in asymptomatic black hypertensive subjects. American Journal of Hypertension. 2015;28(7):924–9.

[35] Karaye KM. Relationship between Tei Index and left ventricular geometric patterns in a hypertensive population: a cross-sectional study. Cardiovascular Ultrasound. 2011;9:21.

[36] Karaye KM, Sai'du H, Shehu MN. Right ventricular dysfunction in a hypertensive population stratified by patterns of left ventricular geometry. Cardiovascular Journal of Africa. 2012;23(9):478–82.

[37] Ojji DB, Lecour S, Atherton JJ, Blauwet LA, Alfa J, Sliwa K. Right ventricular systolic dysfunction is common in hypertensive heart failure: a prospective study in sub-Saharan Africa. PLoS One. 2016;11(4):e0153479.

[38] Stewart S, Libhaber E, Carrington M, Damasceno A, Abbasi H, Hansen C, et al. The clinical consequences and challenges of hypertension in urban-dwelling black Africans: insights from the Heart of Soweto Study. International Journal of Cardiology. 2011;146(1):22–7.

[39] Owusu IK, Adu-Boakye Y, Tetteh LA. Hypertensive heart failure in Kumasi, Ghana. Open Science Journal of Clinical Medicine. 2014;2(1):39–43.

[40] Ogah OS, Sliwa K, Akinyemi JO, Falase AO, Stewart S. Hypertensive heart failure in Nigerian Africans: insights from the Abeokuta Heart Failure Registry. Journal of Clinical Hypertension. 2015;17(4):263–72.

[41] Stewart S, Wilkinson D, Hansen C, Vaghela V, Mvungi R, McMurray J, et al. Predominance of heart failure in the Heart of Soweto Study cohort: emerging challenges for urban African communities. Circulation. 2008;118(23):2360–7.

[42] Ojji DB, Alfa J, Ajayi SO, Mamven MH, Falase AO. Pattern of heart failure in Abuja, Nigeria: an echocardiographic study. Cardiovascular Journal of Africa. 2009;20(6):349–52.

[43] Ojji D, Stewart S, Ajayi S, Manmak M, Sliwa K. A predominance of hypertensive heart failure in the Abuja Heart Study cohort of urban Nigerians: a prospective clinical registry of 1515 de novo cases. European Journal of Heart Failure. 2013;15(8):835–42.

[44] Ogah OS, Stewart S, Falase AO, Akinyemi JO, Adegbite GD, Alabi AA, et al. Contemporary profile of acute heart failure in Southern Nigeria: data from the Abeokuta Heart Failure Clinical Registry. JACC Heart Failure. 2014;2(3):250–9.

[45] Karaye KM, Sani MU. Factors associated with poor prognosis among patients admitted with heart failure in a Nigerian tertiary medical centre: a cross-sectional study. BMC Cardiovascular Disorders. 2008;8:16.

[46] Laabes EP, Thacher TD, Okeahialam BN. Risk factors for heart failure in adult Nigerians. Acta Cardiologica. 2008;63(4):437–43.

[47] Onwuchekwa AC, Asekomeh GE. Pattern of heart failure in a Nigerian teaching hospital. Vascular Health Risk Management. 2009;5:745–50.

[48] Adewuya AO, Ola BA, Ajayi OE, Oyedeji AO, Balogun MO, Mosaku SK. Prevalence and correlates of major depressive disorder in Nigerian outpatients with heart failure. Psychosomatics. 2006;47(6):479–85.

[49] Prevalence, causes and risk factors for left ventricular dysfunction and heart failure in Kenya population [Internet]. 2009 [cited 14 Dec 2014]. Available from: http://spo.escardio.org/eslides/view.aspx?eevtid=40&fp=3567.

[50] Kingue S, Dzudie A, Menanga A, Akono M, Ouankou M, Muna W. [A new look at adult chronic heart failure in Africa in the age of the Doppler echocardiography: experience of the medicine department at Yaounde General Hospital]. In Annales de cardiologie et d'angeiologie 2005 Sep;54(5):276–283.

[51] Tantchou Tchoumi JC, Ambassa JC, Kingue S, Giamberti A, Cirri S, Frigiola A, et al. Occurrence, aetiology and challenges in the management of congestive heart failure in sub-Saharan Africa: experience of the Cardiac Centre in Shisong, Cameroon. The Pan African Medical Journal. 2011;8:11.

[52] Soliman EZ, Juma H. Cardiac disease patterns in northern Malawi: epidemiologic transition perspective. Journal of Epidemiology/Japan Epidemiological Association. 2008;18(5):204–8.

[53] Kuule JK, Seremba E, Freers J. Anaemia among patients with congestive cardiac failure in Uganda—its impact on treatment outcomes. South African Medical Journal = Suid-Afrikaanse tydskrif vir geneeskunde. 2009;99(12):876–80.

[54] Okello S, Rogers O, Byamugisha A, Rwebembera J, Buda AJ. Characteristics of acute heart failure hospitalizations in a general medical ward in Southwestern Uganda. International Journal of Cardiology. 2014;176(3):1233–4.

[55] Owusu IK, Boaky Y. Prevalence and aetiology of heart failure in patients seen at a Teaching Hospital in Ghana. Journal of Cardiovascular Diseases & Diagnosis. 2013;1:131.

[56] Owusu IK. Causes of heart failure as seen in Kumasi, Ghana. Internet J Third world med. 2007;5:201–14.

[57] Habte B, Alemseged F, Tesfaye D. The pattern of cardiac diseases at the cardiac clinic of Jimma University specialised hospital, South West Ethiopia. Ethiopian Journal of Health Sciences. 2010;20(2):99–105.

[58] Makubi A, Hage C, Lwakatare J, Kisenge P, Makani J, Ryden L, et al. Contemporary aetiology, clinical characteristics and prognosis of adults with heart failure observed in a tertiary hospital in Tanzania: the prospective Tanzania Heart Failure (TaHeF) study. Heart. 2014;100(16):1235–41.

[59] Nieminen MS, Brutsaert D, Dickstein K, Drexler H, Follath F, Harjola VP, et al. EuroHeart Failure Survey II (EHFS II): a survey on hospitalized acute heart failure patients: description of population. European Heart Journal. 2006;27(22):2725–36.

[60] Sato N, Kajimoto K, Asai K, Mizuno M, Minami Y, Nagashima M, et al. Acute decompensated heart failure syndromes (ATTEND) registry. A prospective observational multicenter cohort study: rationale, design, and preliminary data. American Heart Journal. 2010;159(6):949–55 e1.

[61] Venskutonyte L, Molyte I, Ablonskyte-Dudoniene R, Mizariene V, Kavoliuniene A. Characteristics and management of acute heart failure patients in a single university hospital center. Medicina. 2009;45(11):855–70.

[62] Sliwa K, Hilfiker-Kleiner D, Petrie MC, Mebazaa A, Pieske B, Buchmann E, Regitz-Zagrosek V, Schaufelberger M, Tavazzi L, Veldhuisen DJ, Watkins H. Current state of knowledge on aetiology, diagnosis, management, and therapy of peripartum cardiomyopathy: a position statement from the Heart Failure Association of the European Society of Cardiology Working Group on peripartum cardiomyopathy. European journal of heart failure. 2010 Aug 1;12(8):767–78.

[63] Pearson GD, Veille J-C, Rahimtoola S, Hsia J, Oakley CM, Hosenpud JD, et al. Peripartum cardiomyopathy: national heart, lung, and blood institute and office of rare diseases (national institutes of health) workshop recommendations and review. Journal of the American Medical Association. 2000;283(9):1183–8.

[64] Sliwa K, Fett J, Elkayam U. Peripartum cardiomyopathy. The Lancet. 2006;368(9536):687–93.

[65] Ford L, Abdullahi A, Anjorin FI, Danbauchi SS, Isa MS, Maude GH, et al. The outcome of peripartum cardiac failure in Zaria, Nigeria. QJM. 1998;91(2):93–103.

[66] Abengowe CU. Cardiovascular disease in Northern Nigeria. Tropical & Geographical Medicine. 1979;31(4):553–60.

[67] Abengowe CU, Das CK, Siddique AK. Cardiac failure in pregnant Northern Nigerian women. International Journal of Gynaecology & Obstetrics: the Official Organ of the International Federation of Gynaecology and Obstetrics. 1980;17(5):467–70.

[68] Isezuo SA, Abubakar SA. Epidemiologic profile of peripartum cardiomyopathy in a tertiary care hospital. Ethnicity & Disease. 2007;17(2):228–33.

[69] Ladipo GO, Froude JR, Parry EH. Pattern of heart disease in adults of the NigerianwSavanna: a prospective clinical study. African Journal of Medicine and Medical Sciences. 1977;6(4):185–92.

[70] Fett JD. Peripartum cardiomyopathy. Insights from Haiti regarding a disease of unknown etiology. Minnesota Medicine. 2002;85(12):46–8.

[71] Fett JD, Carraway RD, Dowell DL, King ME, Pierre R. Peripartum cardiomyopathy in the Hospital Albert Schweitzer District of Haiti. American Journal of Obstetrics & Gynecology. 2002;186(5):1005–10.

[72] Blauwet LA, Libhaber E, Forster O, Tibazarwa K, Mebazaa A, Hilfiker-Kleiner D, et al. Predictors of outcome in 176 South African patients with peripartum cardiomyopathy. Heart. 2013;99(5):308–13.

[73] Isezuo SA, Njoku CH, Airede L, Yaqoob I, Musa AA, Bello O. Case report: acute limb ischaemia and gangrene associated with peripartum cardiomyopathy. Nigerian Postgraduate Medical Journal. 2005;12(3):237–40.

[74] Talle MA, Buba F, Anjorin CO. Prevalence and aetiology of left ventricular thrombus in patients undergoing transthoracic echocardiography at the University of Maiduguri Teaching Hospital. Advances in Medicine. 2014;2014:731936.

[75] Ntusi NB, Badri M, Gumedze F, Sliwa K, Mayosi BM. Pregnancy-associated heart failure: a comparison of clinical presentation and outcome between hypertensive heart failure of pregnancy and idiopathic peripartum cardiomyopathy. PLoS One. 2015;10(8):e0133466

[76] Cenac A, Simonoff M, Moretto P, Djibo A. A low plasma selenium is a risk factor for peripartum cardiomyopathy. A comparative study in Sahelian Africa. International Journal of Cardiology. 1992;36(1):57–9.

[77] Cenac A, Toure K, Diarra MB, Sergeant C, Jobic Y, Sanogo K, et al. Plasma selenium and peripartum cardiomyopathy in Bamako, Mali. Medecine Tropicale (Mars). 2004; 64(2):151–4.

[78] Cenac A, Sacca-Vehounkpe J, Poupon J, Dossou-Yovo-Akindes R, D'Almeida-Massougbodji M, Tchabi Y, et al. [Serum selenium and dilated cardiomyopathy in Cotonou, Benin]. Medecine Tropicale (Mars). 2009;69(3):272–4.

[79] Sliwa K, Forster O, Tibazarwa K, Libhaber E, Becker A, Yip A, et al. Long-term outcome of peripartum cardiomyopathy in a population with high seropositivity for human immunodeficiency virus. International Journal of Cardiology. 2011;147(2):202–8.

[80] Karaye KM, Lindmark K, Henein MY. Electrocardiographic predictors of peripartum cardiomyopathy. Cardiovascular Journal of Africa. 2015;27(2):66–70.

[81] Sliwa K, Wilkinson D, Hansen C, Ntyintyane L, Tibazarwa K, Becker A, et al. Spectrum of heart disease and risk factors in a black urban population in South Africa (the Heart of Soweto Study): a cohort study. The Lancet. 2008;371(9616):915–22.

[82] Karaye KM. Clinical characteristics and prognosis of Peripartum Cardiomyopathy. Print and Media, Umea University, 2016.

[83] Tibazarwa K, Mayosi B, Sliwa K, Carrington M, Stewart S, Lee G. The 12-lead ECG in peripartum cardiomyopathy. Cardiovascular Journal of Africa. 2012;23(6):322–9.

[84] Sliwa K, Forster O, Libhaber E, Fett JD, Sundstrom JB, Hilfiker-Kleiner D, et al. Peripartum cardiomyopathy: inflammatory markers as predictors of outcome in 100 prospectively studied patients. European Heart Journal. 2006;27(4):441–6.

[85] Hilfiker-Kleiner D, Sliwa K. Pathophysiology and epidemiology of peripartum cardiomyopathy. Nature Reviews Cardiology. 2014;11(6):364–70.

[86] WHO. Global update on HIV treatment 2013: results, impact and opportunities. 2013.

[87] HIV/AIDS JUNPo. Global AIDS response progress reporting 2013: construction of core indicators for monitoring the 2011 UN Political Declaration on HIV. AIDS. 2013.

[88] Hakim J, Matenga J, Siziya S. Myocardial dysfunction in human immunodeficiency virus infection: an echocardiographic study of 157 patients in hospital in Zimbabwe. Heart. 1996;76(2):161–5.

[89] Niakara A, Drabo Y, Kambire Y, Nebie L, Kabore N, Simon F. [Cardiovascular diseases and HIV infection: study of 79 cases at the National Hospital of Ouagadougou (Burkina Faso)]. Bulletin de la Societe de Pathologie Exotique (1990). 2002;95(1):23–6.

[90] Longo-Mbenza B, Seghers K, Phuati M, Bikangi FN, Mubagwa K. Heart involvement and HIV infection in African patients: determinants of survival. International Journal of Cardiology. 1998;64(1):63–73.

[91] Twagirumukiza M, Nkeramihigo E, Seminega B, Gasakure E, Boccara F, Barbaro G. Prevalence of dilated cardiomyopathy in HIV-infected African patients not receiving HAART: a multicenter, observational, prospective, cohort study in Rwanda. Current HIV Research. 2007;5(1):129–37.

[92] Patel K, Van Dyke RB, Mittleman MA, Colan SD, Oleske JM, Seage III GR. The impact of HAART on cardiomyopathy among children and adolescents perinatally infected with HIV-1. AIDS (London, England). 2012;26(16):2027.

[93] Barbaro G. WJC. World. 2010;2(3):53–7.

[94] Olusegun-Joseph DA, Ajuluchukwu JN, Okany CC, Mbakwem AC, Oke DA, Okubadejo NU. Echocardiographic patterns in treatment-naive HIV-positive patients in Lagos, south-west Nigeria. Cardiovascular Journal of Africa. 2012;23(8):e1–6.

[95] Ntsekhe M, Mayosi BM. Cardiac manifestations of HIV infection: an African perspective. Nature Clinical Practice Cardiovascular Medicine. 2009;6(2):120–7.

[96] Sliwa K, Carrington MJ, Becker A, Thienemann F, Ntsekhe M, Stewart S. Contribution of the human immunodeficiency virus/acquired immunodeficiency syndrome epidemic to de novo presentations of heart disease in the Heart of Soweto Study cohort. European Heart Journal. 2012;33(7):866–74.

[97] Currie PF, Jacob AJ, Foreman AR, Elton RA, Brettle RP, Boon NA. Heart muscle disease related to HIV infection: prognostic implications. BMJ. 1994;309(6969):1605–7.

[98] Nzuobontane D, Blackett K, Kuaban C. Cardiac involvement in HIV infected people in Yaounde, Cameroon. Postgraduate Medical Journal. 2002;78(925):678–81.

[99] Look M, Rockstroh J, Rao G, Kreuzer K, Barton S, Lemoch H, et al. Serum selenium, plasma glutathione (GSH) and erythrocyte glutathione peroxidase (GSH-Px)-levels in asymptomatic versus symptomatic human immunodeficiency virus-1 (HIV-1)-infection. European Journal of Clinical Nutrition. 1997;51(4):266–72.

[100] Kavanaugh-Mchugh AL, Ruff A, Perlman E, Hutton N, Modlin J, Rowe S. Selenium deficiency and cardiomyopathy in acquired immunodeficiency syndrome. Journal of Parenteral and Enteral Nutrition. 1991;15(3):347–9.

[101] Mondy KE, Gottdiener J, Overton ET, Henry K, Bush T, Conley L, et al. High prevalence of echocardiographic abnormalities among HIV-infected persons in the era of highly active antiretroviral therapy. Clinical Infectious Diseases. 2011;52(3):378–86.

[102] Hsue PY, Deeks SG, Hunt PW. Immunologic basis of cardiovascular disease in HIVinfected adults. Journal of Infectious Diseases. 2012;205(suppl 3):S375–82.

8

Inherited Cardiomyopathies: From Genotype to Phenotype

Marissa Lopez-Pier, Yulia Lipovka,
Eleni Constantopoulos and John P. Konhilas

Abstract

The heart undergoes extensive morphological, metabolic, and energetic remodeling in response to inherited, or familial, hypertrophic cardiomyopathies (FHC). Myocyte contractile perturbations downstream of Ca^{2+}, the so-called sarcomere-controlled mechanisms, may represent the earliest indicators of this remodeling. We can now state that the *dynamics* of cardiac contraction and relaxation during the progression of FHC are governed by downstream mechanisms, particularly the *kinetics* and *energetics* of actin and myosin interaction to drive the trajectory of pathological cardiac remodeling. This notion is unambiguously supported by elegant studies above linking inheritable FHC-causing mutations to cardiomyopathies, known to disturb contractile function and alter the energy landscape of the heart. Although studies examining the biophysical properties of cardiac myocytes with FHC-causing mutations have yielded a cellular and molecular understanding of myofilament function, this knowledge has had limited translational success. This is driven by a critical failure in elucidating an integrated and sequential link among the changing energy landscape, myofilament function, and initiated signaling pathways in response to FHC. Similarly, there continues to be a major gap in understanding the cellular and molecular mechanisms contributing to sex differences in FHC development and progression. The primary reason for this gap is a lack of a "unifying" or "central" hypothesis that integrates signaling cascades, energetics, sex and FHC.

Keywords: hypertrophic cardiomyopathy, sex differences, contractility, sarcomere, mutations

1. Introduction to inherited cardiomyopathies

Cardiomyopathies are a major underlying cause of heart failure (HF) and often have a significant heritable component. Although the origin of the inherited trigger can be traced to a single mutation in a sarcomeric gene, the development and progression of a cardiomyopathic phenotype depends on a complex interaction between initiated cellular signaling pathways, environmental stressors, and individual genotype (including sex/gender). Inherited, or familial, cardiomyopathy (FHC) is a disease of the cardiac sarcomere and can be classified as either a hypertrophic (HCM), dilated (DCM), or restrictive (RCM) cardiomyopathy. Inherited cardiomyopathies, FHC, are relatively common in the general population with a penetrance of 1:500 [1].

Although subjects with an identified genotype are at risk for sudden cardiac death (SCD) or HF, it is clinically heterogeneous with severe, mild, or no symptoms. For example, subjects with severe left ventricular (LV) hypertrophy defined as LV thickness >30 mm are at increased risk for SCD [2]. However, subjects with inherited hypertrophic cardiomyopathy (HCM) may present with little LV hypertrophy but yet still be at risk for SCD and HF. Unlike subjects with non-inherited LV hypertrophy, HCM patients may present with cardiac dysfunction that is not proportional to LV thickness [3–5].

HCM is highly progressive and often transitions to DCM. As the name suggests, DCM is characterized by a dilated LV hypertrophy accompanied by worsening cardiac function [6]. Although primary DCM is less common than HCM, DCM is the most genetically heterogeneous [6]. This is best illustrated by findings that DCM can be linked to genes that are also linked to HCM mutations further highlighting the complex nature of FHC.

HCM with abnormal LV diastolic filling associated with intracellular or interstitial infiltration and/or fibrosis in the absence of LV dilation has been described as a RCM. The prevalence of primary RCM is not known, but RCM is less common than both HCM and DCM with poorer clinical outcomes [5]. Again, co-existent HCM and RCM in the same family illustrates the importance of elucidating the pathogenesis that is not entirely based on genotype. Our ability to develop novel approaches or therapies for FHC will depend on a clear understanding of the genotype-to-phenotype interrelationship and potentially translate into personalized treatment options. Since the primary genetic defect in HCM, DCM, and RCM impacts the biophysics of the cardiac sarcomere, we discuss the genotype-phenotype relationship for inherited cardiomyopathies focusing on cardiomyocyte kinetics and energetics in a sex dimorphic manner.

2. Genotype to phenotype

Approximately 100 genes are genetically linked to FHC with most gene mutations encoding for sarcomeric proteins including β-myosin heavy chain (β-MYHC), cardiac troponin T (cTnT), cardiac myosin binding protein C (cMyBP-C), α-tropomyosin (α-Tm), cardiac troponin I (cTnI), myosin regulatory light chain (RLC), and titin [6–8]. FHC follows an autosomal dominant pattern of inheritance and rarely arises from de novo mutations; although founder mutations are less common, some have been traced to a common ancestor in certain populations and countries [7]. The first identified HCM-causing mutation is a missense in the thick filament gene (*MYH7*) encoding β-MyHC [9]. Since the initial discovery, hundreds of *MYH7* mutations have been genetically linked to HCM and account for 30–40% of all inherited FHCs.

Mutations in *MYBPC3*, a thick filament gene encoding cMyBP-C, is genetically linked to 40–50% distinct HCM-causing mutations, making *MYH7* and *MYBPC3* the most common genes underlying FHC-based disease [3, 10]. Despite the predominance of these gene mutations in HCM, *MYH7* mutations typically result in amino acid substitutions whereas *MYBPC3* variants disrupt the reading frame, leading to a truncated cMyBP-C protein and, often, haploinsufficiency [3]. Considering the role of β-MyHC in cardiomyocyte force generation, a missense mutation within a known critical domain of the *MYH7* gene can be more directly linked to a contractile deficit, usually through a gain-of-function and increased energy cost [11–13]. On the other hand, haploinsufficiency leads to loss of protein or accumulation of truncated protein making it difficult to mechanistically link the mutation to a biophysical effect. In general, patients with *MYBPC3* mutations present with less severe or delayed-onset HCM compared to patients with *MYH7* mutations [3, 6, 10]. Further illustrating profound genetic heterogeneity in FHC-causing mutations, *MYH7* and *MYBPC3* mutations have been linked to inherited DCM as well, even when the mutation is within the same functional domain [2, 6].

Less frequent FHC-causing mutations exist in other thick filament proteins as well. A third thick filament gene linked to FHC, although at a much lower prevalence, is *MLC2*, which encodes for myosin regulatory light chain (RLC). RLC associates with β-MYHC to impact the kinetics of actin-myosin interaction and contractile dynamics [14, 15]. Clinical presentation in patients with *MLC2* mutations is similar to other patients with thick filament mutations, including the phenotypic diversity. Mutations in thin filament proteins (cTnT, α-Tm, and cTnI) have been linked to both HCM, DCM, and RCM [2]. Interestingly, mutations in *TNNT2* (cTnT) and *TPM1* (α-Tm) are potentially more dangerous but with a variable penetrance [4]. For example, subjects are characterized as having "mild hypertrophy" and "less fibrosis", with a significant percentage of SCD patients displaying little to no phenotype [4].

From the above summary, it is clear that a clinical phenotype cannot be categorically assigned to a particular FHC genotype. Still, as a disease of the sarcomere, the prevailing assumption is that FHC-causing mutations perturb the biophysics of muscle contraction. As more sophisticated techniques are available to precisely locate the origins of biophysical abnormalities, investigators remain tasked with detailing the interrelationship between genetic aberrations and basic cardiac sarcomere biology.

3. Sarcomere contractile dynamics

Force generation in a sarcomere is produced by cyclic interactions between myosin and actin, process that is energetically driven by ATP hydrolysis. The myosin-actin interaction is regulated by the tropomyosin and troponin complex; calcium (Ca^{2+}) binding to the troponin complex initiates a macromolecular rearrangement on the thin filament and permits myosin binding to actin [2, 14]. Contractile perturbations downstream of Ca^{2+} cycling, the so-called sarcomere-controlled mechanisms, represent the earliest indicators of HF [16]. We can now state the *dynamics* of cardiac contraction and relaxation during the progression of HF are governed by downstream mechanisms, particularly the *kinetics* and *energetics* of the cross-bridge cycle to drive the trajectory of pathological cardiac remodeling [17]. This notion is unambiguously supported by elegant studies above linking inheritable FHC-causing mutations to cardiomyopathies, known to disturb contractile function and alter the energy landscape of the heart.

The ability to maintain contractile force at a given cytosolic Ca^{2+} concentration (Ca^{2+}-sensitive tension development) provides an index of cardiac contractility and is often used to characterize the impact of FHC-causing mutations on contractile function [18–21]. While Ca^{2+}-sensitive tension development indexes contractility, the rate of cross-bridge (actin-myosin interaction) binding and unbinding can impart knowledge regarding the amount of force that can be extracted from ATP [22].

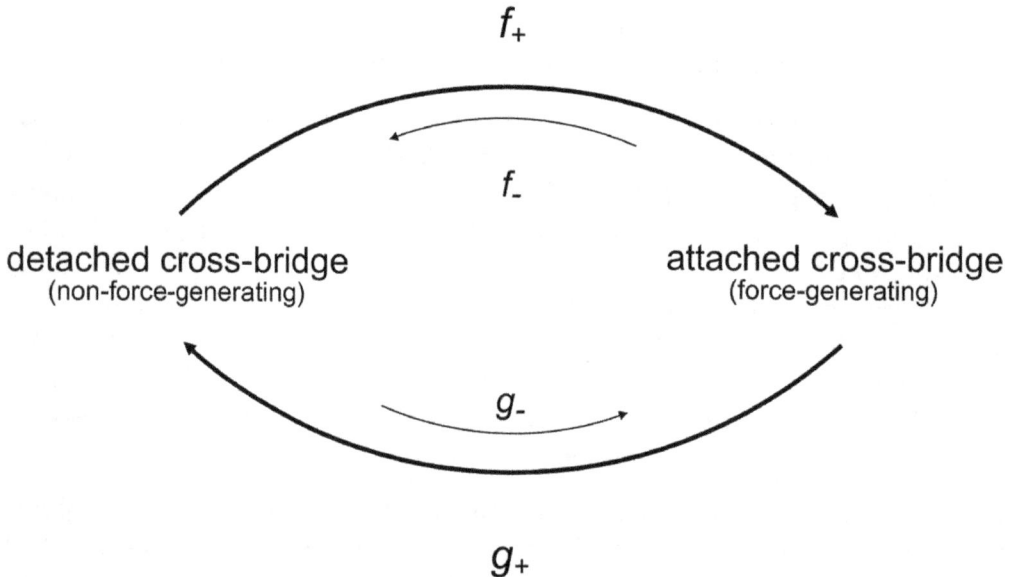

Figure 1. Two-state model of cross-bridge kinetics states that the rate of cross-bridge transition from non-force-generating (detached) to force-generating (attached) is described by f. Similarly, the rate of cross-bridge transition from force generating (attached) to non-force-generating (attached) is described by g. The reverse rate constants, noted as f. and g., are very small. k_{tr} can be defined by $f_+ + g_+$.

The time course of Ca^{2+}-activated tension development following mechanical perturbation (release-restretch protocol) reveals information regarding the kinetics of cycling cross-bridges. Specifically, the rate constant for this time course (k_{tr}) describes the isometric cross-bridge turnover rate, i.e., the sum of the apparent rates of cross-bridges entering and leaving force-generating states using a two-state model system of cross-bridge kinetics [23, 24]. This maneuver can be applied to the muscle at the end of a contraction to measure apparent rate of tension redevelopment (k_{tr}). The recovery of tension toward the isometric steady-state level fitted to a single exponential yields the rate constant k_{tr}. We and others define the rate constant k_{tr} according to the two-state model system. Cross-bridge kinetics of the two-state system can be described by rate constants, f and g, characterizing the making and breaking of cross-bridges [24, 25]. Using this two-state model, k_{tr} can be defined by $f_+ + g_+$ (**Figure 1**).

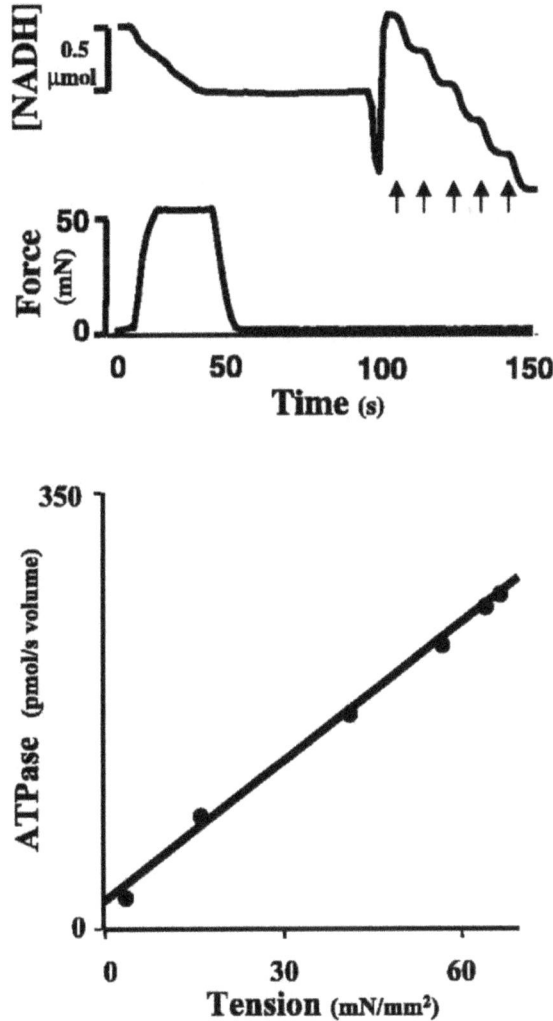

Figure 2. The rate of NADH absorbance is proportional to ATP consumption during isometric steady-state force development (**top panel**). The ATPase rate is plotted against force (**bottom panel**). The slope of this relationship represents the energetic cost (ATPase) of tension generation. Using a two-state model of cross-bridge kinetics, the slope of this line represents the rate of cross-bridge detachment and thus a measure of g. This figure was adapted with permission from Rundell et al. [117].

We have also exploited an apparatus to simultaneously measure force and ATP utilization [26, 27]. Briefly, the bath used for the ATPase assay allows transmission of near-UV light for the measurement of NADH absorbance. The ATPase activity of demembranated cardiac muscle strips or trabecula is measured on-line by means of an enzyme-coupled assay [26, 27]. Formation of ADP by the muscle is stoichiometrically coupled first to the synthesis of pyruvate and ATP from phosphoenolpyruvate, a reaction that is catalyzed by the enzyme pyruvate kinase, and subsequently to synthesis of lactate, a reaction that is catalyzed by the enzyme lactate dehydrogenase and during which NADH is oxidized to NAD$^+$. The breakdown of NADH is determined photometrically by measuring the absorbance of 340 nm near-UV light that is projected through the bath just beneath the preparation. Once the steady-state tension is reached, the first time derivative of this signal, which is proportional to the rate of ATP consumption in the assay bath, is determined off-line by linear regression of the sampled data using custom-designed software (**Figure 2**). The rate of ATP consumption, normalized to fiber volume, is plotted against force (**Figure 2**). This slope reflects the tension cost of contraction [26, 28]. Using the two-state model, this value approximates the rate of detachment (g). The combined measurements of k_{tr} and tension cost can give determinations of cross-bridge attachment (f) and detachment (g) [26].

4. ATP shuttling in the cardiac sarcomere

The hypertrophic heart has long been characterized as energy starved [12], and central to this energy remodeling is an alteration in the production, use, and delivery of ATP. Given the physical barriers to rapid diffusion within the myocyte, the cardiomyocyte utilizes key enzymes and a phosphotransferase system to optimize efficient transfer of phosphoryl groups to ADP [29]. Speaking directly to its significance, disturbances in the creatine kinase (CK)/ adenylate kinase (AK) phosphotransfer system are observed early in CVD and are stronger predictors of heart failure mortality than functional status [30]. The molecular underpinnings of the metabolic derangements reside in changes in the mediators of ATP generation, utilization, and delivery. As seen in Eq. (1) creatine kinase (CK) reversibly and rapidly converts ADP and phosphocreatine (PCr) to ATP and creatine (Cr) [31].

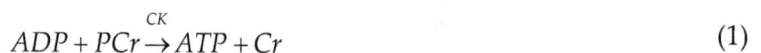

$$ADP + PCr \xrightarrow{CK} ATP + Cr \tag{1}$$

In parallel reactions [Eqs. (1) and (2)], a network of adenylate kinase (AK) enzymes mediates a complementary intracellular phosphotransfer promoting high-energy Pi transfer from ADP to ATP (leaving an increasing AMP pool) via distinct AK isoforms with different cellular localizations [32, 33].

$$ADP + ADP \xrightarrow{AK} ATP + AMP \tag{2}$$

The diseased heart will preferentially recruit phosphotransferase reactions to keep a constant pool of ATP. As cardiac disease ensues, total Cr and PCr decreases and results in elevated ADP and AMP even if ATP is maintained [11]. Further along the disease process, CK activity is reduced leading to a gradual decrease in cellular ATP [34]. Considering the relatively high rate of ATP synthesis in the heart [12], a gradual decrease in ATP can cause disproportionate energetic deficiencies [30, 35]. Such changes in energetics limit contractile reserve and the ability to power myocellular ATPases necessary to support contractile function. Given the physical barriers to rapid diffusion within the myocyte, physical association of CK, AK, and other key enzymes in the phosphotransferase system optimizes efficient transfer of phosphoryl groups to ADP [29]. These phosphotransfer microdomains are localized to sarcomeric myofibrils and act as hubs for energetic "sensing" [32, 36]. During acute or chronic ATP supply–demand imbalance, like the one that occurs during cardiac disease, AK amplifies the amount of AMP within these microdomains to preserve ATP levels for contraction [33].

5. Biophysical impact of inherited cardiomyopathies

5.1. Mutations in β-MyHC

The R403Q point mutation in β-MyHC is the first identified mutation leading to HCM with a heritable component [9]. The R403Q mutation resides in the actin-binding domain and *in vitro* analysis of R403Q myosin kinetics yields inconsistent results such as reduced [37] or enhanced [38] actin filament velocity and reduced [39] or enhanced [40] actin-activated ATPase. On the other hand, human myofibril or multicellular R403Q samples consistently show accelerated tension generation and increased ATP hydrolysis rates [20, 41]. In a recent study, we demonstrated that R403Q male fibers develop tension at an increased energy cost of contraction than WT fibers. This is consistent with a previous study that directly measured cross-bridge kinetics in cardiac myofibrils isolated from a patient carrying the R403Q mutation [41]. In addition, R403Q male cardiac trabeculae show an elevated k_{tr} at submaximal tension, again consistent with the kinetics of human R403Q-expressing myofibrils [41]. These observations show that less mechanical energy can be extracted from ATP suggesting an increase in the energy cost of tension generation in R403Q fibers.

Yet, the role that Ca^{2+}-sensitive tension development as an index of cardiac contractility plays in the progression of HCM is unclear. Studies consistently show that Ca^{2+}-sensitive tension development of cardiac fibers is not different between young (6–20 weeks) WT and R403Q hearts [42–44] even though previous studies show that intact hearts from male mice expressing the R403Q mutation show greater contractility compared to controls [45, 46]. We previously showed that cardiac trabeculae from 10-month-old male R403Q trabeculae were not different from wild-type fibers [21]. At the very least, the presence of the R403Q mutation alters myofilament function and ATP utilization at the level of the sarcomere.

5.2. Mutations in cMyBP-C

Historically, cMyBP-C has been viewed as a modifier of contraction through its direct interaction with myosin. In fact, genetic deletion of cMyBP-C in a murine model results in reduced systolic and diastolic parameters, reduced tension at submaximal activation, and cardiac hypertrophy [47]. Representative of a gain-of-function, myocytes lacking cMyBP-C generate more power and display increased rates of force redevelopment at the submaximal activation [48]. Interestingly, permeabilized myocytes taken from humans harboring *MYBPC3* mutations with evidence of reduced protein expression by haploinsufficiency show reduced maximal force without a change in the kinetics of actin-myosin cycling [49].

In contrast, human samples heterozygous for a missense mutation in *MYBPC3* are more sensitive to activating Ca^{2+}, which may be representative of enhanced contractility [50]. Again, the genetic heterogeneity of *MYBPC3* mutations mirrors the specific impact of each mutation on sarcomeric function. For example, loss of cMyBP-C protein as a result of *MYBPC3* mutations does not necessarily result in "loss-of-function". More recent studies have confirmed that cMyBP-C also interacts with actin to potentially tuning thin filament activation directly while simultaneously maintaining a functional interaction with myosin [51]. The implication for cMyBP-C is a complex regulatory role that imparts novel structural and functional mechanisms during the contractile cycle.

5.3. Mutations in RLC

The myosin regulatory light chain (RLC), also called as the ventricular light chain, is encoded by the *MLC2* gene. The RLC protein forms a non-covalent association with myosin and contains an EF-hand motif implicating functional regulation of myosin and subsequent tension generation [52]. Within this EF-hand "hot spot", the first FHC-causing mutations in the *MLC2* gene were identified, confirming an integral role for the RLC in contractile function [53]. To study the biophysical impact of *MLC2* mutations, mice expressing an E22K RLC transgene were engineered [15, 18]. Hearts from E22K mice display midventricular obstruction due to papillary and septal hypertrophy similar to human counterparts. However, mechanical properties of E22K sarcomeres remain unresolved.

Initial studies using glycerinated cardiac muscle fibers illustrate an increase in Ca^{2+}-sensitivity and Ca^{2+}-activated ATPase of myofibrillar samples from E22K transgenic mice than WT littermate and non-transgenic counterparts [15]. Follow-up studies by the same group report no impact of the E22K RLC mutation on Ca^{2+}-sensitivity of tension and a decrease in maximal ATPase [18]. Inconsistencies in biophysical results from E22K hearts are not surprising, considering the crucial role of RLC phosphorylation in the regulation of myosin mechanics [52, 54]. It is now appreciated that mutations in the *MLC2* gene may impact phosphorylation-dependent changes in force production [54].

5.4. Mutations in cTnT

Along the thin filament, a contractile unit consists of a repeating complex of 7 actin monomers, 1 troponin complex, and 1 α-Tm coil-coil dimer [2]. The heterotrimeric cardiac troponin complex is comprised of cTnI, cTnT, and the Ca^{2+}-binding troponin subunit, cardiac troponin C (cTnC). Myofilament activation hinges on complex molecular interactions between thin filament proteins where Ca^{2+}-binding to cTnC activates the myofilament, changes the position of α-Tm, and removes allosteric inhibition, allowing actin-myosin interaction. Transmission through the contractile unit following Ca^{2+} binding is exquisitely controlled by precise movements of multiple proteins, perhaps predicting a potentially more dangerous phenotype and variable penetrance in patients with FHC mutations residing in thin filament proteins [4].

Missense or splice-site mutations in the *TNNT2* gene result in point mutations or truncated variants resulting in FHC [2, 19]. Unlike *MYBPC3* mutations, truncated cTnT proteins are incorporated into the sarcomere, and early studies in transgenic mice expressing a truncated cTnT modeled after the human condition indicate mild to no cardiac hypertrophy, significant diastolic dysfunction and die more frequently with an increasing allelic expression similar to the human phenotype [55]. Interestingly, cardiac fibers expressing a similar truncated cTnT develop less force at maximum activation [56]. The truncated form of cTnT presumably disrupts the cTnT-cTnI-α-Tm binding domain, but the exact molecular mechanism that leads to the observed phenotype remains unresolved.

Early mapping of cTnT-related FHC alleles intimated the significance of another critical region within the cTnT-α-Tm binding domain [19]. Several FHC-causing substitutions have been identified at residue 92, including R92Q, R92L, and R92W [2]. Hearts taken from mice expressing R92 point mutations are typically smaller, hypercontractile with severe diastolic dysfunction, again, similar to findings in patients with FHC [2, 19, 57]. On the other hand, biophysical studies are inconsistent and depend on experimental approach and the level of molecular resolution. Still, key characteristics can be attributed to R92 mutations, including increased force and actin-myosin cycling at lower Ca^{2+} and less efficient use of ATP to generate force [57–59]. Nevertheless, these biophysical data do not fully explain the phenotypic heterogeneity of cTnT-related FHC arising from genotype-similar patients. Interestingly, a recent work demonstrates significant interplay between cTnT R92 mutations and MyHC isoform [57]. The suggestion from these recent data is that multiple levels of myofilament regulation exist and that specific cTnT FHC mutations cannot be used as surrogates for mutations comprising the functional domain. Clearly, FHC disease progression is a complex integration of myofilament function, cross-bridge kinetics, and cellular signaling, all of which can be modified by environmental and genetic factors such as sex/gender.

6. Sex disparities in FHC

Being male predisposes carriers of FHC-causing mutations to pathological cardiac remodeling [60]. In females, the sharp rise in FHC morbidity and mortality closely aligns with the pre- to post-menopausal transition [60–64]. Despite the longstanding knowledge that pre-menopausal women are protected from developing FHC, our fundamental understanding of the shift in FHC risk with menopause remains inadequate and impedes our ability to develop sex-specific therapeutic strategies to combat FHC and its complications.

The loss of estrogen during menopause positions 17β-estradiol (E2), the predominant naturally occurring estrogen, to play a unique role in cardioprotection. E2 signaling through classical estrogen receptors (ER), ERα and ERβ, and a third, membrane bound and G-protein coupled estrogen receptor (GPER) is initiated by environmental, genetic, and non-genetic cues to impact gene expression and cellular signaling [65–67]. E2-dependent signaling is complex and multiple molecular, and cellular mechanisms have been suggested to underlie protection against CVD [65, 66]. As part of these investigations, studies that utilized gonadectomized rodents subjected to different cardiac pathological stimuli typically demonstrate a benefit of estrogen replacement [68–72]. Unfortunately, the prospective Women's Health Initiative (WHI) and Heart and Estrogen/Progestin Replacement Study (HERS I and II) studies show an increased CVD and stroke risk with estrogen replacement in menopausal women [73, 74].

Our group has spent the past 15 years studying a murine model of HCM, which expresses an autosomal-dominant R403Q mutation in α-myosin heavy chain and exemplifies this sex dimorphism such that R403Q male mice develop progressive left-ventricular dilation, impaired cardiac function, and a number of pathologic indicators well before R403Q female mice [21, 65, 75–80]. The trajectory of HCM due the R403Q FHC model differs between the sexes in an age-dependent manner. As illustrated in **Figure 3**, adolescent (2 month old) males display cardiac hypertrophy whereas females do not; males progress to a worsening phenotype characterized by ventricular dilation by 8 month of age while females maintain ventricular morphometry with mild hypertrophy [27, 75].

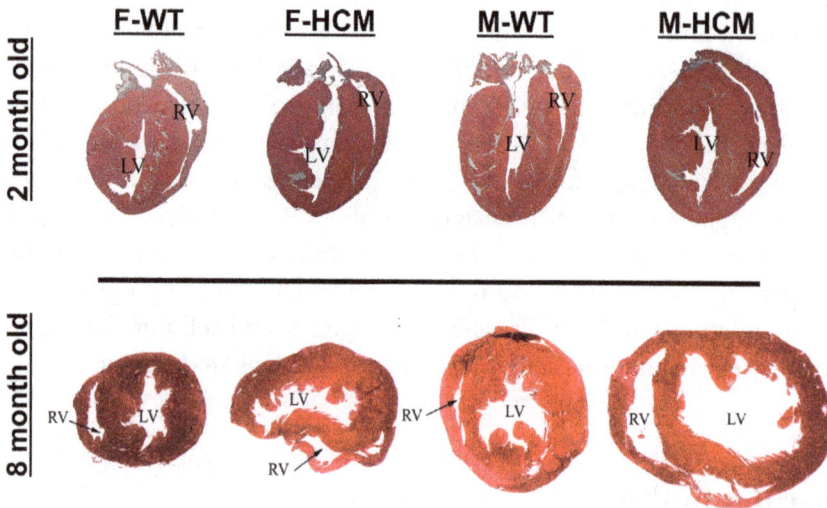

Figure 3. **Cardiac morphometry of R403Q female and male mice. Top panel**: Representative H&E stained longitudinal heart sections from R403Q female and male mice at 2 months of age. **Bottom panel**: Representative H&E stained short axis heart sections from R403Q female and male mice at 8 months of age. This figure was partly adapted with permission from [27].

The biophysical properties of cardiac sarcomeres expressing the R403Q mutation, as for cTnT mutations, depend on the experimental approach. In vitro analysis of R403Q myosin kinetics yields inconsistent results such as reduced [37] or enhanced [38] actin filament velocity and reduced [39] or enhanced [40] actin-activated ATPase. On the other hand, human myofibril or multicellular R403Q samples consistently show accelerated tension generation and increased ATP hydrolysis rates [20, 41]. We and others have reported both age- and sex-dependent effects on Ca^{2+}-sensitivity of tension and the rates of actin and myosin interaction, or k_{tr}. [21, 42, 43]. We further demonstrated that R403Q males show increased cycling (entering and exiting) of cross-bridges at a given force. Furthermore, we find a strong interaction between sex and the R403Q mutation with regard to tension cost. Coupled with measures of k_{tr}, this indicates higher "off" rate and more inefficient use of ATP at a given force in R403Q males with the opposite effect in R403Q females [27].

What is clear from these studies on the biophysics of the R403Q FHC mutation is that male and female myofilament function is perturbed and potentially under energy stress presumably initiated by the FHC mutation. The underlying mechanisms dictating very distinct disease trajectories in males and females are not completely elucidated by these studies necessitating alternative approaches.

6.1. Role of estrogen in FHC

Sex differences are primarily determined by hormonal status. When considering the effect of sex hormones on the progression of FHC, it is imperative to place a special focus on 17β-estradiol (E2) signaling. Estradiol is the main circulating sex hormone in pre-menopausal women. It is mainly synthesized in ovarian follicles, and to a smaller extent in adipose tissue, liver, breast, and neural tissues [81]. It regulates a number of physiological processes including metabolism, cell growth and proliferation, reproduction, and development [82]. It is generally agreed that estrogen plays a protective role in the myocardium and most of the cardio-protective effects have been attributed to E2. For the rest of this discussion, when we mention estrogen (E2), we are referring specifically to 17β-estradiol.

6.2. Estrogen signaling pathways

Estrogen exerts its physiological effects through interaction with intracellular estrogen receptors (ERs). The first described estrogen receptors, also known as classical estrogen receptors, are ERα and ERβ. They are members of the nuclear hormone receptor family (NHR), contain a DNA-binding domain, and share a high degree of homology [83]. In addition, another estrogen receptor has been recently described. GPER1, a membrane-bound G-protein coupled estrogen receptor, formerly known as GPR30, is a seven trans-membrane domain protein that mediates some of the non-transcriptional activity of estrogen [84].

Estrogen signaling pathways fall into two main categories: genomic (also known as classical) and non-genomic signaling. During genomic signaling, classical estrogen receptors act as transcription factors. After binding to estrogen, they undergo a conformational change that leads to the formation of homodimers (ERα/ERα and ERβ/ERβ) or heterodimers (ERα/ERβ). Receptor-dimers then bind to estrogen response elements (ERE), located near promoter regions of genes, and regulate gene transcription [83]. Estrogen signaling can also be initiated at the non-transcriptional level. Estrogen receptors interact with intracellular proteins triggering signal transduction cascades, often mediated by chain-reaction phosphorylation events. The vast array of estrogen non-transcriptional signaling pathways is mediated by ERα, ERβ, and GPER1 [84, 85].

6.3. Molecular mechanisms of estrogen-mediated cardio-protection

It is most widely accepted that the overall effect of cardiac estrogen signaling has a beneficial outcome on cardiac health. Not only does estrogen mediate cardioprotection, but it is also involved in the regulation of physiological processes in the heart. ERα expression, for example, is required to maintain physiological glucose uptake and proper mitochondrial function in the murine heart [86, 87]. Acute E2 injections enhance cardiovascular reflexes and autonomic tone in ovariectomy (OVX) mice [88]. Estrogen receptors interact with AMP-activated protein kinase in neonatal rat cardiomyocytes (NRCM), and potentially mediate its activity [89].

More importantly, there is increasing evidence suggesting that estrogen attenuates the progression of cardiac hypertrophy and prevents HF [70, 90]. The molecular mechanisms behind estrogen effects on cardiomyocyte survival are still under study. However, there are many pieces of evidence pointing to specific molecular pathways bridging estrogen signaling and increased tolerance to hypertrophic stimuli such as those arise from FHC. Some of these findings are explored below.

Estrogen has been shown to reverse agonist-induced cardiomyocyte hypertrophy. In NRCM, E2-treatment counteracts angiotensin II (Ang II)-induced increase in cell surface area, protein synthesis, skeletal muscle actin expression, nuclear translocation, and transcriptional activity of the hypertrophic transcription factor NFAT [85]. An E2-dependent increase in SIRT1 expression levels and AMPK activity protects the cardiomyocyte from Ang II-induced injury [91]. E2 reduces cardiomyocyte apoptosis *in vivo* and *in vitro* through the activation of PI3K/Akt signaling [92]. E2 treatment of OVX mice hearts and NRCM inhibits calcineurin activity and increases its degradation [93, 94]. E2 also limits undesirable extracellular matrix (ECM) remodeling through the modulation of ECM protein expression [95]. The majority of the effects discussed above are mediated by signaling through the classical estrogen receptors.

Limited mechanistic insights are available on E2 cardiac signaling mediated through ERα. Selective ERα agonism attenuates cardiac hypertrophy, increasing cardiac output, left ventricular stroke volume, and cardiac α-MyHC expression [96–98]. Signaling through ERβ has been studied in more depth and has been shown to counteract the development of cardiac hypertrophy by reducing the expression of hypertrophic markers, attenuating fibrosis, apoptosis and inflammation [99–101]. ERβ regulates a network of miRNAs, modulates p38 and ERK signaling, and affects calcineurin expression [102, 103]. In fibroblasts, ERβ blocks TGFβ1 synthesis that signals for the production of fibronectin, vimetin, collagens I and III [104].

At least three different mechanisms by which ERβ modulates hypertrophic gene expression in cardiomyocytes have been described. First, E2 signaling through ERβ induces PI3K activation that upregulates MCIP1 transcription [94]. MCIP1 blocks the Ang II-induced increase in calcineurin activity, preventing NFAT translocation to the nucleus and inhibiting the transcription of hypertrophic genes [105]. Second, ERβ signaling can reverse Ang II-induced inhibitory phosphorylation of glycogen synthase kinase-3β (GSK3B) by Akt. This prevents GATA4 transcription factor activation and also leads to decrease in hypertrophic mRNA expression [106]. The third mechanism involves regulation of histone deacetylases (HDAC). ERβ suppress the production and activation of the pro-hypertrophic HDAC2, while promoting the retention of anti-hypertrophic HDAC in the nucleus to inhibit hypertrophic gene expression [106].

Taking into account the complex and multifaceted nature of cardiac estrogen signaling, it is critical to inquire whether the cardioprotective effect of E2 signaling is sex dependent. In the context of cardiac hypertrophy, females show a better response to E2 than males [100], but that does not necessarily mean that E2 signaling is not beneficial for the male heart. It has been shown that E2 treatment of male rats subjected to chronic volume overload attenuates ventricular remodeling and disease progression [107]. It also improves survival in male mice with TNFα overexpression-induced cardiomyopathy [108]. At the cellular level, E2 stimulation of c-kit-expressing cardiac progenitor cells confers cardioprotection against cardiac injury. When co-cultured, ERα stimulation of c-kit + cells enhances the survival of post-infarct male myocytes [109].

In summary, estrogen signaling plays an important role in preventing cardiac remodeling that occurs during hypertrophy and subsequent heart failure. The exact extent to which the different estrogen-targeted pathways contribute to that is still under study. Better understanding of the mechanisms behind estrogen cardioprotection will help to fully understand the sex differences behind the development of FHC, and therefore lead to better and more specialized therapeutic options.

6.4. Menopause models of estrogen depletion

One obstacle that has stalled translational progression of studies into menopausal hypersensitivity to FHC is the lack of appropriate rodent models mirroring progressive ovarian failure, i.e., one that moves from perimenopause into menopause, similar to humans. Most studies have used the surgical removal of ovaries (ovariectomy) as a model of menopause, yet only 10% of women enter menopause surgically. Our studies have utilized an ovary-intact mouse model of menopause, using the chemical 4-vinylcyclohexene diepoxide (VCD) [110]. Repeated short term daily dosing with VCD selectively targets primordial follicles of the ovaries, accelerating the natural process of follicular atresia, and inducing gradual ovarian failure. This model preserves the important "perimenopause" transitional period and androgen-secreting capacity of residual ovarian tissue, analogous to menopausal women [111, 112]. Preserving endogenous androgens in estrogen-deplete females is particularly critical when studying sex differences in FHC [113]. Although androgen levels drop during menopause, the loss of estrogen in menopause elevates the androgen to estrogen ratio and represents an independent risk factor for FHC [114, 115]. We have used this model to demonstrate that during perimenopause, females were protected from hypertension and adverse cardiac remodeling. However after menopause, hypertension and pathological remodeling, indicative of worse clinical outcomes, is a hallmark of this increase in FHC susceptibility during menopause [116]. Importantly, the worsening phenotype in menopausal females is prevented by estrogen.

7. Conclusions

The assertion that FHC is a complex disease is underscored by the difficulty in attributing a single cause to the disease such as aberrant biophysical function of the myofilament. What is evident from studies of FHC is that although the primary defect may reside in the sarcomere, the development of an HCM, DCM, or RCM phenotype depends on the interaction of the initiated signaling pathways, environmental stressors, and individual genotype (including sex/gender). For example, pathways downstream of Ca^{2+} activation such as Ca^{2+}-sensitivity or actin-myosin cycling kinetics represent functional parameter that is the summation of multiple signals.

Despite an increasing appreciation of sex dimorphisms in the pathophysiology of FHC, many inconsistencies plague the cellular and molecular mechanisms underlying these sex differences. Taken together, there is a clear necessity in elucidating the cellular and molecular actions of estrogen and how this relates to the sex dimorphisms in FHC. Finally, although murine models of FHC do not exactly mimic the human *genotype*, they have proven as useful tools to elucidate the mechanisms underlying the FHC *phenotype*.

Acknowledgements

This work was supported by National Institutes of Health grant (HL098256), by a National Mentored Research Science Development Award (K01 AR052840), and Independent Scientist Award (K02 HL105799) from the NIH awarded to J.P. Konhilas, the Interdisciplinary Training in Cardiovascular Research (HL007249), and the Cardiovascular Biomedical Engineering Training Grant (HL007955). Support was received from the Sarver Heart Center at the University of Arizona and the Steven M. Gootter Foundation.

Author details

Marissa Lopez-Pier[1,3], Yulia Lipovka[2,3], Eleni Constantopoulos[2,3] and John P. Konhilas[2,3*]

*Address all correspondence to: konhilas@arizona.edu

1 Department of Biomedical Engineering, University of Arizona, Tucson, Arizona

2 Department of Physiology, University of Arizona, Tucson, Arizona

3 Sarver Molecular Cardiovascular Research Program, University of Arizona, Tucson, Arizona

References

[1]   Maron BJ. Hypertrophic cardiomyopathy: a systematic review. JAMA 287: 1308-1320, 2002.

[2] Tardiff JC. Thin filament mutations: developing an integrative approach to a complex disorder. Circ Res 108: 765-782, 2011.

[3] Behrens-Gawlik V, Mearini G, Gedicke-Hornung C, Richard P, and Carrier L. MYBPC3 in hypertrophic cardiomyopathy: from mutation identification to RNA-based correction. Pflugers Arch 466: 215-223, 2014.

[4] Keren A, Syrris P, and McKenna WJ. Hypertrophic cardiomyopathy: the genetic determinants of clinical disease expression. Nat Clin Pract Cardiovasc Med 5: 158-168, 2008.

[5] Sen-Chowdhry S, Syrris P, and McKenna WJ. Genetics of restrictive cardiomyopathy. Heart Fail Clin 6: 179-186, 2010.

[6] McNally EM, Barefield DY, and Puckelwartz MJ. The genetic landscape of cardiomyopathy and its role in heart failure. Cell Metab 21: 174-182, 2015.

[7] Claes GR, van Tienen FH, Lindsey P, Krapels IP, Helderman-van den Enden AT, Hoos MB, Barrois YE, Janssen JW, Paulussen AD, Sels JW, Kuijpers SH, van Tintelen JP, van den Berg MP, Heesen WF, Garcia-Pavia P, Perrot A, Christiaans I, Salemink S, Marcelis CL, Smeets HJ, Brunner HG, Volders PG, and van den Wijngaard A. Hypertrophic remodelling in cardiac regulatory myosin light chain (MYL2) founder mutation carriers. Eur Heart J 37: 1815-1822, 2016.

[8] Kensler RW, Shaffer JF, and Harris SP. Binding of the N-terminal fragment C0-C2 of cardiac MyBP-C to cardiac F-actin. J Struct Biol 174: 44-51, 2011.

[9] Geisterfer-Lowrance AA, Kass S, Tanigawa G, Vosberg HP, McKenna W, Seidman CE, and Seidman JG. A molecular basis for familial hypertrophic cardiomyopathy: a beta cardiac myosin heavy chain gene missense mutation. Cell 62: 999-1006, 1990.

[10] Maron BJ, Niimura H, Casey SA, Soper MK, Wright GB, Seidman JG, and Seidman CE. Development of left ventricular hypertrophy in adults in hypertrophic cardiomyopathy caused by cardiac myosin-binding protein C gene mutations. J Am Coll Cardiol 38: 315-321, 2001.

[11] Ingwall JS. ATP and the Heart. Boston: Kluwer Academic Publishers, 2002.

[12] Ingwall JS. Energy metabolism in heart failure and remodelling. Cardiovasc Res 81: 412-419, 2009.

[13] Walsh R, Rutland C, Thomas R, and Loughna S. Cardiomyopathy: a systematic review of disease-causing mutations in myosin heavy chain 7 and their phenotypic manifestations. Cardiology 115: 49-60, 2010.

[14] Scruggs SB and Solaro RJ. The significance of regulatory light chain phosphorylation in cardiac physiology. Arch Biochem Biophys 510: 129-134, 2011.

[15] Szczesna-Cordary D, Guzman G, Zhao J, Hernandez O, Wei J, and Diaz-Perez Z. The E22K mutation of myosin RLC that causes familial hypertrophic cardiomyopathy

increases calcium sensitivity of force and ATPase in transgenic mice. J Cell Sci 118: 3675-3683, 2005.

[16] Yar S, Monasky MM, and Solaro RJ. Maladaptive modifications in myofilament proteins and triggers in the progression to heart failure and sudden death. Pflugers Arch 466: 1189-1197, 2014.

[17] Stehle R and Iorga B. Kinetics of cardiac sarcomeric processes and rate-limiting steps in contraction and relaxation. J Mol Cell Cardiol 48: 843-850, 2010.

[18] Szczesna-Cordary D, Jones M, Moore JR, Watt J, Kerrick WG, Xu Y, Wang Y, Wagg C, and Lopaschuk GD. Myosin regulatory light chain E22K mutation results in decreased cardiac intracellular calcium and force transients. FASEB J 21: 3974-3985, 2007.

[19] Tardiff JC, Hewett TE, Palmer BM, Olsson C, Factor SM, Moore RL, Robbins J, and Leinwand LA. Cardiac troponin T mutations result in allele-specific phenotypes in a mouse model for hypertrophic cardiomyopathy. J Clin Invest 104: 469-481, 1999.

[20] Witjas-Paalberends ER, Ferrara C, Scellini B, Piroddi N, Montag J, Tesi C, Stienen GJ, Michels M, Ho CY, Kraft T, Poggesi C, and van der Velden J. Faster cross-bridge detachment and increased tension cost in human hypertrophic cardiomyopathy with the R403Q MYH7 mutation. J Physiol 592: 3257-3272, 2014.

[21] McKee LA, Chen H, Regan JA, Behunin SM, Walker JW, Walker JS, and Konhilas JP. Sexually dimorphic myofilament function and cardiac troponin I phosphospecies distribution in hypertrophic cardiomyopathy mice. Arch Biochem Biophys 535: 39-48, 2013.

[22] Tesi C, Colomo F, Nencini S, Piroddi N, and Poggesi C. The effect of inorganic phosphate on force generation in single myofibrils from rabbit skeletal muscle. Biophys J 78: 3081-3092, 2000.

[23] Hill TL, Eisenberg E, and Greene L. Theoretical model for the cooperative equilibrium binding of myosin subfragment 1 to the actin-troponin-tropomyosin complex. Proc Natl Acad Sci U S A 77: 3186-3190, 1980.

[24] Huxley AF. Muscle structure and theories of contraction. Prog Biophys 7: 255-318, 1957.

[25] Podolsky RJ, Nolan AC, and Zaveler SA. Cross-bridge properties derived from muscle isotonic velocity transients. Proc Natl Acad Sci U S A 64: 504-511, 1969.

[26] de Tombe PP and Stienen GJ. Impact of temperature on cross-bridge cycling kinetics in rat myocardium. J Physiol 584: 591-600, 2007.

[27] Birch CL, Behunin SM, Lopez-Pier MA, Danilo C, Lipovka Y, Saripalli C, Granzier H, and Konhilas JP. Sex dimorphisms of crossbridge cycling kinetics in transgenic hypertrophic cardiomyopathy mice. Am J Physiol Heart Circ Physiol 311: H125-136, 2016.

[28] de Tombe PP and Stienen GJ. Protein kinase A does not alter economy of force maintenance in skinned rat cardiac trabeculae. Circ Res 76: 734-741, 1995.

[29] Ingwall JS and Shen W. On energy circuits in the failing myocardium. Eur J Heart Fail 12: 1268-1270, 2010.

[30] Neubauer S. The failing heart—an engine out of fuel. N Engl J Med 356: 1140-1151, 2007.

[31] Nascimben L, Ingwall JS, Pauletto P, Friedrich J, Gwathmey JK, Saks V, Pessina AC, and Allen PD. Creatine kinase system in failing and nonfailing human myocardium. Circulation 94: 1894-1901, 1996.

[32] Aksentijevic D, Lygate CA, Makinen K, Zervou S, Sebag-Montefiore L, Medway D, Barnes H, Schneider JE, and Neubauer S. High-energy phosphotransfer in the failing mouse heart: role of adenylate kinase and glycolytic enzymes. Eur J Heart Fail 12: 1282-1289, 2010.

[33] Dzeja P and Terzic A. Adenylate kinase and AMP signaling networks: metabolic monitoring, signal communication and body energy sensing. Int J Mol Sci 10: 1729-1772, 2009.

[34] Weiss RG, Gerstenblith G, and Bottomley PA. ATP flux through creatine kinase in the normal, stressed, and failing human heart. Proc Natl Acad Sci U S A 102: 808-813, 2005.

[35] Shen W, Asai K, Uechi M, Mathier MA, Shannon RP, Vatner SF, and Ingwall JS. Progressive loss of myocardial ATP due to a loss of total purines during the development of heart failure in dogs: a compensatory role for the parallel loss of creatine. Circulation 100: 2113-2118, 1999.

[36] Koons S and Cooke R. Function of creatine kinase localization in muscle contraction. Adv Exp Med Biol 194: 129-137, 1986.

[37] Cuda G, Fananapazir L, Epstein ND, and Sellers JR. The in vitro motility activity of beta-cardiac myosin depends on the nature of the beta-myosin heavy chain gene mutation in hypertrophic cardiomyopathy. J Muscle Res Cell Motil 18: 275-283, 1997.

[38] Palmiter KA, Tyska MJ, Haeberle JR, Alpert NR, Fananapazir L, and Warshaw DM. R403Q and L908V mutant beta-cardiac myosin from patients with familial hypertrophic cardiomyopathy exhibit enhanced mechanical performance at the single molecule level. J Muscle Res Cell Motil 21: 609-620, 2000.

[39] Sweeney HL, Straceski AJ, Leinwand LA, Tikunov BA, and Faust L. Heterologous expression of a cardiomyopathic myosin that is defective in its actin interaction. J Biol Chem 269: 1603-1605, 1994.

[40] Yamashita H, Tyska MJ, Warshaw DM, Lowey S, and Trybus KM. Functional consequences of mutations in the smooth muscle myosin heavy chain at sites implicated in familial hypertrophic cardiomyopathy. J Biol Chem 275: 28045-28052, 2000.

[41] Belus A, Piroddi N, Scellini B, Tesi C, D'Amati G, Girolami F, Yacoub M, Cecchi F, Olivotto I, and Poggesi C. The familial hypertrophic cardiomyopathy-associated myosin mutation R403Q accelerates tension generation and relaxation of human cardiac myofibrils. J Physiol 586: 3639-3644, 2008.

[42] Palmer BM, Fishbaugher DE, Schmitt JP, Wang Y, Alpert NR, Seidman CE, Seidman JG, VanBuren P, and Maughan DW. Differential cross-bridge kinetics of FHC myosin mutations R403Q and R453C in heterozygous mouse myocardium. Am J Physiol Heart Circ Physiol 287: H91-99, 2004.

[43] Palmer BM, Wang Y, Teekakirikul P, Hinson JT, Fatkin D, Strouse S, Vanburen P, Seidman CE, Seidman JG, and Maughan DW. Myofilament mechanical performance is enhanced by R403Q myosin in mouse myocardium independent of sex. Am J Physiol Heart Circ Physiol 294: H1939-1947, 2008.

[44] Blanchard E, Seidman C, Seidman JG, LeWinter M, and Maughan D. Altered cross-bridge kinetics in the alphaMHC403/+ mouse model of familial hypertrophic cardio-myopathy. Circ Res 84: 475-483, 1999.

[45] Semsarian C, Ahmad I, Giewat M, Georgakopoulos D, Schmitt JP, McConnell BK, Reiken S, Mende U, Marks AR, Kass DA, Seidman CE, and Seidman JG. The L-type calcium channel inhibitor diltiazem prevents cardiomyopathy in a mouse model. J Clin Invest 109: 1013-1020, 2002.

[46] Georgakopoulos D, Christe ME, Giewat M, Seidman CM, Seidman JG, and Kass DA. The pathogenesis of familial hypertrophic cardiomyopathy: early and evolving effects from an alpha-cardiac myosin heavy chain missense mutation. Nat Med 5: 327-330, 1999.

[47] Harris SP, Bartley CR, Hacker TA, McDonald KS, Douglas PS, Greaser ML, Powers PA, and Moss RL. Hypertrophic cardiomyopathy in cardiac myosin binding protein-C knockout mice. Circ Res 90: 594-601, 2002.

[48] Korte FS, McDonald KS, Harris SP, and Moss RL. Loaded shortening, power output, and rate of force redevelopment are increased with knockout of cardiac myosin binding protein-C. Circ Res 93: 752-758, 2003.

[49] van Dijk SJ, Boontje NM, Heymans MW, Ten Cate FJ, Michels M, Dos Remedios C, Dooijes D, van Slegtenhorst MA, van der Velden J, and Stienen GJ. Preserved cross-bridge kinetics in human hypertrophic cardiomyopathy patients with MYBPC3 mutations. Pflugers Arch 466: 1619-1633, 2014.

[50] Sequeira V, Witjas-Paalberends ER, Kuster DW, and van der Velden J. Cardiac myosin-binding protein C: hypertrophic cardiomyopathy mutations and structure-function relationships. Pflugers Arch 466: 201-206, 2014.

[51] van Dijk SJ, Bezold KL, and Harris SP. Earning stripes: myosin binding protein-C interactions with actin. Pflugers Arch 466: 445-450, 2014.

[52] Declercq JP, Evrard C, Lamzin V, and Parello J. Crystal structure of the EF-hand parvalbumin at atomic resolution (0.91 Å) and at low temperature (100 K). Evidence for conformational multistates within the hydrophobic core. Protein Sci 8: 2194-2204, 1999.

[53] Flavigny J, Richard P, Isnard R, Carrier L, Charron P, Bonne G, Forissier JF, Desnos M, Dubourg O, Komajda M, Schwartz K, and Hainque B. Identification of two novel mutations in the ventricular regulatory myosin light chain gene (MYL2) associated with familial and classical forms of hypertrophic cardiomyopathy. J Mol Med 76: 208-214, 1998.

[54] Karabina A, Kazmierczak K, Szczesna-Cordary D, and Moore JR. Myosin regulatory light chain phosphorylation enhances cardiac beta-myosin in vitro motility under load. Arch Biochem Biophys 580: 14-21, 2015.

[55] Tardiff JC, Factor SM, Tompkins BD, Hewett TE, Palmer BM, Moore RL, Schwartz S, Robbins J, and Leinwand LA. A truncated cardiac troponin T molecule in transgenic mice suggests multiple cellular mechanisms for familial hypertrophic cardiomyopathy. J Clin Invest 101: 2800-2811., 1998.

[56] Watkins H, Seidman CE, Seidman JG, Feng HS, and Sweeney HL. Expression and functional assessment of a truncated cardiac troponin T that causes hypertrophic cardiomyopathy. Evidence for a dominant negative action. J Clin Invest 98: 2456-2461, 1996.

[57] Ford SJ, Mamidi R, Jimenez J, Tardiff JC, and Chandra M. Effects of R92 mutations in mouse cardiac troponin T are influenced by changes in myosin heavy chain isoform. J Mol Cell Cardiol 53: 542-551, 2012.

[58] Chandra M, Tschirgi ML, and Tardiff JC. Increase in tension-dependent ATP consumption induced by cardiac troponin T mutation. Am J Physiol Heart Circ Physiol 289: H2112-2119, 2005.

[59] Javadpour MM, Tardiff JC, Pinz I, and Ingwall JS. Decreased energetics in murine hearts bearing the R92Q mutation in cardiac troponin T. J Clin Invest 112: 768-775, 2003.

[60] Helms AS and Day SM. Hypertrophic cardiomyopathy: single gene disease or complex trait? Eur Heart J, 2015.

[61] Lima R, Wofford M, and Reckelhoff JF. Hypertension in postmenopausal women. Curr Hypertens Rep 14: 254-260, 2012.

[62] Rosano GM, Vitale C, Marazzi G, and Volterrani M. Menopause and cardiovascular disease: the evidence. Climacteric 10 Suppl 1: 19-24, 2007.

[63] Dubey RK, Oparil S, Imthurn B, and Jackson EK. Sex hormones and hypertension. Cardiovasc Res 53: 688-708, 2002.

[64] Olivotto I, Maron MS, Adabag AS, Casey SA, Vargiu D, Link MS, Udelson JE, Cecchi F, and Maron BJ. Gender-related differences in the clinical presentation and outcome of hypertrophic cardiomyopathy. J Am Coll Cardiol 46: 480-487, 2005.

[65] Konhilas JP and Leinwand LA. The effects of biological sex and diet on the development of heart failure. Circulation 116: 2747-2759, 2007.

[66] Yang XP and Reckelhoff JF. Estrogen, hormonal replacement therapy and cardiovascular disease. Curr Opin Nephrol Hypertens 20: 133-138, 2011.

[67] Thomas P, Pang Y, Filardo EJ, and Dong J. Identity of an estrogen membrane receptor coupled to a G protein in human breast cancer cells. Endocrinology 146: 624-632, 2005.

[68] Widder J, Pelzer T, von Poser-Klein C, Hu K, Jazbutyte V, Fritzemeier KH, Hegele-Hartung C, Neyses L, and Bauersachs J. Improvement of endothelial dysfunction by selective estrogen receptor-alpha stimulation in ovariectomized SHR. Hypertension 42: 991-996, 2003.

[69] Cavasin MA, Sankey SS, Yu AL, Menon S, and Yang XP. Estrogen and testosterone have opposing effects on chronic cardiac remodeling and function in mice with myocardial infarction. Am J Physiol Heart Circ Physiol 284: H1560-1569, 2003.

[70] van Eickels M, Grohe C, Cleutjens JP, Janssen BJ, Wellens HJ, and Doevendans PA. 17beta-estradiol attenuates the development of pressure-overload hypertrophy. Circulation 104: 1419-1423, 2001.

[71] Sharkey LC, Holycross BJ, Park S, Shiry LJ, Hoepf TM, McCune SA, and Radin MJ. Effect of ovariectomy and estrogen replacement on cardiovascular disease in heart failure-prone SHHF/Mcc- fa cp rats. J Mol Cell Cardiol 31: 1527-1537, 1999.

[72] de Jager T, Pelzer T, Muller-Botz S, Imam A, Muck J, and Neyses L. Mechanisms of estrogen receptor action in the myocardium. Rapid gene activation via the ERK1/2 pathway and serum response elements. J Biol Chem 276: 27873-27880, 2001.

[73] Grady D, Applegate W, Bush T, Furberg C, Riggs B, and Hulley SB. Heart and Estrogen/progestin Replacement Study (HERS): design, methods, and baseline characteristics. Control Clin Trials 19: 314-335, 1998.

[74] Rossouw JE, Anderson GL, Prentice RL, LaCroix AZ, Kooperberg C, Stefanick ML, Jackson RD, Beresford SA, Howard BV, Johnson KC, Kotchen JM, and Ockene J. Risks and benefits of estrogen plus progestin in healthy postmenopausal women: principal results from the Women's Health Initiative randomized controlled trial. JAMA 288: 321-333, 2002.

[75] Vikstrom KL, Factor SM, and Leinwand LA. Mice expressing mutant myosin heavy chains are a model for familial hypertrophic cardiomyopathy. Mol Med 2: 556-567, 1996.

[76] Stauffer BL, Konhilas JP, Luczak ED, and Leinwand LA. Soy diet worsens heart disease in mice. J Clin Invest 116: 209-216, 2006.

[77] Konhilas JP, Watson PA, Maass A, Boucek DM, Horn T, Stauffer BL, Luckey SW, Rosenberg P, and Leinwand LA. Exercise can prevent and reverse the severity of hypertrophic cardiomyopathy. Circ Res 98: 540-548, 2006.

[78] Geisterfer-Lowrance AA, Christe M, Conner DA, Ingwall JS, Schoen FJ, Seidman CE, and Seidman JG. A mouse model of familial hypertrophic cardiomyopathy. Science 272: 731-734, 1996.

[79] Haines CD, Harvey PA, Luczak ED, Barthel KK, Konhilas JP, Watson PA, Stauffer BL, and Leinwand LA. Estrogenic compounds are not always cardioprotective and can be lethal in males with genetic heart disease. Endocrinology 153: 4470-4479, 2012.

[80] Konhilas JP. What we know and do not know about sex and cardiac disease. J Biomed Biotechnol 2010: 562051, 2010.

[81] Simpson ER. Sources of estrogen and their importance. J Steroid Biochem Mol Biol 86: 225-230, 2003.

[82] Thomas MP and Potter BV. The structural biology of oestrogen metabolism. J Steroid Biochem Mol Biol 137: 27-49, 2013.

[83] Lipovka Y and Konhilas JP. The complex nature of estrogen signaling in breast cancer: enemy or ally. Biosci Rep, 2016.

[84] Revankar CM, Cimino DF, Sklar LA, Arterburn JB, and Prossnitz ER. A transmembrane intracellular estrogen receptor mediates rapid cell signaling. Science 307: 1625-1630, 2005.

[85] Pedram A, Razandi M, and Levin ER. Nature of functional estrogen receptors at the plasma membrane. Mol Endocrinol 20: 1996-2009, 2006.

[86] Arias-Loza PA, Kreissl MC, Kneitz S, Kaiser FR, Israel I, Hu K, Frantz S, Bayer B, Fritzemeier KH, Korach KS, and Pelzer T. The estrogen receptor-alpha is required and sufficient to maintain physiological glucose uptake in the mouse heart. Hypertension 60: 1070-1077, 2012.

[87] Rattanasopa C, Phungphong S, Wattanapermpool J, and Bupha-Intr T. Significant role of estrogen in maintaining cardiac mitochondrial functions. J Steroid Biochem Mol Biol 147: 1-9, 2015.

[88] Saleh TM, Connell BJ, and Saleh MC. Acute injection of 17beta-estradiol enhances cardiovascular reflexes and autonomic tone in ovariectomized female rats. Auton Neurosci 84: 78-88, 2000.

[89] Lipovka Y and Konhilas JP. AMP-activated protein kinase signalling in cancer and cardiac hypertrophy. Cardiovasc Pharm Open Access 4, 2015.

[90] Satoh M, Matter CM, Ogita H, Takeshita K, Wang CY, Dorn GW, 2nd, and Liao JK. Inhibition of apoptosis-regulated signaling kinase-1 and prevention of congestive heart failure by estrogen. Circulation 115: 3197-3204, 2007.

[91] Shen T, Ding L, Ruan Y, Qin W, Lin Y, Xi C, Lu Y, Dou L, Zhu Y, Cao Y, Man Y, Bian Y, Wang S, Xiao C, and Li J. SIRT1 functions as an important regulator of estrogen-mediated cardiomyocyte protection in angiotensin II-induced heart hypertrophy. Oxid Med Cell Longev 2014: 713894, 2014.

[92] Patten RD, Pourati I, Aronovitz MJ, Baur J, Celestin F, Chen X, Michael A, Haq S, Nuedling S, Grohe C, Force T, Mendelsohn ME, and Karas RH. 17beta-estradiol reduces cardiomyocyte apoptosis in vivo and in vitro via activation of phospho-inositide-3 kinase/Akt signaling. Circ Res 95: 692-699, 2004.

[93] Donaldson C, Eder S, Baker C, Aronovitz MJ, Weiss AD, Hall-Porter M, Wang F, Ackerman A, Karas RH, Molkentin JD, and Patten RD. Estrogen attenuates left ventricular and cardiomyocyte hypertrophy by an estrogen receptor-dependent pathway that increases calcineurin degradation. Circ Res 104: 265-275, 211p following 275, 2009.

[94] Pedram A, Razandi M, Aitkenhead M, and Levin ER. Estrogen inhibits cardiomyocyte hypertrophy in vitro. Antagonism of calcineurin-related hypertrophy through induction of MCIP1. J Biol Chem 280: 26339-26348, 2005.

[95] Voloshenyuk TG and Gardner JD. Estrogen improves TIMP-MMP balance and collagen distribution in volume-overloaded hearts of ovariectomized females. Am J Physiol Regul Integr Comp Physiol 299: R683-693, 2010.

[96] Pelzer T, Loza PA, Hu K, Bayer B, Dienesch C, Calvillo L, Couse JF, Korach KS, Neyses L, and Ertl G. Increased mortality and aggravation of heart failure in estrogen receptor-beta knockout mice after myocardial infarction. Circulation 111: 1492-1498, 2005.

[97] Bolego C, Rossoni G, Fadini GP, Vegeto E, Pinna C, Albiero M, Boscaro E, Agostini C, Avogaro A, Gaion RM, and Cignarella A. Selective estrogen receptor-alpha agonist provides widespread heart and vascular protection with enhanced endothelial progenitor cell mobilization in the absence of uterotrophic action. FASEB J 24: 2262-2272, 2010.

[98] Westphal C, Schubert C, Prelle K, Penkalla A, Fliegner D, Petrov G, and Regitz-Zagrosek V. Effects of estrogen, an ERalpha agonist and raloxifene on pressure overload induced cardiac hypertrophy. PLoS One 7: e50802, 2012.

[99] Babiker FA, Lips D, Meyer R, Delvaux E, Zandberg P, Janssen B, van Eys G, Grohe C, and Doevendans PA. Estrogen receptor beta protects the murine heart against left ventricular hypertrophy. Arterioscler Thromb Vasc Biol 26: 1524-1530, 2006.

[100] Fliegner D, Schubert C, Penkalla A, Witt H, Kararigas G, Dworatzek E, Staub E, Martus P, Ruiz Noppinger P, Kintscher U, Gustafsson JA, and Regitz-Zagrosek V. Female sex and estrogen receptor-beta attenuate cardiac remodeling and apoptosis in pressure overload. Am J Physiol Regul Integr Comp Physiol 298: R1597-1606, 2010.

[101] Kararigas G, Fliegner D, Gustafsson JA, and Regitz-Zagrosek V. Role of the estrogen/ estrogen-receptor-beta axis in the genomic response to pressure overload-induced hypertrophy. Physiol Genom 43: 438-446, 2011.

[102] Queiros AM, Eschen C, Fliegner D, Kararigas G, Dworatzek E, Westphal C, Sanchez Ruderisch H, and Regitz-Zagrosek V. Sex- and estrogen-dependent regulation of a miRNA network in the healthy and hypertrophied heart. Int J Cardiol 169: 331-338, 2013.

[103] Gurgen D, Hegner B, Kusch A, Catar R, Chaykovska L, Hoff U, Gross V, Slowinski T, da Costa Goncalves AC, Kintscher U, Gustafsson JA, Luft FC, and Dragun D. Estrogen receptor-beta signals left ventricular hypertrophy sex differences in normotensive deoxycorticosterone acetate-salt mice. Hypertension 57: 648-654, 2011.

[104] Pedram A, Razandi M, O'Mahony F, Lubahn D, and Levin ER. Estrogen receptor-beta prevents cardiac fibrosis. Mol Endocrinol 24: 2152-2165, 2010.

[105] Pedram A, Razandi M, Lubahn D, Liu J, Vannan M, and Levin ER. Estrogen inhibits cardiac hypertrophy: role of estrogen receptor-beta to inhibit calcineurin. Endocrinology 149: 3361-3369, 2008.

[106] Pedram A, Razandi M, Narayanan R, Dalton JT, McKinsey TA, and Levin ER. Estrogen regulates histone deacetylases to prevent cardiac hypertrophy. Mol Biol Cell 24: 3805-3818, 2013.

[107] Gardner JD, Murray DB, Voloshenyuk TG, Brower GL, Bradley JM, and Janicki JS. Estrogen attenuates chronic volume overload induced structural and functional remodeling in male rat hearts. Am J Physiol Heart Circ Physiol 298: H497-504, 2010.

[108] Kadokami T, McTiernan CF, Higuichi Y, Frye CS, Kubota T, and Feldman AM. 17 Beta-estradiol improves survival in male mice with cardiomyopathy induced by cardiac-specific tumor necrosis factor-alpha overexpression. J Interferon Cytokine Res 25: 254-260, 2005.

[109] Brinckmann M, Kaschina E, Altarche-Xifro W, Curato C, Timm M, Grzesiak A, Dong J, Kappert K, Kintscher U, Unger T, and Li J. Estrogen receptor alpha supports cardio-myocytes indirectly through post-infarct cardiac c-kit + cells. J Mol Cell Cardiol 47: 66-75, 2009.

[110] Brinckmann M, Kaschina E, Altarche-Xifro W, Curato C, Timm M, Grzesiak A, Dong J, Kappert K, Kintscher U, Unger T, and Li J. Estrogen receptor alpha supports cardio-myocytes indirectly through post-infarct cardiac c-kit+ cells. J Mol Cell Cardiol 47: 66-75, 2009.

[111] Rivera Z, Christian PJ, Marion SL, Brooks HL, and Hoyer PB. Steroidogenic capacity of residual ovarian tissue in 4-vinylcyclohexene diepoxide-treated mice. Biol Reprod 80: 328-336, 2009.

[112] Mayer LP, Devine PJ, Dyer CA, and Hoyer PB. The follicle-deplete mouse ovary produces androgen. Biol Reprod 71: 130-138, 2004.

[113] Morris PD and Channer KS. Testosterone and cardiovascular disease in men. Asian J Androl 14: 428-435, 2012.

[114] Erickson GF, Magoffin DA, Dyer CA, and Hofeditz C. The ovarian androgen producing cells: a review of structure/function relationships. Endocr Rev 6: 371-399, 1985.

[115] Liu Y, Ding J, Bush TL, Longenecker JC, Nieto FJ, Golden SH, and Szklo M. Relative androgen excess and increased cardiovascular risk after menopause: a hypothesized relation. Am J Epidemiol 154: 489-494, 2001.

[116] Pollow DP, Jr., Romero-Aleshire MJ, Sanchez JN, Konhilas JP, and Brooks HL. ANG II-induced hypertension in the VCD mouse model of menopause is prevented by estrogen replacement during perimenopause. Am J Physiol Regul Integr Comp Physiol 309: R1546-1552, 2015.

[117] Rundell VL, Geenen DL, Buttrick PM, and de Tombe PP. Depressed cardiac tension cost in experimental diabetes is due to altered myosin heavy chain isoform expression. Am J Physiol Heart Circ Physiol 287: H408-413, 2004.

9

Novel Insights into the Pathophysiology of Chagas' Cardiomyopathy

Philipp Stahl and Thomas Meyer

Abstract

The protozoan hemoflagellate *Trypanosoma cruzi* (*T. cruzi*) is the etiologic agent of the zoonotic Chagas' disease that affects approximately six to seven million people in Central and South America, causing dilated cardiomyopathy and megavisceral disease. Although Chagas' disease is the leading cause of heart failure in Latin America among people living in poverty and places an immense socioeconomic burden on society, it is still currently classified as a neglected tropical disease (NTD). The disease is typically transmitted by *reduviid* bugs or orally by contaminated food, while the transmission of parasitic organisms by other routes such as blood transfusion, organ transplantation, and transplacental infection is relatively rare. Given the wide cellular tropism infecting virtually all nucleated cells, the protozoan is able to persist asymptomatically for decades until ultimately causing organ-specific symptoms of chronic Chagas' disease such as chronic heart failure. The acute phase of the disease triggers an immune response that often does not restrict the dissemination of the parasite and may cause skin lesions, fever, enlarged lymph nodes, pallor, swelling, and abdominal and chest pain. Despite recent advances in our knowledge about the pathogenesis of this disease, the complex host-parasite interactions are not completely understood and, in particular, the persistence of parasites in host cells for such a long time remains largely undefined. In this book chapter, we focus on the pathophysiology of American trypanosomiasis and emphasize the role of host-specific transcription factors executing antiparasitic immune reactions.

Keywords: *Trypanosoma cruzi*, Chagas' disease, dilated cardiomyopathy, immune response, STAT transcription factors, apoptosis

1. Introduction

The pathogenic protozoan *Trypanosoma cruzi* (*T. cruzi*) is the causative agent of Chagas' disease, and more than 150 species of mammals are affected by this unicellular parasite, including humans. The parasite was discovered in 1909 by the Brazilian physician Carlos Chagas, while dissecting assassin bugs (*Reduviidae*) from the subfamily *Triatominae* that act as vectors and hosts for the parasite, and was later named after Chagas' scientific mentor Oswaldo Cruz [1].

Chagas' disease, also termed American trypanosomiasis, causes the third largest disease burden of the tropics after malaria and schistosomiasis [2] and is responsible for higher morbidity and mortality than any other parasitic infection in America [3]. According to surveys of the World Health Organization (WHO) from 2014, six to seven million people worldwide are estimated to be infected with *T. cruzi*, while around 14,000 patients die annually as a result of the parasitosis. An overview of the geographic distribution of Chagas' disease is presented in **Figure 1**.

The link between poverty and dissemination of Chagas' disease is striking, as it particularly affects people living in simple huts made of mud and wood with roofs of straw or palm leaves in rural areas of Latin America, where the predatory bugs have easy access. In the most important endemic areas, vectors include *Panstrongylus megistus, Triatoma infestans, T. dimidiata, T. pallidipennis,* and *Rhodnius prolixus* [4] (**Figure 2**). Non-vectorial transmission, such as the ingestion of *T. cruzi*-contaminated food and congenital transmission from the mother to the fetus [5] as well as blood transfusion and organ transplantation, increase the number of people at risk, estimated at 100 million worldwide. Owing to international migration, isolated cases of Chagas' disease in nonendemic countries are increasingly being recognized.

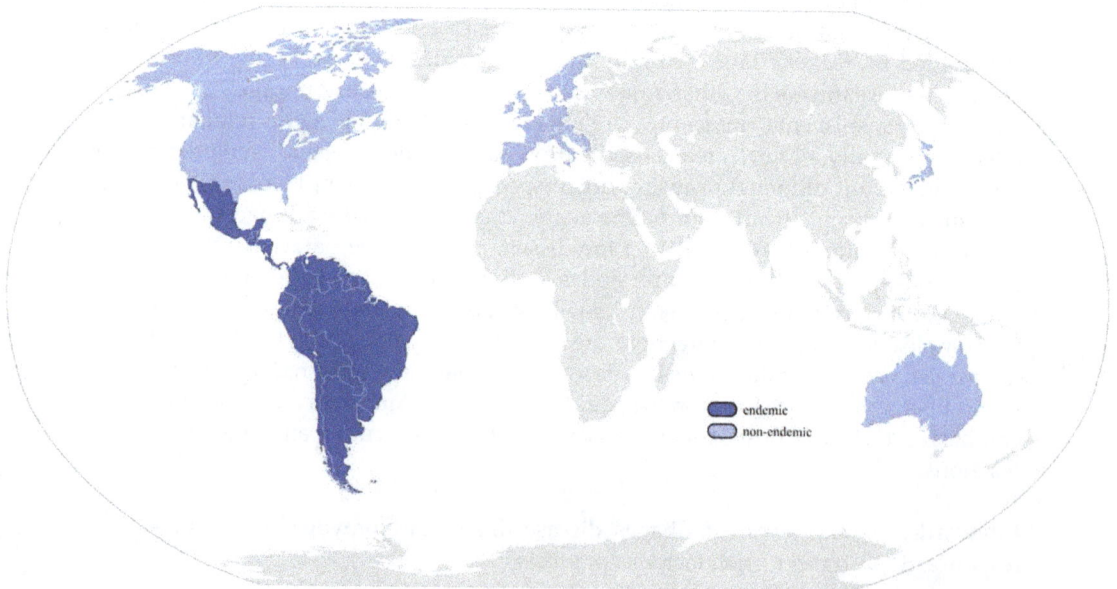

Figure 1. Geographical distribution of Chagas' disease. Dark blue indicates endemic countries and light blue nonendemic countries.

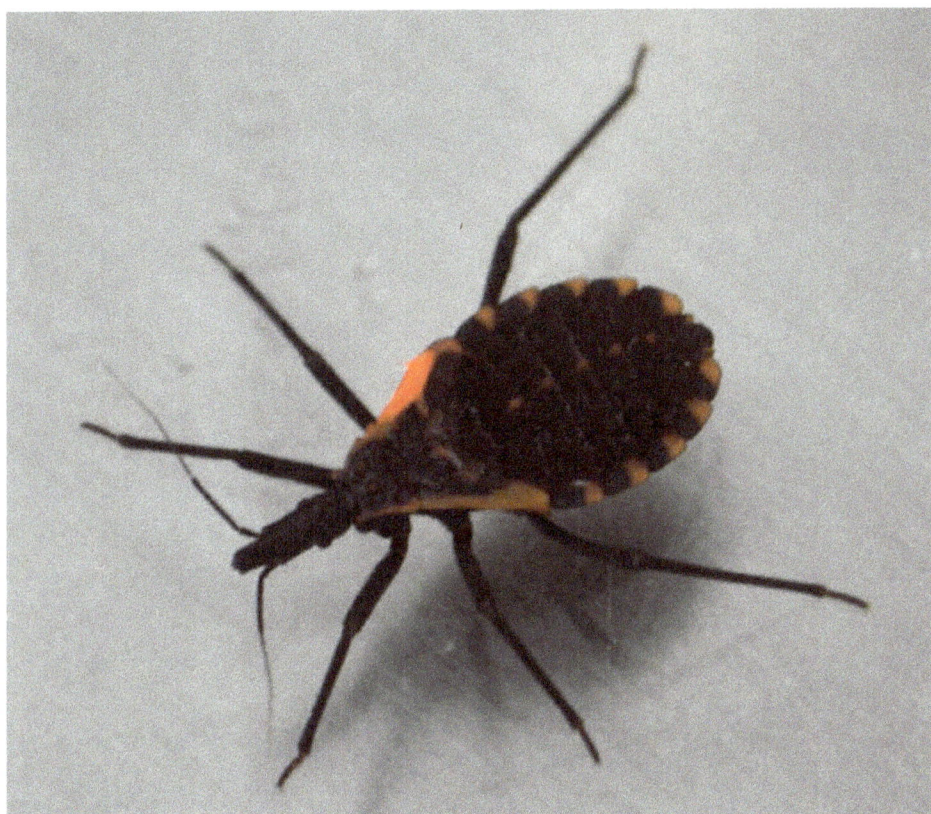

Figure 2. *Meccus pallidipennis* (syn. *Triatoma pallidipennis*, Hemiptera: *Reduviidae*) from the subfamily *Triatominae* as a vector for *T. cruzi*.

2. Biology and life cycle of *T. cruzi*

Assassin bugs infected with *T. cruzi* preferably sting sleeping victims and usually suck their blood unnoticed. After the blood meal, the pressure in the bug's gastrointestinal tract increases and the insect defecates on the skin near the wound. This behavior of *Triatominae* is crucial for their ability to act as a vector for *T. cruzi*, since infective stages of *T. cruzi* reach the stab wound only when the bugs defecate during food intake. The assassin bug transmits the parasites to the definitive host, by spreading excrement on the wound while escaping. When the pathogen-containing feces are rubbed into the fresh puncture wound by the victim or when the pathogen penetrates into uninjured mucosa, especially those of the eye, highly infectious and very motile metacyclic trypomastigotes of *T. cruzi* are transmitted into the blood flow of the host [6, 7] (**Figure 3**). The trypomastigotes are then disseminated successively into the organism of the host, and preferably infect cells of the reticuloendothelial and mononuclear phagocytic system [8]. A parasitophorous vacuole is formed only briefly during the life cycle of *T. cruzi*, while the intracellular parasites multiply in the cytoplasm of the host cell by binary division [9, 10].

T. cruzi can infect any nucleated cell but predominantly replicates in cardiac muscle cells as well as in cells of the nervous system, gonads, intestinal mucosa, and placenta [11]. After penetration into the cytoplasm of the host cell, the morphology of the metacyclic trypomastigotes

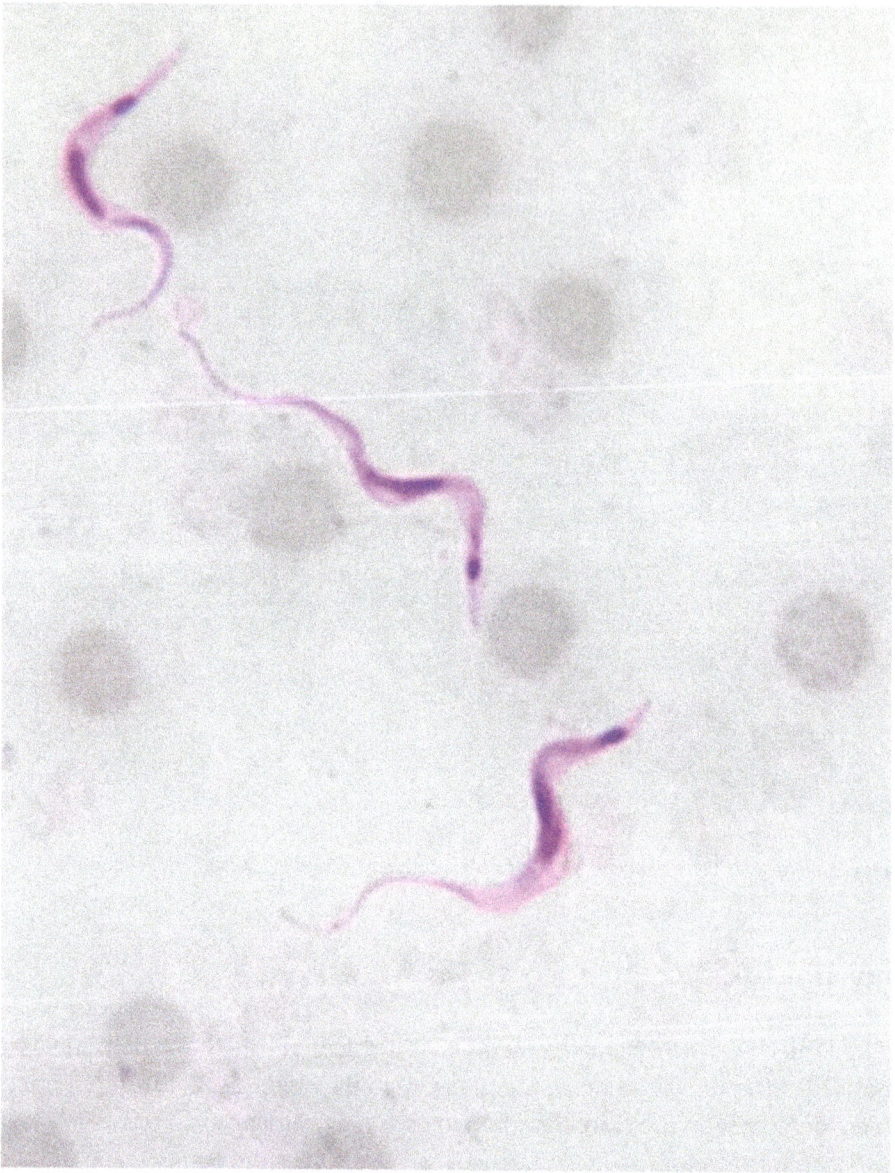

Figure 3. *Trypanosoma cruzi* metacyclic trypomastigotes on a peripheral blood smear shown by Giemsa staining.

changes to intracellular amastigotes with diameters of 3–5 μm, when they lose their undulating membrane which is a characteristic feature of mobile trypomastigotes [9, 12] (**Figure 4**). Intracellular amastigotes undergo several rounds of division and are then transformed into trypomastigotes, approximately 20-μm long, which leave the host cell and spread further into the organism to infect new host cells [13]. Unlike the African sleeping sickness caused by *T. brucei*, intracellular replication of *T. cruzi* in host cells is mandatory, since the pathogenic agent of American trypanosomiasis is not able to divide in the blood. For this reason, the intracellular amastigote form of *T. cruzi* is always present and can be histopathologically detected in tissue samples from spleen, liver, brain, and heart muscle. The life cycle of *T. cruzi* continues when the bug takes a blood meal from an infected host, and the parasites transform in the

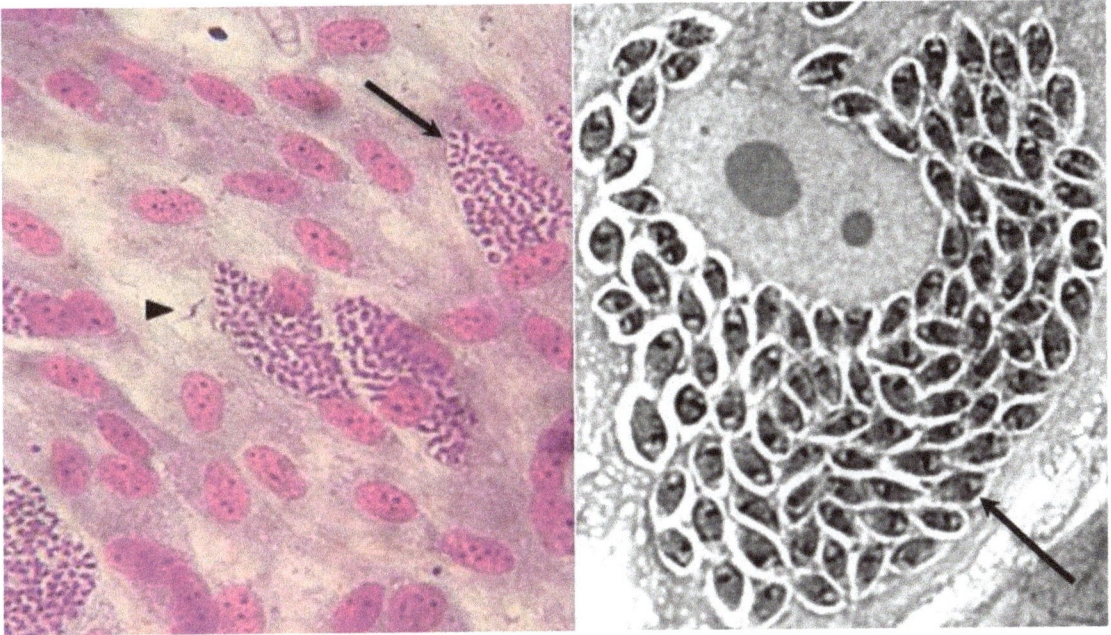

Figure 4. Intracytoplasmic localization of *T. cruzi* amastigotes in cultured fibroblasts stained with Giemsa at low (left) and high (right) magnification. Arrows mark intracellular amastigotes, and the arrow head (left) indicates an extracellular trypomastigote.

bug's midgut to epimastigote forms and multiply by binary fission. Finally, the highly infectious metacyclic trypomastigotes develop in the rectum of the bug, and will be passed again with the feces during a subsequent second blood meal [14].

3. Epidemiology

Following a decline in incidence in endemic countries of Latin America, recorded in the mid-1990s up to the beginning of this millennium due to vector-eradication campaigns, Chagas' disease is currently worldwide on the rise again even in Europe [15–21]. Alternative transmission modes of Chagas' disease, such as congenital infection and infection through contaminated blood and organ donations, now play a major role both in classical endemic areas and in countries outside Latin America due to an increase in worldwide migration. The disease is, therefore, increasingly being detected in Europe, since more than 14 million people have left the endemic areas of South America, four to five million for Europe [22]. In a statement from the WHO for Chagas' disease in Europe in 2010, the number of *T. cruzi*-infected individuals in Europe is estimated at 80,000–100,000. Switzerland is home to a group of people at risk, and it is estimated that of the approximately 40,000 legal immigrants from Latin America, 2000–4000 people may have become infected with this pathogen [23]. In Spain, the estimated number of people infected with *T. cruzi*, most of these being legal immigrants from South America, is 25,000–48,000 [17, 18].

Chagas' disease can also pose a threat to Germany. The data collection among the approximately 85,000 immigrants coming from endemic areas is, however, incomplete. It is estimated that the prevalence of seropositive immigrants is 1.3–1.7% (1100–1450-infected individuals); however, it is assumed that the number of patients is significantly underdiagnosed with Chagas' disease [18, 24]. Epidemiological data from the United States of America estimated up to a million people infected with T. cruzi, and for the entire American continent including Mexico up to seven million [25]. In South America, Bolivia is the country with by far the highest infection rate, and serological screening in maternity hospitals detected up to 23.6% pregnant women infected with the parasite [26]. Recent data also underline the spread with increasing prevalence of Chagas' disease in Australia and New Zealand [27].

4. Symptomatology of Chagas' disease

Infection with T. cruzi can be divided into three distinct phases: the acute, indeterminate (latent), and chronic phase. The acute phase is characterized by the detection of circulating trypomastigotes in the blood. The majority of patients infected in adulthood are asymptomatic or show only mild and nonspecific symptoms. Children, however, are much more susceptible to a recognizable acute infection with T. cruzi and often have a higher parasitemia than adults. After an incubation period of 1–3 weeks, local inflammatory reactions develop at the entry point. In about half of all cases, the eye is the primary portal of entry. Parasites penetrate transconjunctivally into mesenchymal cells or are phagocytosed by macrophages and cause a local inflammatory reaction. Characteristic for acute Chagas' disease is a periorbital edema accompanied by conjunctivitis, which is termed Româna's sign.

Inflammatory lesions or nodules on the puncture wound in the face are less frequently observed manifestations of the acute stage (Chagoma), indicating a local inflammatory response with tissue destruction. Invasion of neutrophils and activation of tissue macrophages result in the secretion of pro-inflammatory cytokines such as tumor necrosis factor-α (TNF-α) and interferon-γ (IFN-γ). After a further 1–2 weeks, the stage of hematogenous and lymphatic spread is achieved, and further clinical symptoms of the acute phase may develop such as fever, anemia, muscle and bone pain, fatigue, diarrhea, lymphadenopathy, and hepatosplenomegaly. Whereas these symptoms typically disappear after 3–4 months, a small number of individuals, especially children, die from complications such as myocarditis or meningoencephalitis. The fatal course is highly dependent on the immune system and nutritional status of the host as well as the parasite load during transmission. The subsequent indeterminate phase is characterized by a very low parasitemia in the blood and can last for decades. Cellular immunity is at this stage an important endogenous strategy of the host to keep the parasites under control. Usually, 20–30% of seropositive patients develop the chronic phase of Chagas' disease [28]. In 40–50% of the affected patients, a progressive cardiomyopathy and less frequently neuronal dysfunction of the autonomic nerves of the gastrointestinal tract can develop [29]. These symptoms are often found clinically only at a later stage, as many patients are initially asymptomatic. During routine analysis, radiological signs of left heart failure and cardiomegaly can be found. Damage to the heart may result in atrioventricular (AV), His-bundle or intraventricular blocks with Adam-Stokes seizures and syncopes [30]. Cellular hypertrophy and subsequent chamber enlargement lead to systolic heart failure and may result in arrhythmias. Patients often die of sudden cardiac death induced by ventricular tachycardia and congestive heart failure [31]. Histopathologic examination of endomyocardial biopsies shows myocardial fibrosis, resulting from cell lysis by trypanosomes and/or immune-pathological mechanisms. Development of gastrointestinal mega-syndrome, particularly the esophagus and colon, are additional clinical manifestations of chronic Chagas' disease. The formation of mega-organs results from the destruction of the parasympathetic ganglia of the Meissner and Auerbach plexus in the gastrointestinal tract, which critically impairs peristalsis and leads to the ballooning of the organs. Clinically, these patients show symptoms of dysphagia, regurgitation, constipation, and secondary achalasia resulting from the dysfunction of the lower esophageal sphincter.

5. Diagnosis and treatment

Based on the aforementioned clinical signs of *T. cruzi* infection, chronic Chagas' disease is diagnosed using conventional methods in clinical cardiology. The electrocardiogram (ECG) is the diagnostic tool of choice in the question of Chagas' cardiomyopathy. Magnetic resonance imaging (MRI) allows noninvasive and accurate assessment of inflammatory infiltrates of the heart muscle and the identification of an apical ventricular aneurysm. To confirm the diagnosis, a series of laboratory tests should be employed. The classic laboratory diagnostic measure to confirm an acute infection is a blood smear, which is stained after fixation with Giemsa and typically shows motile trypanomastigotes. The serological diagnosis comprises detection of both immunoglobulin (Ig) M and IgG antibodies against *T. cruzi* using enzyme-linked immunosorbent assay (ELISA), indirect hemagglutination assay (IHA) or indirect immunofluorescence assay (IFA). For suspected Chagas' disease, the WHO recommends two mutually independent tests [32]. The polymerase chain reaction (PCR) for the detection of nucleic acid sequences of parasites can be used to detect parasites in organ transplants, as well as to test the parasite load during and after chemotherapy. Finally, in unclear serological cases and when the blood smear is repeatedly negative, the xenodiagnosis developed by the French parasitologist Alexander Joseph Émile Brumpt may be applied using confirmed *T. cruzi*-negative assassin bugs, which take a blood meal on the patient's skin. After 10–30 days, in the case of an infection of the patient with *T. cruzi*, even at low parasitemia, metacyclic trypomastigotes of *T. cruzi* can be demonstrated in the intestine of the bug and confirm the diagnosis [33].

In principle, two drugs for the treatment of acute Chagas' disease are available, nifurtimox and benznidazole, which require prolonged treatment and may cause significant side effects [34]. Nifurtimox, a nitrofuran with antiparasitic activity against both life cycle stages in the host, causes the accumulation of free radicals and superoxides and is generally genotoxic [35]. The nitroimidazole derivate benznidazole is an antiparasitic medication equally effective against the two life-cycle stages. This drug inhibits the synthesis of RNA and generates the accumulation of superoxides [35]. Although the parasite burden can be reduced below the detection limit in about 70% of all pharmacologically treated cases in acute Chagas' disease, there is still no evidence that antiparasitic treatment can cure the patient completely from *T. cruzi* [36–38]. Data for the treatment of patients with chronic Chagas' heart disease are not sufficiently validated to recommend a basic chemotherapy for these patients due to the unfavorable side-effect profile. In nonrandomized clinical or animal studies, some authors conclude that treatment with benznidazole may also be of benefit during the chronic phase, since thus severe courses of Chagas' cardiomyopathy can be avoided [39, 40]. However, results from the multicenter, randomized Benznidazole Evaluation for Interrupting Trypanosomiasis (BENEFIT) trial to assess the efficacy and safety of benznidazole treatment in patients with chronic Chagas' cardiomyopathy demonstrated that anti-trypanocidal therapy does not significantly reduce clinical deterioration through 5 years of follow-up as compared to placebo, despite reductions in the parasite load in serum samples [41]. These findings emphasize the urgent need for the development of new pharmacological agents against chronic Chagas' disease.

6. Prevention

Hitherto, the only sure prevention of the disease is the exposure prophylaxis by aerial spraying of insecticides and by modernization of traditional huts in rural areas. *T. cruzi*-infected pets, especially dogs and cats, provide a large reservoir of pathogens. Some countries perform an obligatory blood bank screening for the pathogen of Chagas' disease. These include, for example, Brazil, Uruguay, Argentina, Colombia, and the United States, but also Spain and Portugal. A vaccination against *T. cruzi* does not yet exist. Surface components of the parasite, particularly glycolipids such as glycosylphosphatidylinositol (GPI) anchors, have been well studied for their role in infectivity [42]. Trypanosomal trans-sialidase, belonging to the family of GPI-anchored proteins which transfer sialic acids from the cell membrane of the host to glycoproteins on the parasite surface, is involved in the infection of the host cell, and trans-sialidase inhibitors have been successfully tested *in vitro* [43].

7. Innate immune response to infections with *T. cruzi*

The innate immune system is essential in order to control the spread of *T. cruzi* parasites in the body and to ensure the survival of the host [44]. Pattern recognition receptors (PRRs), particularly the transmembrane toll-like receptors (TLRs), recognize the so-called pathogen-associated molecular patterns (PAMPs) in microorganisms [45]. Binding of glycoinositol-phospholipids (GIPL), GPI anchors, DNA, and RNA fragments of *T. cruzi* to TLR2, TLR4, TLR7, and TLR9 initiates a signaling cascade that finally activates important pro-inflammatory processes [46–52]. In myocarditis, genes for the endogenous TLR-7 and TLR-9 receptors are upregulated and their gene products serve as potential biomarkers for inflammatory heart disease [53]. Through the adapter molecule myeloid differentiation factor 88 (MyD88), a signal pathway is activated that finally leads to the upregulation of pro-inflammatory genes, such as interleukin-(IL)-1β [54], IL-6 [55], IL-12 [56–60], TNF-α [57, 58, 61], IFN-β [62–64], and IFN-γ [54, 59–61, 65–67].

Activation of these pathways is critical for resistance to infection with *T. cruzi*. Mice functionally deficient in MyD88 expression are more susceptible to infection by this protozoan, which is probably due to a defect in the production of pro-inflammatory cytokines [68]. In *T. cruzi*-infected macrophages, the expression of pro-inflammatory cytokines is mediated by two transcription factors: nuclear factor-κB (NF-κB) [69–71] and interferon-regulatory factor 3 (IRF3) [64]. NF-kB also activates inducible NO synthase (iNOS) which catalyzes the production of microbicidal nitric oxide (NO). Mice with a deficiency of iNOS or IFN-γ receptor are sensitive to infection with *T. cruzi*, showing a high rate of parasitemia, and, furthermore, macrophages from these mice have impaired trypanocidal activity due to lower amounts of NO [72].

8. Apoptosis of cardiac myocytes in Chagas' disease

The chronic stage of Chagas' disease usually leads to symptoms of dilated cardiomyopathy, which is characterized by an enlargement of the heart muscle with a steadily progressive loss of systolic function. The decrease in the biventricular ejection volume is presumably reflecting altered heart muscle remodeling and may include apoptotic cell death. Apoptosis is a form of programmed cell death which differs from necrosis by actively carrying out a cell-death program [73]. Apoptosis-regulating genes such as Bax and Apaf-1 are involved in the execution of apoptosis, whereas Bcl-2 is an antiapoptotic protein.

Proteolytic enzymes termed caspases play a central role in the execution of apoptotic cell death. The activation of the caspase cascade can be initiated by both intra- and extracellular stimuli. Extracellular stimuli induce the activation of caspases 8 and 10 through the Fas ligand and TNF receptors, whereas the intracellular pathway consists of the cytochrome C-regulated apoptosome which activates caspase 9. The JAK-STAT-signaling pathway regulates apoptosis via STAT3 (signal transducer and activator of transcription 3) by promoting the expression of antiapoptotic genes coding for the Bcl-2 protein family [74]. Cytotoxic T lymphocytes (CTLs, CD8+ T-cells) activate caspases 3 and 7. These are key caspases in which caspases 8 and 9 converge and henceforth result in a common final pathway of the signaling cascade. Apoptosis of cardiomyocytes in the context of *T. cruzi* infection is a potential mechanism of the host to limit the spread of parasites.

In autopsy samples from Chagas' cardiomyopathy patients, signs of apoptotic cell death were detected post mortem in cardiac myocytes [75], confirming earlier results that *T. cruzi*-infected cardiomyocytes undergo fibrosis and apoptotic cell death [76, 77]. Zhang and colleagues detected apoptosis in a canine model of acute chagasic myocarditis characterized by the presence of amastigotes and trypomastigotes of *T. cruzi* within the cytoplasm of cardiac muscle cells [76]. In a gene expression study, Manque and colleagues showed that the infection of murine cardiomyocytes with *T. cruzi* resulted in the upregulation of the two classical proapoptotic genes *bid*, encoding BH3-interacting domain death agonist, and *fas* which encodes a member of the TNF receptor gene. In addition, the *gadd45b* gene engaged in cell cycle control, DNA repair, and apoptosis was upregulated upon infection [78].

However, there are conflicting results on the role of apoptosis in murine cardiomyocytes during infection with *T. cruzi* trypomastigotes. De Souza et al. reported that cardiomyocytes became apoptotic after infection with different strains of *T. cruzi* [79], whereas Aoki et al.

showed that the cysteine protease cruzipain on the surface of *T. cruzi* appears to have a protective effect on the host cell and serves as a survival factor supporting the propagation of the parasites [80]. Our group demonstrated apoptotic rat cardiomyocytes upon infection with either trypomastigote or amastigote stages of *T. cruzi* [81]. Petersen et al. showed that both *T. cruzi* infection and activation of NF-κB prevented apoptotic cell death in isolated neonatal rat cardiomyocytes [82]. Another study reported that amastigotes presented higher rates of apoptosis-like cell death as compared to trypomastigotes [83].

The JAK-STAT-signaling pathway has an important role in cardiomyopathy, myocarditis, and myocardial infarction [84]. Cardiomyocytes express various receptors for cytokines and growth factors (among others, TNFα and EGF) on their surface. Secreted cytokines or growth factors may be involved in the apoptotic cell death of cardiomyocytes and chronic cardiomyopathy. Specifically, the balance in the activation state of the two related transcription factors STAT1 and STAT3 may determine the outcome between cell death and survival of cardiac muscle cells during infection with *T. cruzi* [85].

In the context of chronic Chagas' disease, which can develop up to 25 years after parasitic infection, the question arises as to how the parasite can persist and replicate for such a long period of time in the host without causing an exacerbating immune response. The most obvious explanation is that the parasite has developed effective mechanisms to circumvent the immune response which affects the steady balance between parasite load and apoptosis-induced destruction of host cells. Various parasitological studies highlight the dogma that the replication of parasites in the cardiac myocytes is required to initiate the complete picture of Chagas' heart disease ranging from acute myocarditis to chronic cardiomyopathy [86].

9. The role of STAT proteins in Chagas' cardiomyopathy

There is growing evidence that not only NF-kB but also STAT transcription factors are engaged in *T. cruzi* infection. Recently, we have demonstrated that serine phosphorylation of STAT1 at position 727 is targeted by *T. cruzi*, suggesting that the parasite inhibits the antiparasitic effects of STAT1 [87] (**Figure 5**). Ponce and coworkers reported that the secretion of endogenous IL-6 or the addition of recombinant IL-6 protects cardiomyocytes from cell death by apoptosis during an infection with *T. cruzi* [88]. Furthermore, the authors showed the phosphorylation of STAT3 at tyrosine 705 by IL-6 in response to infection with *T. cruzi*. In cardiac tissues, the expression of the STAT3-regulated antiapoptotic factor Bcl-2 was increased, suggesting that, during the acute phase of infection with *T. cruzi*, tyrosine-phosphorylated STAT3 acts as a mediator of cell survival. In summary, the results of this important study suggest that STAT3 executes pro-survival effects in cardiac muscle cells evoked by the parasite.

In addition, Ponce et al. demonstrated that, in *T. cruzi*-infected cells, the release of IL-6 via a TLR2-dependent pathway is required to induce survival of cardiomyocytes [88]. The enzymatic activity of cruzipain, the main cysteine protease secreted by this parasite, critically interferes with IL-6-mediated STAT3 phosphorylation by means of cleavage of the ectodomain of glycoprotein gp130, which is the shared receptor of several IL-6-type cytokines [89]. The parasite cysteine protease inhibitor chagasin inhibits cruzipain-induced gp130 cleavage,

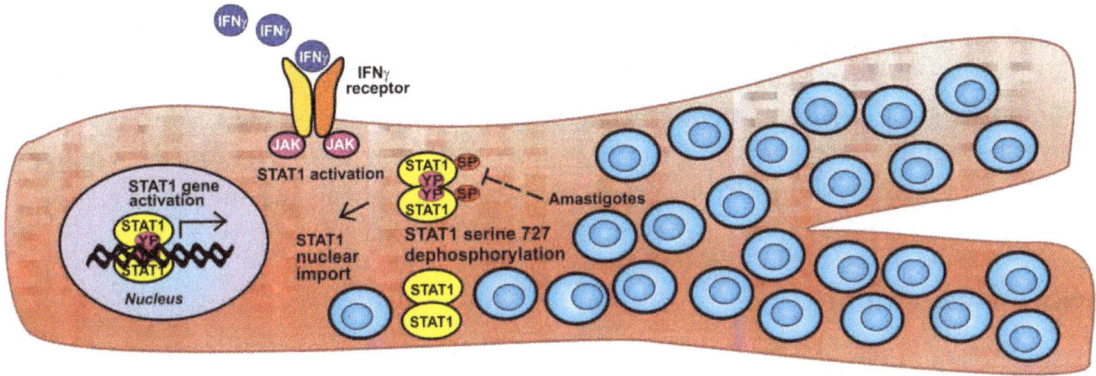

Figure 5. Illustration of a cardiac myocyte showing replicating intracellular *T. cruzi* parasites that evade the protective role of IFN-γ signaling by targeting essential components of the JAK-STAT pathway such as the dephosphorylation of STAT1 at serine 727. While phosphorylation of STAT1 serine 727 is required for full transcriptional activity, its dephosphorylation inhibits antiparasitic effects of STAT1.

suggesting that the pro-inflammatory IL-6 response in *T. cruzi*-infected cells is modified by cysteine protease activity. In addition, it has been well established that STAT transcription factors activate genes whose products have been identified as suppressors of cytokine signaling (SOCS) which act as inhibitors of the JAK-STAT pathway in a negative feedback loop [90].

Previous studies have described how STAT3 is activated by the two cytokines IL-6 or IL-10 [91, 92] and how the expression of SOCS3 is upregulated by the anti-inflammatory IL-10 in *T. cruzi*-infected cardiomyocytes [71]. During chronic infection with *T. cruzi*, the expression of SOCS2 is upregulated and most probably plays a significant role in the etiopathogenesis of Chagas' heart disease by influencing heart muscle damage [93].

Another member of the STAT family, the transcription factor STAT4, is activated in response to the cytokine IL-12, which acts as a pro-inflammatory cytokine and drives Th cells along a Th1 lineage. STAT6 is activated by receptor binding of two cytokines with anti-inflammatory properties, IL-4 and IL-13, which provide an alternative signal for the development along a Th2 lineage. Tarleton and coworkers demonstrated that STAT4-deficient mice were highly susceptible to infection with *T. cruzi*, whereas STAT6-deficient mice showed enhanced resistance with lower parasitemia and little or no evidence of inflammatory processes in the heart muscle as compared to their wild-type littermates [94]. The apparent absence of disease in chronically infected STAT6-deficient mice is remarkable despite their inability to achieve entire parasite clearance. The findings in this investigation suggest that the severity of inflammation critically depends on STAT4- and STAT6-mediated cytokine-driven immune reactions which modulate tissue parasite load [94]. Finally, the authors infer that the clearance of intracellular parasites may not be required to prevent the progression of the disease to cardiomyopathy.

10. Concluding remarks

In summary, the pathogenic protozoan *T. cruzi* has evolved complex and still undefined mechanisms to circumvent an effective immune response in the human myocardium. The bypassing of protective signaling pathways by the parasite such as the JAK-STAT pathway may account for the intracellular multiplication and long-lasting persistence of *T. cruzi* in the host. Amastigotes of *T. cruzi* proliferating in the cytoplasm of infected cardiomyocytes have developed effective strategies to counteract the attack executed by STAT proteins, which are crucial for an effective immune defense against the protozoan. Further research efforts are required to elucidate the role of cytokine-driven gene expression in the fight against the parasite.

Acknowledgement

The research on this subject was funded by grants from Deutsche Forschungsgemeinschaft (DFG), Deutsche Gesellschaft für Kardiologie (DGK), and Deutsches Zentrum für Herz- und Kreislaufforschung (DZHK).

Author details

Philipp Stahl[1, 2] and Thomas Meyer[3, 4*]

*Address all correspondence to: thomas.meyer@med.uni-goettingen.de

1 Institute of Virology, Parasitology Unit, University of Marburg, Marburg, Germany

2 Department of Internal Medicine, Section of Gastroenterology and Infectious Diseases, University Hospital Gießen and Marburg, Marburg, Germany

3 Department of Psychosomatic Medicine and Psychotherapy, University of Göttingen, Göttingen, Germany

4 German Center for Cardiovascular Research, partner site Göttingen, Göttingen, Germany

References

[1] Chagas C. Nova tripanozomiase humana. Estudos sobre a morfologia e o ciclo evolutivo do Schizotrypanum cruzi n. gen., n. sp., agente etiológico de nova entidade mórbida do homem. Mem. Inst. Oswaldo Cruz 1909;**1**:159–218.

[2] Moncayo A. Progress towards the elimination of transmission of Chagas disease in Latin America. World Health Stat. Q. 1997;**50**:195–198.

[3] Rassi A Jr, Rassi A, Marin-Neto JA. Chagas disease. Lancet 2010;**375**:1388–1402.

[4] Schaub GA. Pathogenicity of trypanosomatids on insects. Parasitol. Today 1994; **10**:463–468.

[5] Sánchez LV, Ramírez JD. Congenital and oral transmission of American trypanosomiasis: an overview of physiopathogenic aspects. Parasitology 2013;**140**:147–159.

[6]   Brener Z. Biology of *Trypanosoma cruzi*. Annu. Rev. Microbiol. 1973;**27**:347–382.

[7]   Vickerman K. Developmental cycles and biology of pathogenic trypanosomes. Br. Med. Bull. 1985:**41**:105–114.

[8]   De Souza W. Basic cell biology of *Trypanosoma cruzi*. Curr. Pharm. Des. 2002;**8**:269–285.

[9]   Andrews NW. Living dangerously: how *Trypanosoma cruzi* uses lysosomes to get inside host cells, and then escapes into the cytoplasm. Biol. Res. 1993:**26**:65–67.

[10] Tan H, Andrews NW. Don't bother to knock—the cell invasion strategy of *Trypanosoma cruzi*. Trends Parasitol. 2002;**18**:427–428.

[11] Burleigh BA, Andrews NW. The mechanisms of *Trypanosoma cruzi* invasion of mammalian cells. Annu. Rev. Microbiol. 1995;**49**:175–200.

[12] Tyler KM, Engman DM. The life cycle of *Trypanosoma cruzi* revisited. Int. J. Parasitol. 2001;**31**:472–481.

[13] Ferreira ER, Bonfim-Melo A, Mortara RA, Bahia D. *Trypanosoma cruzi* extracellular amastigotes and host cell signaling: more pieces to the puzzle. Front. Immunol. 2012;**3**:363.

[14] De Souza W. Cell biology of *Trypanosoma cruzi*. Int. Rev. Cytol. 1984;**86**:197–283.

[15] Schofield CJ, Dias JC. The Southern Cone Initiative against Chagas disease. Adv. Parasitol. 1999;**42**:1–27.

[16] Moncayo A, Silveira AC. Current epidemiological trends for Chagas disease in Latin America and future challenges in epidemiology, surveillance and health policy. Mem. Inst. Oswaldo Cruz 104 Suppl 2009;**1**:17–30.

[17] Gascon J, Bern C, Pinazo MJ. Chagas disease in Spain, the United States and other nonendemic countries. Acta Trop. 2010;**115**:22–27.

[18] Basile L, Jansá JM, Carlier Y, Salamanca DD, Angheben A, Bartoloni A, Seixas J, Van Gool T, Canavate C, Flores-Chávez M, Jackson Y, Chiodini PL, Albajar-Vinas P, and Working Group on Chagas Disease. Chagas disease in European countries: the challenge of a surveillance system. Euro. Surveill. 2011;**16**.

[19] Angheben A, Anselmi M, Gobbi F, Marocco S, Monteiro G, Buonfrate D, Tais S, Talamo M, Zavarise G, Strohmeyer M, Bartalesi F, Mantella A, Di Tommaso M, Aiello KH, Veneruso G, Graziani G, Ferrari M, Spreafico I, Bonifacio E, Gaiera G, Lanzafame M, Mascarello M, Cancrini G, Albajar-Vinas P, Bisoffi Z, Bartoloni A. Chagas disease in Italy: breaking an epidemiological silence. Euro. Surveill. 2011:**16**.

[20] Perez-Molina JA, Perez-Ayala A, Parola P, Jackson Y, Odolini S, Lopez-Velez R, and EuroTravNet Network. EuroTravNet: imported Chagas disease in nine European countries, 2008 to 2009. Euro Surveill. Bull. 2011;**16**.

[21] Albajar-Vinas P, Jannin J. The hidden Chagas disease burden in Europe. Euro Surveill. 2011;**16***.

[22] Schmunis GA, Yadon ZE. Chagas disease: a Latin American health problem becoming a world health problem. Acta Trop. 2010;**115**:14–21.

[23] Jackson Y, Chappuis F. Chagas disease in Switzerland: history and challenges. Euro. Surveill. 2011;**16**.

[24] Strasen J, Williams T, Ertl G, Zoller T, Stich A, Ritter O. Epidemiology of Chagas disease in Europe: many calculations, little knowledge. Clin. Res. Cardiol. 2014;**103**:1–10.

[25] Hotez PJ, Dumonteil E, Betancourt Cravioto M, Bottazzi ME, Tapia-Conyer R, Meymandi S, Karunakara U, Ribeiro I, Cohen RM, Pecoul B. An unfolding tragedy of Chagas disease in North America. PLoS Negl. Trop. Dis. 2013;**7**:e2300.

[26] Salas Clavijo NA, Postigo JR, Schneider D, Santalla JA, Brutus L, Chippaux JP. Prevalence of Chagas disease in pregnant women and incidence of congenital transmission in Santa Cruz de la Sierra, Bolivia. Acta Trop. 2012;**124**:87–91.

[27] Jackson Y, Pinto A, Pett S. Chagas disease in Australia and New Zealand: risks and needs for public health interventions. Trop. Med. Int. Health 2014,**19**:212–218.

[28] Rossi MA, Bestetti RB. The challenge of chagasic cardiomyopathy. The pathologic roles of autonomic abnormalities, autoimmune mechanisms and microvascular changes, and therapeutic implications. Cardiology 1995;**86**:1–7.

[29] Rassi A Jr, Rassi A, Marcondes de Rezende J. American Trypanosomiasis (Chagas Disease). Infect. Dis. Clin. North Am. 2012;**26**:275–291.

[30] Marin-Neto JA, Cunha-Neto E, Maciel BC, Simões MV. Pathogenesis of chronic Chagas heart disease. Circulation 2007;**115**:1109–1123.

[31] de Lourdes Higuchi M, Benvenuti LA, Martins Reis M, Metzger M. Pathophysiology of the heart in Chagas' disease: current status and new developments. Cardiovasc. Res. 2003;**60**:96–107.

[32] Otani MM, Vinelli E, Kirchhoff LV, del Pozo A, Sands A, Vercauteren G, Sabino EC. WHO comparative evaluation of serologic assays for Chagas disease. Transfusion (Paris) 2009;**49**:1076–1082.

[33] Brumpt E. Le xenodiagnostic. Application au diagnostic de quelques infections parasitaires et en particulier à la trypanosome de Chagas. Bull. Soc. Path. Exot. 1914;**77**:706–710.

[34] Lattes R, Lasala MB. Chagas disease in the immunosuppressed patient. Clin. Microbiol. Infect. 2014;**20**:300–309.

[35] Le Loup G, Pialoux G, Lescure FX. Update in treatment of Chagas disease. Curr. Opin. Infect. Dis. 2011;**24**:428–434.

[36] Marin-Neto JA, Rassi A, Avezum A, Mattos AC, Rassi A, Morillo CA, Sosa-Estani S, Yusuf S, and BENEFIT Investigators. The BENEFIT trial: testing the hypothesis that trypanocidal therapy is beneficial for patients with chronic Chagas heart disease. Mem. Inst. Oswaldo Cruz 104 Suppl 2009;**1**:319–324.

[37] Apt W. Current and developing therapeutic agents in the treatment of Chagas disease. Drug Des. Devel. Ther. 2010;**4**:243–253.

[38] Bern C. Chagas' Disease. N. Engl. J. Med. 2015;**373**:456–466.

[39] Garcia S, Ramos CO, Senra JFV, Vilas-Boas F, Rodrigues MM, Campos-de-Carvalho AC, Ribeiro-dos-Santos R, Soares MBP. Treatment with benznidazole during the chronic phase of experimental Chagas' disease decreases cardiac alterations. Antimicrob. Agents Chemother. 2005;**49**:1521–1528.

[40] Viotti R, Vigliano C, Lococo B, Bertocchi G, Petti M, Alvarez MG, Postan M, Armenti A. Long-term cardiac outcomes of treating chronic Chagas disease with benznidazole versus no treatment: a nonrandomized trial. Ann. Intern. Med. 2006:**144**:724–734.

[41] Morillo CA, Marin-Neto JA, Avezum A, Sosa-Estani S, Rassi A Jr, Rosas F, Villena E, Quiroz R, Bonilla R, Britto C, Guhl F, Velazquez E, Bonilla L, Meeks B, Rao-Melacini P, Pogue J, Mattos A, Lazdins J, Rassi A, Connolly SJ, Yusuf S, and BENEFIT Investigators. Randomized trial of benznidazole for chronic Chagas' cardiomyopathy. N. Engl. J. Med. 2015;**373**:1295–1306.

[42] Debierre-Grockiego F. Glycolipids are potential targets for protozoan parasite diseases. Trends Parasitol. 2010;**26**:404–411.

[43] Schauer R, Kamerling JP. The chemistry and biology of trypanosomal trans-sialidases: virulence factors in Chagas disease and sleeping sickness. ChemBioChem 2011;**12**:2246–2264.

[44] Machado FS, Dutra WO, Esper L, Gollob KJ, Teixeira MM, Factor SM, Weiss LM, Nagajyothi F, Tanowitz HB, Garg NJ. Current understanding of immunity to *Trypanosoma cruzi* infection and pathogenesis of Chagas disease. Semin. Immunopathol. 2012;**34**:753–770.

[45] Takeda K, Akira S. Toll-like receptors in innate immunity. Int. Immunol. 2005;**17**:1–14.

[46] Campos MA, Almeida IC, Takeuchi O, Akira S, Valente EP, Procópio DO, Travassos LR, Smith JA, Golenbock DT, Gazzinelli RT. Activation of Toll-like receptor-2 by glycosylphosphatidylinositol anchors from a protozoan parasite. J. Immunol. 2001;**167**:416–423.

[47] Ropert C, Gazzinelli RT. Regulatory role of Toll-like receptor 2 during infection with *Trypanosoma cruzi*. J. Endotoxin Res. 2004;**10**:425–430.

[48] Oliveira AC, Peixoto JR, de Arruda LB, Campos MA, Gazzinelli RT, Golenbock DT, Akira S, Previato JO, Mendonça-Previato L, Nobrega A, Bellio M. Expression of functional TLR4 confers proinflammatory responsiveness to *Trypanosoma cruzi* glycoinositolphospholipids and higher resistance to infection with *T. cruzi*. J. Immunol. 2004;**173**:5688–5696.

[49] Bafica A, Santiago HC, Goldszmid R, Ropert C, Gazzinelli RT, Sher A. Cutting edge: TLR9 and TLR2 signaling together account for MyD88-dependent control of parasitemia in *Trypanosoma cruzi* infection. J. Immunol. 2006;**177**:3515–3519.

[50] Medeiros MM, Peixoto JR, Oliveira AC, Cardilo-Reis L, Koatz VLG, Van Kaer L, Previato JO, Mendonça-Previato L, Nobrega A, Bellio M. Toll-like receptor 4 (TLR4)-dependent proinflammatory and immunomodulatory properties of the glycoinositolphospholipid (GIPL) from *Trypanosoma cruzi*. J. Leukoc. Biol. 2007;**82**:488–496.

[51] Caetano BC, Carmo BB, Melo MB, Cerny A, dos Santos SL, Bartholomeu DC, Golenbock DT, Gazzinelli RT. Requirement of UNC93B1 reveals a critical role for TLR7 in host resistance to primary infection with *Trypanosoma cruzi*. J. Immunol. 2011;**187**:1903–1911.

[52] Gravina HD, Antonelli L, Gazzinelli RT, Ropert C. Differential use of TLR2 and TLR9 in the regulation of immune responses during the infection with *Trypanosoma cruzi*. PloS One 2013;**8**:e63100.

[53] Heidecker B, Kittleson MM, Kasper EK, Wittstein IS, Champion HC, Russell SD, Hruban RH, Rodriguez ER, Baughman KL, Hare JM. Transcriptomic biomarkers for the accurate diagnosis of myocarditis. Circulation 2011;**123**:1174–1184.

[54] Gonçalves VM, Matteucci KC, Buzzo CL, Miollo BH, Ferrante D, Torrecilhas AC, Rodrigues MM, Alvarez JM, Bortoluci KR. NLRP3 controls *Trypanosoma cruzi* infection through a caspase-1-dependent IL-1R-independent NO production. PLoS Negl. Trop. Dis. 2013;**7**:e2469.

[55] Truyens C, Angelo-Barrios A, Torrico F, Van Damme J, Heremans H, Carlier Y. Interleukin-6 (IL-6) production in mice infected with *Trypanosoma cruzi*: effect of its paradoxical increase by anti-IL-6 monoclonal antibody treatment on infection and acute-phase and humoral immune responses. Infect. Immun. 1994:**62**:692–696.

[56] Aliberti JC, Cardoso MA, Martins GA, Gazzinelli RT, Vieira LQ, Silva, JS. Interleukin-12 mediates resistance to *Trypanosoma cruzi* in mice and is produced by murine macrophages in response to live trypomastigotes. Infect. Immun. 1996;**64**:1961–1967.

[57] Camargo MM, Almeida IC, Pereira ME, Ferguson MA, Travassos LR, Gazzinelli RT. Glycosylphosphatidylinositol-anchored mucin-like glycoproteins isolated from *Trypanosoma cruzi* trypomastigotes initiate the synthesis of proinflammatory cytokines by macrophages. J. Immunol. 1997;**158**:5890–5901.

[58] Almeida IC, Camargo MM, Procópio DO, Silva LS, Mehlert A, Travassos LR, Gazzinelli RT, Ferguson MA. Highly purified glycosylphosphatidylinositols from *Trypanosoma cruzi* are potent proinflammatory agents. EMBO J. 2000;**19**:1476–1485.

[59] Antúnez MI, Cardoni RL. IL-12 and IFN-γ production, and NK cell activity, in acute and chronic experimental *Trypanosoma cruzi* infections. Immunol. Lett. 2000;**71**:103–109.

[60] Michailowsky V, Silva NM, Rocha CD, Vieira LQ, Lannes-Vieira J, Gazzinelli RT. Pivotal role of interleukin-12 and interferon-gamma axis in controlling tissue parasitism and inflammation in the heart and central nervous system during *Trypanosoma cruzi* infection. Am. J. Pathol. 2001;**159**:1723–1733.

[61] Bastos KRB, Barboza R, Sardinha L, Russo M, Alvarez JM, Lima MRD. Role of endogenous IFN-γ in macrophage programming induced by IL-12 and IL-18. J. Interferon Cytokine Res. 2007;**27**:399–410.

[62] Kierszenbaum F, Sonnenfeld G. Beta-interferon inhibits cell infection by *Trypanosoma cruzi*. J. Immunol. 1984;**132**:905–908.

[63] Koga R, Hamano S, Kuwata H, Atarashi K, Ogawa M, Hisaeda H, Yamamoto M, Akira S, Himeno K, Matsumoto M, Takeda K. TLR-dependent induction of IFN-β mediates host defense against *Trypanosoma cruzi*. J. Immunol. 2006;**177**:7059–7066.

[64] Chessler ADC, Ferreira LRP, Chang TH, Fitzgerald KA, Burleigh BA. A novel IFN regulatory factor 3-dependent pathway activated by trypanosomes triggers IFN-β in macrophages and fibroblasts. J. Immunol. 2008;**181**:7917–7924.

[65] Wirth JJ, Kierszenbaum F, Sonnenfeld G, Zlotnik A. Enhancing effects of gamma interferon on phagocytic cell association with and killing of *Trypanosoma cruzi*. Infect. Immun. 1985:**49**:61–66.

[66] Müller U, Köhler G, Mossmann H, Schaub GA, Alber G, Di Santo JP, Brombacher F, Hölscher C. IL-12-independent IFN-γ production by T cells in experimental Chagas' disease is mediated by IL-18. J. Immunol. 2001;**167**:3346–3353.

[67] Rodrigues AA, Saosa JSS, da Silva GK, Martins FA, da Silva AA, da Silva Souza Neto CP, Horta CV, Zamboni DS, da Silva JS, Ferro EAV, da Silva CV. IFN-γ plays a unique role in protection against low virulent *Trypanosoma cruzi* strain. PLoS Negl. Trop. Dis. 2012;**6**:e1598.

[68] Campos MA, Closel M, Valente EP, Cardoso JE, Akira S, Alvarez-Leite JI, Ropert C, Gazzinelli RT. Impaired production of proinflammatory cytokines and host resistance to acute infection with *Trypanosoma cruzi* in mice lacking functional myeloid differentiation factor 88. J. Immunol. 2004;**172**:1711–1718.

[69] Huang H, Calderon TM, Berman JW, Braunstein VL, Weiss LM, Wittner M, Tanowitz HB. Infection of endothelial cells with *Trypanosoma cruzi* activates NF-kappaB and induces vascular adhesion molecule expression. Infect. Immun. 1999;**67**:5434–5440.

[70] Hall BS, Tam W, Sen R, Pereira ME. Cell-specific activation of nuclear factor-kappaB by the parasite *Trypanosoma cruzi* promotes resistance to intracellular infection. Mol. Biol. Cell 2000;**11**:153–160.

[71] Hovsepian E, Penas F, Siffo S, Mirkin GA, Goren NB. IL-10 inhibits the NF-κB and ERK/MAPK-mediated production of pro-inflammatory mediators by up-regulation of SOCS-3 in *Trypanosoma cruzi*-infected cardiomyocytes. PloS One 2013;**8**:e79445.

[72] Hölscher C, Köhler G, Müller U, Mossmann H, Schaub GA, Brombacher F. Defective nitric oxide effector functions lead to extreme susceptibility of *Trypanosoma cruzi*-infected mice deficient in gamma-interferon receptor or inducible nitric oxide synthase. Infect. Immun. 1998;**66**:1208–1215.

[73] Böhm I, Schild H. Apoptosis: the complex scenario for a silent cell death. Mol. Imaging Biol. 2003;**5**:2–14.

[74] Fukada T, Hibi M, Yamanaka Y, Takahashi-Tezuka M, Fujitani Y, Yamaguchi T, Nakajima K, Hirano T. Two signals are necessary for cell proliferation induced by a cytokine receptor gp130: involvement of STAT3 in anti-apoptosis. Immunity. 1996;**5**:449–460.

[75] Tostes S Jr, Bertulucci Rocha-Rodrigues D, de Araujo Pereira G, Rodrigues V Jr. Myocardiocyte apoptosis in heart failure in chronic Chagas' disease. Int. J. Cardiol. 2005;**99**:233–237.

[76] Zhang J, Andrade ZA, Yu ZX, Andrade SG, Takeda K, Sadirgursky M, Ferrans VJ. Apoptosis in a canine model of acute Chagasic myocarditis. J. Mol. Cell. Cardiol. 1999;**31**:581–596.

[77] Henriques-Pons A, Oliveira GM, Paiva MM, Correa AFS, Batista MM, Bisaggio RC, Liu CC, Cotta-de-Almeida V, Coutinho CMLM, Persechini PM, Araújo-Jorge. Evidence for a perforin-mediated mechanism controlling cardiac inflammation in *Trypanosoma cruzi* infection. Int. J. Exp. Pathol. 2002;**83**:67–79.

[78] Manque PA, Probst CM, Probst CM, Pereira MCS, Rampazzo RCP, Ozaki LS, Ozaki LS, Pavoni DP, Silva Neto DT, Carvalho MR, Xu P, Serrano MG, Alves JMP, de Nazareth SL Meirelles M, Goldenberg S, Krieger MA, Buck GA. *Trypanosoma cruzi* infection induces a global host cell response in cardiomyocytes. Infect. Immun. 2011;**79**:1855–1862.

[79] De Souza EM, Araújo-Jorge TC, Bailly C, Lansiaux A, Batista MM, Oliveira GM, Soeiro MN. Host and parasite apoptosis following *Trypanosoma cruzi* infection in in vitro and in vivo models. Cell Tissue Res. 2003;**314**:223–235.

[80] Aoki MP, Guiñazú NL, Pellegrini AV, Gotoh T, Masih DT, Gea S. Cruzipain, a major *Trypanosoma cruzi* antigen, promotes arginase-2 expression and survival of neonatal mouse cardiomyocytes. Am. J. Physiol. Cell Physiol. 2004;**286**:C206–212.

[81] Stahl P, Ruppert V, Meyer T, Schmidt J, Campos MA, Gazzinelli RT, Maisch B, Schwarz RT, Debierre-Grockiego F. Trypomastigotes and amastigotes of *Trypanosoma cruzi* induce apoptosis and STAT3 activation in cardiomyocytes in vitro. Apoptosis 2013;**18**:653–663.

[82] Petersen CA, Krumholz KA, Carmen J, Sinai AP, Burleigh BA. *Trypanosoma cruzi* infection and nuclear factor kappa B activation prevent apoptosis in cardiac cells. Infect. Immun. 2006;**74**:1580–1587.

[83] De Souza EM, Nefertiti ASG, Bailly C, Lansiaux A, Soeiro MN. Differential apoptosis-like cell death in amastigote and trypomastigote forms from *Trypanosoma cruzi*-infected heart cells in vitro. Cell Tissue Res. 2010;**341**:173–180.

[84] Barry SP, Townsend PA, Latchman DS, Stephanou A. Role of the JAK-STAT pathway in myocardial injury. Trends Mol. Med. 2007;**13**:82–89.

[85] Stahl P, Schwarz RT, Debierre-Grockiego F, Meyer T. *Trypanosoma cruzi* parasites fight for control of the JAK-STAT pathway by disarming their host. JAK-STAT 2015;**3**:e1012964.

[86] Tarleton RL, Zhang L. Chagas disease etiology: autoimmunity or parasite persistence? Parasitol. Today 1999;**15**:94–99.

[87] Stahl P, Ruppert V, Schwarz RT, Meyer T. *Trypanosoma cruzi* evades the protective role of interferon-gamma-signaling in parasite-infected cells. PLoS One 2014;**9**:e110512.

[88] Ponce NE, Cano RC, Carrera-Silva EA, Lima AP, Gea S, Aoki MP. Toll-like receptor-2 and interleukin-6 mediate cardiomyocyte protection from apoptosis during *Trypanosoma cruzi* murine infection. Med. Microbiol. Immunol. 2012;**201**:145–155.

[89] Ponce NE, Carrera-Silva EA, Pellegrini AV, Cazorla SI, Malchiodi EL, Lima AP, Gea S, Aoki MP. *Trypanosoma cruzi*, the causative agent of Chagas disease, modulates interleukin-6-induced STAT3 phosphorylation via gp130 cleavage in different host cells. Biochim. Biophys. Acta 2013;**1832**:485–494.

[90] Starr R, Willson TA, Viney EM, Murray LJ, Rayner JR, Jenkins BJ, Gonda TJ, Alexander WS, Metcalf D, Nicola NA, Hilton DJ. A family of cytokine-inducible inhibitors of signalling. Nature 1997;**387**:917–921.

[91] Zhong Z, Wen Z, Darnell JE Jr. Stat3: a STAT family member activated by tyrosine phosphorylation in response to epidermal growth factor and interleukin-6. Science 1994;**264**:95–98.

[92] Riley JK, Takeda K, Akira S, Schreiber RD. Interleukin-10 receptor signaling through the JAK-STAT pathway. Requirement for two distinct receptor-derived signals for anti-inflammatory action. J. Biol. Chem. 1999;**274**:16513–16521.

[93] Esper L, Roman-Campos D, Lara A, Brant F, Castro LL, Barroso A, Araujo RRS, Vieira LQ, Mukherjee S, Gomes ERM, Rocha NN, Ramos IPR, Lisanti MP, Campos CF, Arantes RME Guatimosim S, Weiss LM, Cruz JS, Tanowitz HB, Teixeira MM, Machado FS. Role of SOCS2 in modulating heart damage and function in a murine model of acute Chagas disease. Am. J. Pathol. 2012;**181**:130–140.

[94] Tarleton RL, Grusby MJ, Zhang L. Increased susceptibility of Stat4-deficient and enhanced resistance in Stat6-deficient mice to infection with *Trypanosoma cruzi*. J. Immunol. 2000;**165**:1520-1525.

10

Left Ventricular Noncompaction

Ana G. Almeida

Abstract

Left ventricular noncompaction (LVNC) is accepted as an unclassified (the American Heart Association) or a genetic cardiomyopathy (the European Society of Cardiology), but some argue that this phenotype may be a morphologic trait shared by different cardiomyopathies. This chapter covers the state of the art on the pathology, underlying mechanisms, its clinical manifestations, and diagnosis and treatment modalities of LVNC. LVNC may be defined as follows: an inner non-compacted layer with prominent left ventricular trabeculae and deep intertrabecular recesses and a thin outer compacted layer. Mechanisms are still debatable, with the hypothesis of compaction arrest during embryogenesis as the most accepted theory. Genetic data support LVNC as a distinct cardiomyopathy, although evidence for LVNC as a shared morphological trait is not ruled out, since LVNC may be associated with other cardiomyopathies, congenital heart diseases and in some cases may be acquired. Diagnosis is based on imaging and may be confirmed by the use of genetics. Clinical picture and prognosis and the management options are discussed.

Keywords: cardiomyopathy, Noncompaction, Echocardiography, cardiovascular magnetic resonance, prognosis

1. Introduction

Left ventricular noncompaction (LVNC) is a myocardial disorder that has been thought to occur due to the failure of left ventricle (LV) compaction during embryogenesis, leading to distinct morphological characteristics in the ventricular chamber [1]. In its first description, about 80 years ago, LVNC occurred in association with complex congenital heart diseases. More recently, an isolated form of LVNC was described [2], followed by many other reports. The involvement of the right ventricle in the noncompaction process has been increasingly identified, and the condition is now included among the cardiomyopathies, but currently there is an intense debate whether LVNC is a distinct entity or a trait common to several cardiac conditions [3].

2. Anatomy and pathology

Left ventricular noncompaction (LVNC) is defined by essential markers: an inner noncompacted layer with prominent left ventricular (LV) trabeculae and deep intertrabecular recesses, and a thin compacted layer. There is a spectrum of morphologic variability, ranging from hearts with different degrees of noncompaction extension and amount, and right ventricular involvement.

From hearts obtained from autopsies or transplantation, LVNC diagnosis is based on the presence of a two-layered ventricular wall, comprising a thinner compact epicardial layer and an inner noncompacted layer, with prominent trabeculations associated with deep, intertrabecular recesses that communicate with the ventricular cavity but not with the coronary circulation [2, 3].

Noncompacted areas are commonly located at the LV apex and mid-apical wall segments, but typically spares the interventricular septum. When associated with hypertrophic cardiomyopathy phenotype (HCM), the hypertrophied septum coexists with the LVNC phenotype. Other described associations include dilated cardiomyopathy (DCM) and, more rarely, restrictive cardiomyopathy (RCM) or arrhythmogenic right ventricular cardiomyopathy (ARVC). Besides the relationship of LVNC with other cardiomyopathies, which may share the same genetic basis, there has been considerable controversy regarding the differentiation from normal LV trabeculation, which seems to occur in some normal asymptomatic individuals as found in analysis from the MESA study [4].

Histopathology has shown continuity between the endothelium of inter-trabecular recesses and that of the endocardium, distinguishing LVNC from persistent sinusoids. Other findings have included loosely organised myocytes and endocardial and subendocardial replacement fibrosis suggestive of ischaemic necrosis, which has been demonstrated by imaging techniques *in vivo* [5].

LV dilatation and ischemia are frequently present, and thrombus formation in the recesses may occur, which may be associated with possible thromboembolic events.

3. Aetiology and mechanisms

There are several etiologic hypotheses for LVNC. It may occur as an isolated disease (isolated LVNC) or in association with genetic diseases and congenital defects, as observed more commonly in infancy. The condition may also be sporadic and acquired, in physiological or pathologic conditions, and may also be permanent or transient. Thus, LVNC can originate during embryonic development or be acquired later in life.

The theory that supports the embryogenic hypothesis has been based in observational foetal studies showing the coexistence of LVNC with heart block and congenital heart diseases and from experimental studies on LVNC [6]. In humans, the embryonic myocardium is composed of a loose meshwork of interwoven fibres separated by deep recesses, which communicate with the LV cavity, allowing an increase in the myocardial surface area and the exchange diffusion from the cavity. From the 5th–8th weeks of embryogenesis, LV trabecular compaction occurs simultaneously with the invasion of the myocardium by the coronary vasculature coming from the epicardium. The LV compaction progresses from the heart base to the apex and from the epicardium to the endocardium [1]. LVNC is thus thought to result from the arrest of trabecular compaction during this phase of embryogenesis. A second embryogenic hypothesis suggests that LVNC results from the inhibition of the regression of embryonic structures that would maintain the looseness of cells or of cell bundles [7].

On the other hand, evidence supports the hypothesis that the pathogenetic mechanisms leading to noncompaction may occur in adult life, ending in acquired forms of LVNC and supporting a non-embryogenic theory. This is the case of young athletes, pregnant women, patients with sickle cell disease, and renal failure, which may present the phenotype of LVNC. In athletes, the phenotype seems to relate to intensive training, but in a small proportion of 0.9% has been found to develop ultimately LV dysfunction suggestive of a LVNC cardiomyopathy [8]. In pregnancy, an important proportion of women, described as up to 25% were found to develop LVNC phenotype de novo, which was reversible. This pattern was not shown to be associated with deleterious clinical events and has been proposed to result from a response to increased loading conditions [9]. Also, in sickle cell disease, this pattern has been found and hypothesised to result from chronic anaemia and increased preload, resulting in a stimulus for hypertrabeculation [10].

4. Genetics

The LVNC trait may be familial, inherited, or non-familial, sporadic. Non-familial forms are diagnosed when LVNC is proven absent in relatives. As presented above, sporadic LVNC can be acquired and may be transient, as in highly trained athletes, sickle cell anaemia patients, and pregnancy. Many familial cases identified to date are associated with mutations in the same genes that cause other types of cardiomyopathies but may also occur isolated.

In fact, several studies suggest that noncompaction of the LV myocardium is a genetically heterogeneous disorder [11], with a familial and a sporadic form. Studies of the familial form have shown that LVNC may be transmitted as an autosomal dominant inheritance with incomplete penetrance, as an autosomal recessive, and as X-linked traits. Sporadic cases of LVNC and de novo mutations have also been recognised. To date, several disease loci have been identified.

The Barth syndrome was the first recognised genetic LVNC, characterised by dilated cardiomyopathy associated with LVNC. It is an X-linked disease with mutations in the G4.5 gene, located at Xq28, which encodes the tafazzins (a family of proteins) with acetyltransferase functions in the mitochondria. This mutation was also identified in an X-linked severe neonatal LVNC, allelic with the Barth syndrome.

Another mutation, located in the α-dystrobrevin gene, was identified subsequently in patients with LVNC and associated with congenital heart diseases. [12]; α-dystrobrevin is a cytoskeletal protein component of the dystrophin associated glycoprotein complex, which links the extracellular matrix to the dystrophin cytoskeleton of the muscle fibre. This mutation was associated with a significant phenotypic variability with variable severity.

Mutations in the Z-line protein Cypher/ZASP have been identified in association with LVNC and dilated cardiomyopathy. This protein appears to play an important role in the maintenance of the normal myocyte architecture of cardiac and skeletal muscle.

Another LVNC phenotype has been reported in association with a mutation in the Lamin A/C protein, which has been linked to dilated cardiomyopathy, conduction system diseases, and muscular dystrophy.

Recently, LVNC has been linked to sarcomere gene mutations, causing hypertrophic cardiomyopathy. In a study of 247 families with cardiomyopathy, a mutation in the α-cardiac actin gene, essential for cell maintenance, was associated with LVNC, apical hypertrophic cardiomyopathy, and septal defects. Moreover, in a large study of patients with phenotype of LVNC, nine heterozygous mutations were identified in a proportion of the probands in genes encoding α-myosin heavy chain (MYH7), β-cardiac actin (ACTC), and cardiac troponin T (TNNT2), with 100% penetrance in the family members [13]. Another study identified a mutation in the sarcomeric TPM1 gene, at 15q22.1, in a family with LVNC and a history of sudden death.

Some studies have suggested that the phenotype for isolated LVNC may appear during adult life in patients with muscular dystrophy and with myocarditis. Nevertheless, these cases were not followed serially clinically and with an imaging modality, and the significance of the LV hypertrabeculation described is still unclear.

Although, many genes associated with LVNC are associated with additional phenotypes, like hypertrophic or dilated cardiomyopathies or congenital heart defects, several mutations were described in association with isolated LVNC. For instance, mutations in gene MIB1 were identified in two families with LVNC and autosomal dominant inheritance [14]. Recently, an important role in trabeculation for endocardial expression of a Notch ligand, Fkbp1a, was reported, [15] which was confirmed in a mouse model, suggesting its direct involvement in the LVNC phenotype.

A large number of genes have been identified in relation with the LVNC phenotype in association with other cardiomyopathies, congenital and acquired heart diseases, as well as part of syndromes; specific genetic mutations have been related with the LVNC phenotype, and there is a need for large databases and systematic follow-up with clinical and imaging to obtain definite conclusions on the clinical and prognostic significance of LVNC phenotype in relation with the genotype.

The role of modifying genes or epigenetics and load changes may influence the relationship of genotype-phenotype and contribute to explain the phenotype variability.

5. Epidemiology

LVNC has been considered rare, and its incidence and prevalence are uncertain, but is commonly diagnosed, due to increased awareness and more accurate imaging methods.

LVNC has been described to occur in infants (0.81 per 100,000 infants/year), children (0.12 cases per 100,000 children/year), and adults (prevalence suggested as 0.014% of patients referred for echocardiography and 0.05% among all adult echocardiograms in a large institution) [16, 17]. In a large population of patients with LV ejection fraction <45%, the prevalence was 3.7% [18]. However, LVNC can occur as an isolated myocardial trait or be associated with cardiomyopathies (hypertrophic, restrictive, dilated, and arrhythmogenic), congenital heart diseases, and complex syndromes affecting multiple organs and tissues, including mitochondrial diseases caused by mutations in both nuclear and mitochondrial genes, leading to increased uncertainty on the prevalence.

In fact, given the variability of clinical presentation, the prevalence of LVNC is largely unknown.

6. Clinical manifestations

Heart failure, ventricular and atrial arrhythmias, and systemic embolic events comprise the typical complications in patients with LVNC and may occur at any age. However, the initial presentation is variable and the patient may be asymptomatic (frequently diagnosed during a family screening) or present any of the clinical features and complications, including sudden death.

In its severe neonatal form, LVNC may manifest as heart failure or ventricular arrhythmias, which may lead to sudden death [2]. Studies of older children and adults have reported a high incidence of severe manifestations [7, 17, 19–22] such as LV dysfunction, thromboembolic events, which probably originate in the deep intertrabecular recesses, arrhythmias, and sudden death. Other studies, however, have found a much lower incidence of complications, suggesting subclinical or milder cases [23]. **Table 1** presents clinical findings from published studies.

There is no agreement so far on the natural history and outcomes in LVNC because most studies are retrospective, populations are limited and use distinct study methods.

Heart failure seems to occur frequently, as over 50% of symptomatic patients, and most researchers also report ventricular arrhythmias, cardiovascular deaths, and sudden cardiac death. A recent registry of a large population of adult patients with LVNC found heart failure in 74%, LV systolic dysfunction in 88%, strokes in 10%, and syncope episodes in 9%, [20] suggesting the need for long term surveillance of LVNC patients. Other series have found a more benign prognosis [23]. A recent published series describe a mean freedom from death or transplantation of 97% at 46 months in adults with LVNC.

Author	Chin	Ichida	Oechslin	Murphy	Lofiego	Aras	Stanton	Greutmann
Patients (N)	8	27	34	45	65	67	30	132
Population	Paediatric	Paediatric	Adult	Adult	Adult	Adult	Adult	>14 years-old
Follow-up	≤5 years	≤17 years	44 months	46 months	46 months	30 months	2.5 years	2.7 years
Family history (%)	50	44	18	51	31	33	–	23
Embolic events (%)	38	0	21	4	5	9	0	4
Ventricular tachycardia (%)	38	0	41	20	6	36	27	4
Heart failure (%)	63	30	68	67	34	34	–	13
CV death or transplantation (%)	0	11	47	2	24	15	10	23
Sudden death (%)	13	0	18	2	5	9	10	9

LVNC, left ventricle noncowmpaction; CV, cardiovascular.

Table 1. LVNC clinical characteristics and outcomes.

Predictors of death and heart transplantation have been difficult to assess due to the variability of the phenotype and the variable underlying pathophysiological scenarios. However, the presence of heart failure, history of sustained ventricular tachycardia or systemic thromboembolism seem to be associated with an unfavourable prognosis among other phenotypes with distinct outcomes [21, 22]. In a recent study, mortality did not differ significantly between patients with isolated LVNC and control patients with dilated cardiomyopathy, [24] suggesting that LV dysfunction rather than the phenotype itself is the risk-increasing mechanism. However, this finding has not been confirmed by others [17].

7. Diagnosis

Cardiac imaging is essential for establishing the diagnosis of LVNC, not only to detect the characteristic features and application of the diagnostic criteria, but to assess the systolic and diastolic function, valve regurgitation, pulmonary hypertension, the presence of thrombus in the ventricular recesses. However, there is still a lack of agreement from the medical community regarding the best technique and the most reliable diagnostic criterion. **Table 2** summarises the most frequently used imaging criteria for LVNC diagnosis.

7.1. Echocardiography

Cardiac ultrasound is a first-line technique for diagnosing LVNC, since it is a bedside modality, uses no radiation and is readily available. This modality allows the detection, location,

Jenni et al. [25]	Stlöberger et al. [26]	Petersen et al. [30]	Jacquier et al. [31]
Echo	Echo	CMR	CMR
- Ratio noncompacted/ compacted >2.0	- Three trabeculations protruding from the LV wall, apically to the papillary muscles, visible in one image plane	- Ratio noncompacted/ compacted >2.3	- Trabecular LV mass >20% of global LV mass,
- Intratrabecular recesses filled by blood flow from the LV cavity	- Intertrabecular spaces perfused from the ventricular cavity on colour Doppler imaging	- Acquisition: long-axis end-diastolic images	- Acquisition: end-diastolic images
- Acquisition: short-axis; end-systolic images	- Trabeculations with the same echogenicity as the myocardium and synchronous with LV - Acquisition: oblique views to differentiate false chords, aberrant bands, trabeculations		
LV, left ventricle.			

Table 2. The most frequently used diagnostic criteria in left ventricle noncompaction.

and confirmation of this condition. The first criterion was proposed by Chin et al. [2], who recommended the assessment of the ratio of X/Y dimensions in diastole—where X is the distance from the epicardial surface to the trough of the trabecular recesses, and Y the distance from the epicardial surface to the peak of the trabeculation. An X/Y ratio of up to 0.5 would be required for the diagnosis. The more widely used criterion, however, was proposed by Jenni et al. in which the ratio of noncompacted and compacted myocardium, measured from end systolic short-axis images. If the ratio is >2, the criterion for LVNC is considered fulfilled [25] (**Figures 1** and **2**). Additionally, observation and quantification of the apical trabeculations are available by echocardiography, although sometimes challenging, and permit the use of the LVNC criterion proposed by Stöllberger et al. [26].

The inherent limitation of echocardiography in evaluating the LV apex and, often, other LV walls poses a diagnostic issue. If the image quality is poor, LVNC can be confused with apical cardiomyopathy, thrombus or fibroelastosis. The use of contrast echocardiography, which permits the visualisation of the trabeculations and the recesses that communicate with the cavity, may help in clarifying the diagnosis [27]. Additional information with prognostic impact may be derived from the evaluation of LV systolic and diastolic function, mitral regurgitation, pulmonary hypertension. Systolic dysfunction is frequently present in LVNC. It has been hypothesised that microvascular disease with impaired coronary flow reserve and myocardial necrosis, as well as a primary myocardial disease, is responsible for the functional abnormalities [5], although in other cases a DCM may be associated, The presence of thrombus in the ventricular recesses, although rare, has been described.

More recently, speckle tracking has revealed abnormal LV rotation and twist, and these findings are promising for diagnosis even in patients with normal ejection fraction [28]. Three-dimension echocardiography has been proposed as an alternative for detecting LVNC due to

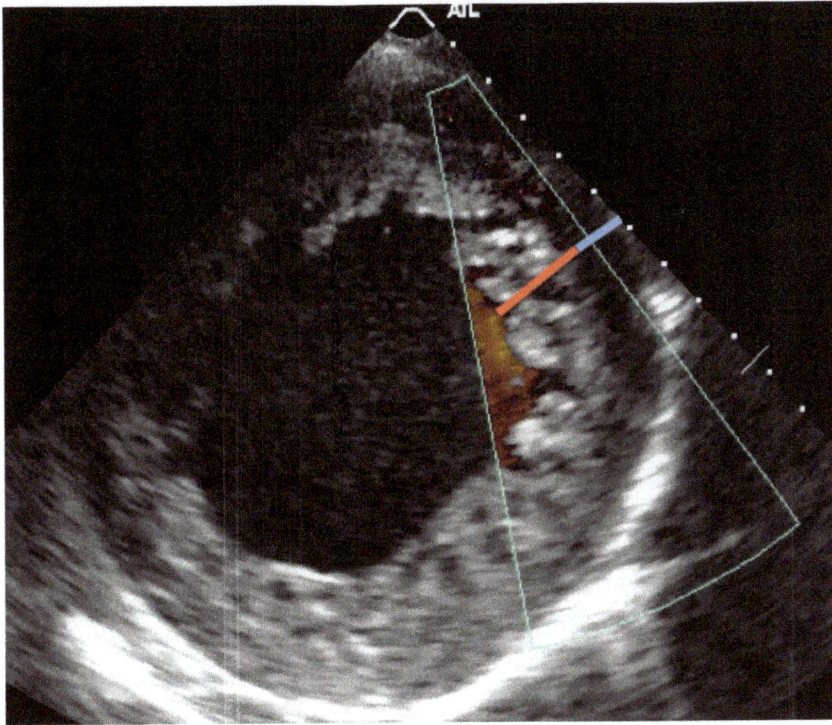

Figure 1. A systolic short-axis image from an echocardiogram of a 27-year-old patient with LVNC, showing the ratio measurement of compacted layer (blue line) to noncompacted layer (red line) of >2; Doppler colour shows the blood flow in the recesses.

the lower dependence on the observer for image acquisition and higher reproducibility [29]. However, the image quality and resolution may be compromised in comparison with the conventional 2D, remaining uncertain its real value.

7.2. Cardiovascular magnetic resonance (CMR)

CMR is a non-ionising high-resolution technique without acoustic limitations, which reveals a wider extent of disease, particularly at the LV apex and the poorly observed segments, which are often problematic with echocardiography.

This modality confirms the presence of the anatomic features of LVNC, as well as an accurate and reproducible measurement of the noncompacted and compacted myocardial layers (**Figures 3** and **4**). The diagnosis is supported if the end-diastolic thickness of the noncompacted layer is ≥2.3 times the compacted one, as proposed by Petersen et al. [30]. This criterion yielded >43% of positive subjects in MESA study, although this population included only asymptomatic individuals, with low pretest probability of disease [4].

CMR confirmation of trabeculated LV mass >20% of global LV mass fulfils the criterion proposed by Jacquier et al. [31] although the feasibility and reproducibility of this methodology have been debated.

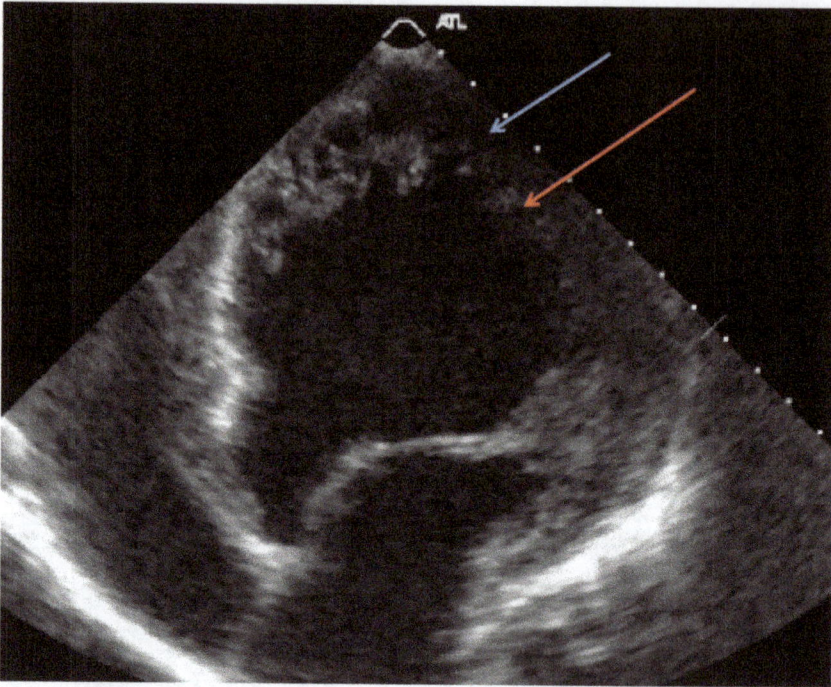

Figure 2. A diastolic four-chamber image from an echocardiogram of a patient with LVNC. Blue arrow—compacted layer; red arrow—noncompacted layer.

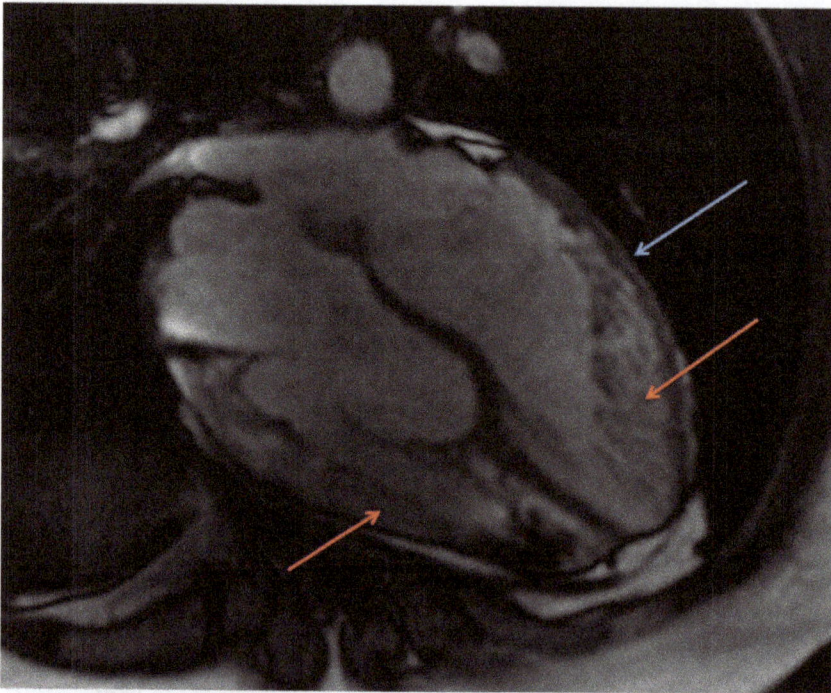

Figure 3. A diastolic four-chamber view from a magnetic resonance cine study of a 23-year-old patient with LVNC, showing biventricular noncompaction. Blue arrow—compacted layer; red arrows—noncompacted layers.

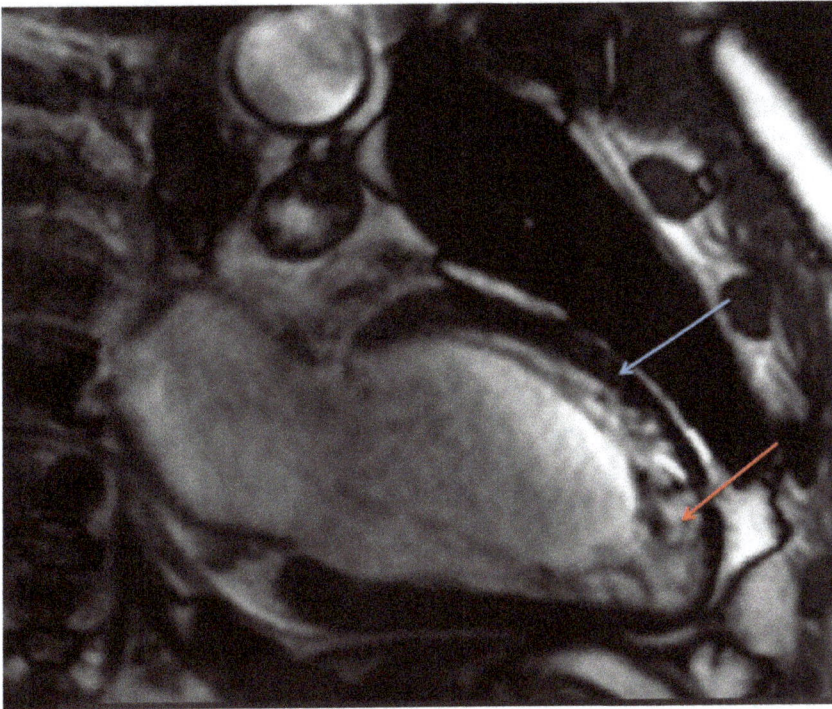

Figure 4. A diastolic two-chamber view from a magnetic resonance cine study of a patient with LVNC and arrhythmia. Blue arrow—compacted layer; red arrows—noncompacted layer.

Fractal analysis was also used to quantify LV trabeculae. In a study of 30 patients of Captur et al., the combination of end-diastolic measurements at basal, mid, and apical segments was found to be the best selector of LVNC cases from the normal population [32].

The combined use of echocardiography and CMR may contribute to lessening the risk of over diagnosing LVNC, which can occur with the isolated use of ultrasound, and overcome the limitations on reproducibility of echocardiography [33], but such an approach has not yet been validated.

Reliable evaluation of LV function is an additional advantage offered by CMR. Involvement of the right ventricle remains controversial because echocardiography presents inherent difficulties in analysing this chamber, but CMR has been increasingly detecting biventricular LVNC, although no specific criteria have been proposed so far.

Late gadolinium enhancement (LGE) CMR, as a surrogate marker of fibrosis, has been detected in patients with LVNC and confirmed by histology. A recent study suggests that the presence and amount of LGE is associated with more severe clinical [34]. Abnormal T2-weighting myocardial intensity and perfusion defects have been described as additional information obtained from CMR but its usefulness is not established so far.

7.3. Cardiac computed tomography

This modality has been proposed as an alternative to patients that have acoustic limitations to echocardiography and contra-indications for CMR, due to the high spatial resolution provided by this technique [35].

7.4. Electrocardiogram

Electrocardiogram (ECG) may be normal. ECG changes, when present, are non-specific and include LV hypertrophy and repolarisation abnormalities. Left bundle branch block is common, especially in patients with LV dysfunction. Wolff–Parkinson–White has been frequently detected in paediatric patients [36].

8. Management and prognosis

The true significance of noncompaction still remains a matter of debate, due to the genetic heterogeneity, the overlapping phenotype with other cardiomyopathies sharing the same genetic background, the high prevalence in neuromuscular diseases. These findings suggest that other factors may play a role in the development of LVNC disease [37]. Another important challenge is the clear differentiation of the LVNC phenotype from the normal heart, since this is associated with the risk of overdiagnosis.

There are no specific guidelines for management of LVNC since evidence supporting the management is limited. First of all, management includes confirmation of the diagnosis by echocardiography or CMR.

Guidelines suggest that familial LVNC should be diagnosed by echocardiographic screening of family members [38]. Echocardiographic screening is recommended for family members, given that the symptoms are variable and the risks include heart failure and sudden cardiac death.

According to current guidelines, mutation-specific genetic testing is recommended for family members and appropriate relatives, following the identification of an LVNC causative mutation in the index case. Moreover, this testing may be useful for patients where the cardiologist has established a clinical diagnosis of LV noncompaction based on examination of the patient's clinical manifestations (namely with increased pre-test probability or left ventricular dysfunction [39]) and family history, electrocardiographic and echocardiographic phenotype or when associated with another cardiomyopathy or congenital heart disease. Following genetic and imaging assessment, the possibility of an early diagnosis of LVNC increases, ensuring appropriate monitoring and prophylactic measures.

According to recent American Heart Association/American College of Cardiology Scientific Statement on Eligibility and Disqualification Recommendations for Competitive Athletes With Cardiovascular Abnormalities, "until more clinical information is available, participation in competitive sports may be considered for asymptomatic patients with a diagnosis of LVNC and normal systolic function, without important ventricular tachyarrhythmias on ambulatory monitoring or exercise testing, and specifically with no prior history of unexplained syncope (Class IIb; Level of Evidence C)" [40].

The main therapeutic objectives are the prevention and treatment of complications, using conventional measures. Thromboembolism, heart failure, and arrhythmias constitute the typical clinical features of LVNC to be addressed.

Anticoagulation for prevention of thromboembolism is probably only indicated in cases of LV dilatation and dysfunction, or when a previous history of embolic events is present, although to date no data are available to support these options. For symptomatic ventricular arrhythmias, particularly the ones associated with LV and for heart failure, the treatment should follow current guidelines. In patients with severe LV dysfunction, ICD implantation and CRT therapy are measures to improve heart failure and prevent sudden death. In some cases, heart transplantation may be the option for patients with refractory heart failure [41].

9. Conclusion

The pathogenesis and diagnosis of LVNC remains a challenge. The disease may be secondary to genetic mutations that induce the myocardial pathology. However, phenotypes are heterogeneous, are frequently shared with other cardiomyopathy, suggesting the influence of additional modifiers or a common aetiology.

The detection of new genetic mutations and the evaluation of its relationship with phenotypes may shed light on the pathogenesis of this condition, which may have an impact on follow-up and management.

The current awareness of the disease and the availability of high-resolution imaging, namely CMR, have increased the number of diagnosed patients. There is, however, a risk of overdiagnoses. The genotype and phenotype heterogeneity suggests the need for multicentre studies involving large populations, allowing more

robust conclusions regarding all the important areas of LVNC including the clinical ground, genetics, pathogenesis, diagnosis, and management.

Acknowledgements

Funding source: Cardiovascular Centre of Lisbon University.

Author details

Ana G. Almeida

Address all correspondence to: anagalmeida@gmail.com; amalmeida@medicina.ulisboa.pt

Faculty of Medicine of Lisbon University, University Hospital Santa Maria/CHLN/Academic Centre of Lisbon University, Cardiovascular Centre of Lisbon University (FCT), Lisbon, Portugal.

References

[1] Sedmera D, Pexieder T, Vuillemin M, et al. Developmental patterning of the myocardium. Anat Rec. 2000;258:319–37.

[2]   Chin TK, Perloff JK, Williams RG, et al. Isolated noncompaction of left ventricular myo-cardium. A study of eight cases. Circulation. 1990;82:507–13.

[3]   Arbustini E, Weidemann F, Hall JL. Left ventricular noncompaction: a distinct car-diomyopathy or a trait shared by different cardiac diseases? J Am Coll Cardiol. 2014;64:1840–50.

[4]   Zemrak F, Ahlman MA, Captur G, Mohiddin SA, Kawel-Boehm N, Prince MR, Moon JC, Hundley WG, Lima JA, Bluemke DA, Petersen SE. The relationship of left ventricular trabeculation to ventricular function and structure over a 9.5-year follow-up: the MESA study. J Am Coll Cardiol. 2014 ;64:1971–80.

[5]   Jenni R, Wyss CA, Oechslin EN, et al. Isolated ventricular noncompaction is associated with coronary microcirculatory dysfunction. J Am Coll Cardiol. 2002;39:450–4.

[6]   Vinograd CA, Srivastava S, Panesar LE. Fetal diagnosis of left-ventricular noncompac-tion cardiomyopathy in identical twins with discordant congenital heart disease. Pediatr Cardiol. 2013;34:1503–7.

[7]   Oechslin EN, Attenhofer Jost CH, Rojas JR, et al. Long-term follow-up of 34 adults with isolated left ventricular noncompaction: a distinct cardiomyopathy with poor prognosis. J Am Coll Cardiol 2000;36:493–500.

[8]   Gati S, Chandra N, Bennett RL, et al. Increased left ventricular trabeculation in highly trained athletes: do we need more stringent criteria for the diagnosis of left ventricular non-compaction in athletes? Heart. 2013;99:401–8.

[9]   Gati S, Papadakis M, Papamichael ND, et al. Reversible de novo left ventricular trabecu-lations in pregnant women: implications for the diagnosis of left ventricular noncompac-tion in low-risk populations. Circulation. 2014;130:475–83.

[10] Gati S, Papadakis M, Van Niekerk N, et al. Increased left ventricular trabecula-tion in individuals with sickle cell anaemia: physiology or pathology? Int J Cardiol. 2013;168:1658–60.

[11] Oechslin E, Jenni R. Left ventricular non-compaction revisited: a distinct phenotype with genetic heterogeneity? Eur Heart J. 2011;32:1446–56.

[12] Ichida F, Tsubata S, Bowles KR, et al. Novel gene mutations in patients with left ventricu-lar noncompaction or Barth syndrome. Circulation. 2001;103:1256–63.

[13] Klaassen S, Probst S, Oechslin E, et al. Mutations in sarcomere protein genes in left ven-tricular noncompaction. Circulation. 2008;117:2893–90.

[14] Luxan G, Casanova JC, Martinez-Poveda B, et al. Mutations in the NOTCH pathway regulator MIB1 cause left ventricular noncompaction cardiomyopathy. Nat Med. 2013;19:193–201.

[15] Chen H, Zhang W, Sun X, et al. Fkbp1a controls ventricular myocardium trabecu-lation and compaction by regulating endocardial Notch1 activity. Development. 2013;140:1946–57.

[16] Ritter M, Oechslin E, Sütsch G, Attenhofer C, Schneider J, Jenni R. Isolated noncompaction of the myocardium in adults. Mayo Clin Proc. 1997; 72:26–31.

[17] Aras D, Tufekcioglu O, Ergun K, et al. Clinical features of isolated ventricular noncompaction in adults long-term clinical course, echocardiographic properties, and predictors of left ventricular failure. J Card Fail. 2006;12:726–33.

[18] Sandhu R, Finkelhor RS, Gunawardena DR, Bahler RC. Prevalence and characteristics of left ventricular noncompaction in a community hospital cohort of patients with systolic dysfunction. Echocardiography. 2008;25:8–12.

[19] Ichida F, Hamamichi Y, Miyawaki T, et al. Clinical features of isolated noncompaction of the ventricular myocardium: long-term clinical course, hemodynamic properties, and genetic background. J Am Coll Cardiol. 1999;34:233–40.

[20] Habib G, Charron P, Eicher JC, et al. Isolated left ventricular non-compaction in adults: clinical and echocardiographic features in 105 patients. Results from a French registry. Eur J Heart Fail. 2011;13:177–85.

[21] Lofiego C, Biagini E, Pasquale F, et al. Wide spectrum of presentation and variable outcomes of isolated left ventricular noncompaction. Heart. 2007;93:65–71.

[22] Greutmann M, Mah ML, Silversides CK, et al. Predictors of adverse outcome in adolescents and adults with isolated left ventricular noncompaction. Am J Cardiol. 2012;109:276–81.

[23] Murphy RT, Thaman R, Blanes JG, et al. Natural history and familial characteristics of isolated left ventricular noncompaction. Eur Heart J. 2005;26:187–92.

[24] Stanton C, Bruce C, Connolly H, et al. Isolated left ventricular noncompaction syndrome. Am J Cardiol. 2009;104:1135–8.

[25] Jenni R, Oechslin E, Schneider J, et al. Echocardiographic and pathoanatomical characteristics of isolated left ventricular non-compaction: a step towards classification as a distinct cardiomyopathy. Heart. 2001;86:666–71.

[26] Stöllberger C, Finsterer J, Blazek G. Left ventricular hypertrabeculation, noncompaction and association with additional cardiac abnormalities and neuromuscular disorders. Am J Cardiol. 2002;90:899–902.

[27] Chow CM, Lim KD, Wu L, et al. Images in cardiovascular medicine. Isolated left ventricular noncompaction enhanced by echocontrast agent. Circulation. 2007;116:e90–1.

[28] Bellavia D, Michelena HI, Martinez M, et al. Speckle myocardial imaging modalities for early detection of myocardial impairment in isolated left ventricular non-compaction. Heart. 2010;96:440–7.

[29] Caselli S, Autore C, Serdoz A, et al. Three-dimensional echocardiographic characterization of patients with left ventricular noncompaction. J Am Soc Echocardiogr. 2012;25:203–9.

[30] Petersen SE, Selvanayagam JB, Wiesmann F, et al. Left ventricular non-compaction: insights from cardiovascular magnetic resonance imaging. J Am Coll Cardiol. 2005;46:101–5.

[31] Jacquier A, Thuny F, Jop B, et al. Measurement of trabeculated left ventricular mass using cardiac magnetic resonance imaging in the diagnosis of left ventricular non-compaction. Eur Heart J. 2010;31:1098–104.

[32] Captur G, Muthurangu V, Cook C, et al. Quantification of left ventricular trabeculae using fractal nalysis. J Cardiovasc Magn Reson. 2013;15:36.

[33] Stöllberger C, Gerecke B, Engberding R, et al. Interobserver agreement of the echocardiographic diagnosis of LV hypertrabeculation/noncompaction. J Am Coll Cardiol Img. 2015;8:1252–1257.

[34] Nucifora G, Aquaro GD, Pingitore A, et al. Myocardial fibrosis in isolated left ventricular noncompaction and its relation to disease severity. Eur J Heart Fail. 2011;13:170–6.

[35] Sidhu MS, Uthamalingam, Ahmed SW, et al. Defining left ventricular noncompaction using cardiac computed tomography. J Thorac Imaging. 2014;29:60–6.

[36] Petersen SE. Left ventricular noncompaction. A clinically useful diagnostic label? JACC Cardiovasc Imaging. 2015;8:947–8.

[37] Almeida AG, Pinto FJ. Non-compaction cardiomyopathy. Heart. 2013;99:1535–1542.

[38] Hershberger RE, Lindenfeld J, Mestroni L, et al. Genetic evaluation of cardiomyopathy—a Heart Failure Society of America practice guideline. J Card Fail. 2009;15:83–97.

[39] Aung N, Zemrak F, Mohiddin SA, Petersen SB. LV noncompaction cardiomyopathy or just a lot of trabeculations? JACC Cardiovasc Imaging. 2016 Aug 20.

[40] Maron BJ, Udelson JE, Bonow RO, et al. Eligibility and disqualification recommendations for competitive athletes with cardiovascular abnormalities: Task Force 3: hypertrophic cardiomyopathy, arrhythmogenic right ventricular cardiomyopathy and other cardiomyopathies, and myocarditis: a scientific statement from the American Heart Association and American College of Cardiology. J Am Coll Cardiol. 2015;66:2362–71.

[41] Arbustini E, Favalli V, Narula N, Serio A, Grasso M. Left ventricular noncompaction: a distinct genetic cardiomyopathy? J Am Coll Cardiol. 2016;68:949–66.

Permissions

All chapters in this book were first published in CARDIOMYOPATHIES, by InTech Open; hereby published with permission under the Creative Commons Attribution License or equivalent. Every chapter published in this book has been scrutinized by our experts. Their significance has been extensively debated. The topics covered herein carry significant findings which will fuel the growth of the discipline. They may even be implemented as practical applications or may be referred to as a beginning point for another development.

The contributors of this book come from diverse backgrounds, making this book a truly international effort. This book will bring forth new frontiers with its revolutionizing research information and detailed analysis of the nascent developments around the world.

We would like to thank all the contributing authors for lending their expertise to make the book truly unique. They have played a crucial role in the development of this book. Without their invaluable contributions this book wouldn't have been possible. They have made vital efforts to compile up to date information on the varied aspects of this subject to make this book a valuable addition to the collection of many professionals and students.

This book was conceptualized with the vision of imparting up-to-date information and advanced data in this field. To ensure the same, a matchless editorial board was set up. Every individual on the board went through rigorous rounds of assessment to prove their worth. After which they invested a large part of their time researching and compiling the most relevant data for our readers.

The editorial board has been involved in producing this book since its inception. They have spent rigorous hours researching and exploring the diverse topics which have resulted in the successful publishing of this book. They have passed on their knowledge of decades through this book. To expedite this challenging task, the publisher supported the team at every step. A small team of assistant editors was also appointed to further simplify the editing procedure and attain best results for the readers.

Apart from the editorial board, the designing team has also invested a significant amount of their time in understanding the subject and creating the most relevant covers. They scrutinized every image to scout for the most suitable representation of the subject and create an appropriate cover for the book.

The publishing team has been an ardent support to the editorial, designing and production team. Their endless efforts to recruit the best for this project, has resulted in the accomplishment of this book. They are a veteran in the field of academics and their pool of knowledge is as vast as their experience in printing. Their expertise and guidance has proved useful at every step. Their uncompromising quality standards have made this book an exceptional effort. Their encouragement from time to time has been an inspiration for everyone.

The publisher and the editorial board hope that this book will prove to be a valuable piece of knowledge for researchers, students, practitioners and scholars across the globe.

List of Contributors

Carolina Gálvez-Montón
ICREC Research Program, Germans Trias i Pujol Health Science Research Institute, Badalona, Spain

Santiago Roura
ICREC Research Program, Germans Trias i Pujol Health Science Research Institute, Badalona, Spain
Center of Regenerative Medicine in Barcelona, Barcelona, Spain

Josep Lupón
Cardiology Service, Germans Trias i Pujol University Hospital, Badalona, Spain
Department of Medicine, Autonomous University of Barcelona, Barcelona, Spain

Antoni Bayes-Genis
ICREC Research Program, Germans Trias i Pujol Health Science Research Institute, Badalona, Spain
Cardiology Service, Germans Trias i Pujol University Hospital, Badalona, Spain
Department of Medicine, Autonomous University of Barcelona, Barcelona, Spain

Jordi Camps, Tristan Pulinckx and Robin Duelen
Translational Cardiomyology Lab, Stem Cell Biology and Embryology Unit, Department of Development and Regeneration, KU Leuven, Leuven, Belgium

Enrico Pozzo and Maurilio Sampaolesi
Translational Cardiomyology Lab, Stem Cell Biology and Embryology Unit, Department of Development and Regeneration, KU Leuven, Leuven, Belgium
Division of Human Anatomy, Department of Public Health, Experimental and Forensic Medicine, University of Pavia, Pavia, Italy

Kazumasu Sasaki
Department of Functional Brain Imaging and Preclinical Evaluation, Institute of Development, Aging and Cancer, Tohoku University, Sendai, Japan
Sendai Animal Care and Research Center, Sendai, Japan

Tatsushi Mutoh
Department of Nuclear Medicine and Radiology, Institute of Development, Aging and Cancer, Tohoku University, Sendai, Japan
Department of Surgical Neurology, Research Institute for Brain and Blood Vessels-AKITA, Akita, Japan

Kinji Shirota
Department of Veterinary Pathology, School of Veterinary Medicine, Azabu University, Kanagawa, Japan

Ryuta Kawashima
Department of Functional Brain Imaging, Institute of Development, Aging and Cancer, Tohoku University, Sendai, Japan

Bandar Al-Ghamdi
Heart Centre, King Faisal Specialist Hospital and Research Centre, Alfaisal University, Riyadh, Saudi Arabia

Tanıl Özer and Mustafa Mert Özgür
Department of Cardiac Transplantation and Ventricular Assist Device, Kartal Koşuyolu YIEA Hospital, Istanbul, Turkey

Kaan Kırali
Department of Cardiac Transplantation and Ventricular Assist Device, Kartal Koşuyolu YIEA Hospital, Istanbul, Turkey
Department of Cardiovascular Surgery, Faculty of Medicine, Sakarya University, Sakarya, Turkey

Sara Nunes and Flávio Reis
Laboratory of Pharmacology and Experimental Therapeutics, Institute for Biomedical Imaging and Life Sciences (IBILI), Faculty of Medicine and CNC.IBILI Consortium, University of Coimbra, Coimbra, Portugal

Anabela Pinto Rolo and Carlos Manuel Palmeira
Department of Life Sciences and Center for Neurosciences and Cell Biology, University of Coimbra, Coimbra, Portugal

Okechukwu S. Ogah and Ayodele O. Falase
Division of Cardiology, Department of Medicine, University College Hospital, Ibadan, Nigeria

Marissa Lopez-Pier
Department of Biomedical Engineering, University of Arizona, Tucson, Arizona
Sarver Molecular Cardiovascular Research Program, University of Arizona, Tucson, Arizona

Yulia Lipovka, Eleni Constantopoulos and John P. Konhilas
Department of Physiology, University of Arizona, Tucson, Arizona
Sarver Molecular Cardiovascular Research Program, University of Arizona, Tucson, Arizona

Philipp Stahl
Institute of Virology, Parasitology Unit, University of Marburg, Marburg, Germany
Department of Internal Medicine, Section of Gastroenterology and Infectious Diseases, University Hospital Gießen and Marburg, Marburg, Germany

Thomas Meyer
Department of Psychosomatic Medicine and Psychotherapy, University of Göttingen, Göttingen, Germany
German Center for Cardiovascular Research, partner site Göttingen, Göttingen, Germany

Ana G. Almeida
Faculty of Medicine of Lisbon University, University Hospital Santa Maria/CHLN/ Academic Centre of Lisbon University, Cardiovascular Centre of Lisbon University (FCT), Lisbon, Portugal

Index

www.ingramcontent.com/pod-product-compliance
Lightning Source LLC
Chambersburg PA
CBHW061951190326
41458CB00009B/2848